Prostate Brachytherapy
MADE COMPLICATED

Prostate Brachytherapy
MADE COMPLICATED

Kent Wallner
John Blasko
Michael J. Dattoli

SmartMedicine Press
Seattle, Washington

First Edition

Library of Congress Catalog Card Number: 97-69257
ISBN: 0-9648991-1-6

Published by SmartMedicine Press, Seattle, Washington
Printed by Marrakech Express, Tarpon Springs, Florida

Page design & typesetting by Kent Wallner
Copy-editing by Lindsay Elliott
Cover design by Deborah Rust

Dedicated to our patients.
By choosing brachytherapy and by their willingness
to inform us of their progress, they are pioneers
in prostate brachytherapy.

Acknowledgements

The following people share credit for this book. Their comments and suggestions during the preparation of the manuscript were invaluable.

Robert Amdur
Lowell Anderson
Jennifer Cash
William Cavanagh
Adam Dicker
Kathryn Elliott
Lindsay Elliott
Jay Friedland
Paul Gaudin
Susan Giles Godsey
David Gregg
Steven Howard
Christine Jacobs
Mick Langdon
Brad Prestidge
Linda Lively, M.H.A. & James Hugh, M.H.A. (AMAC)
Greg Lawrence
Clifton Ling
Felix Mick™
Mack Roach
Raymond Ross
David L. Schwartz
Richard Stock
Anthony Zeitman

Kent Wallner, M.D.
Chief, Radiation Oncology
Puget Sound Health Care System
Department of Veterans Affairs
Associate Professor
Department of Radiation Oncology
University of Washington Medical Center
Seattle, Washington

John Blasko, M.D.
Professor
Director, Prostate Brachytherapy Program
Department of Radiation Oncology
University of Washington Medical Center
Seattle, Washington

Michael J. Dattoli, M.D.
Chief, Brachytherapy Division
University Community Hospital, Tampa
Tampa, Florida

Contents

Chapter 1

Why this book

TOO MANY BOOKS AND JOURNALS, BUT...

Prostate brachytherapy is experiencing a rebirth -- it is rapidly regaining popularity. Despite its rapidly growing use, there is still little published information regarding the techniques and the results. Although physician mail boxes and bookshelves are already overpopulated with medical journals and text books, we are adding this text to the crowded shelves because there is no other comprehensive current text for I-125 and Pd-103 prostate brachytherapy.

IMPLANTS ARE TRICKY

Achieving good results with brachytherapy requires substantial technical skill. Although implant quality variation has not been well documented, the technical and clinical results can vary substantially from one practitioner to the next. The dependence on physician skill is much greater than for external beam radiation therapy (EBRT), and probably greater than for surgery. The necessity for substantial technical expertise has lead some to criticize the modality, in that not all patients will receive the same results as those treated by highly specialized brachytherapists. This book should help to disseminate the techniques of prostate brachytherapy, and help all brachytherapists to perform the highest quality implant procedures possible.

TOUGH POLITICS

Prostate brachytherapy has always been controversial. There is almost a visceral dislike of it among many mainstream, otherwise rational radiation oncologists and urologists. The reasons are varied and include skepticism that has arisen from inferior results with older retropubic techniques, as well as a natural disdain toward a newer modality that is viewed as competition for more established procedures. Whatever the reason, it is sometimes unduly difficult to get even good quality articles on the topic of brachytherapy accepted for publication in mainstream journals. In this book, we can share our experiences without concern for "getting past the reviewer." In addition to our desire to circumvent some of the editorial bias in mainstream cancer literature, much of the detail included in the pages ahead is beyond that which is appropriate for journal publications.

IMPLANTS AREN'T FOR EVERY PATIENT

While cancer control rates look good and morbidity rates are relatively low, prostate brachytherapy is not for every patient. This is something that we have sometimes learned the hard way. In the pages ahead, we provide detailed information about potential complications and who is more likely to experience them. Considerable effort is made throughout this text to help determine which patients are not good brachytherapy candidates.

IMPLANTS AREN'T FOR EVERY PHYSICIAN

Performing good prostate brachytherapy requires skill, attention to detail, and tolerance for tedium. Given the current technological limits, there is still a substantial dependence on manual dexterity and familiarity with the physics of brachytherapy. Physicians who are too busy with other responsibilities to put substantial effort into a brachytherapy practice should leave prostate brachytherapy to someone else. The title of this book was chosen to emphasize this point.

PERMANENT VS TEMPORARY IMPLANTS

The placing of permanent implants is the primary prostate brachytherapy method used in the United States. It is currently favored over temporary, Ir-192 brachytherapy due to convenience and encouraging tumor control rates with I-125 and Pd-103. Because of the current overwhelming preference for permanent implants, we have chosen not to include much information about temporary implants. That may change with future editions of this book.

THIS BOOK SHOULD HELP

There is a bright future for prostate brachytherapy. This text gives us a platform to share our experiences and advice. The descriptions, data, opinions and ruminations ahead should be helpful to brachytherapists who are just getting started, and to those who have established practices and are looking for ways to improve their techniques. We hope that this book helps you to improve your brachytherapy practice.

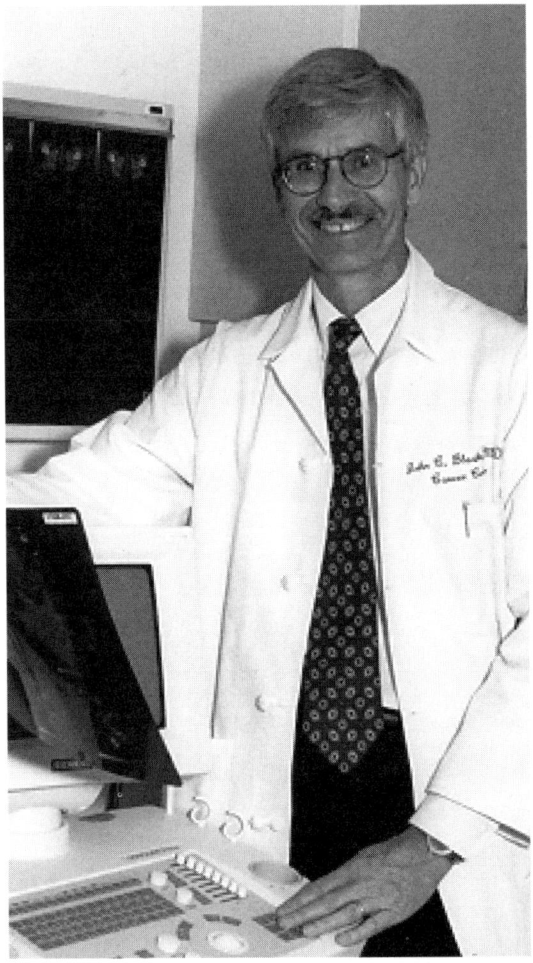

John Blasko

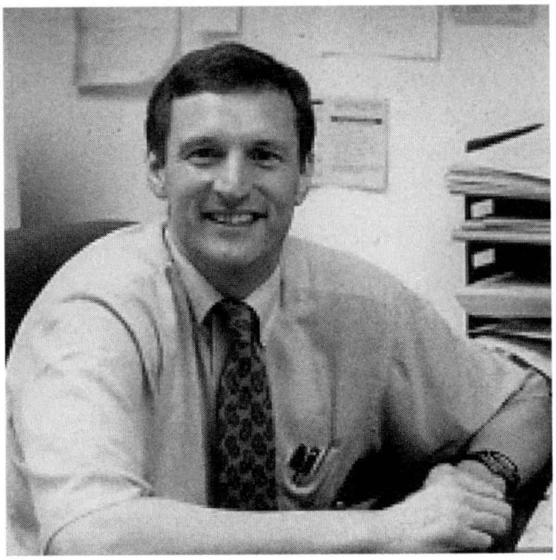

Kent Wallner

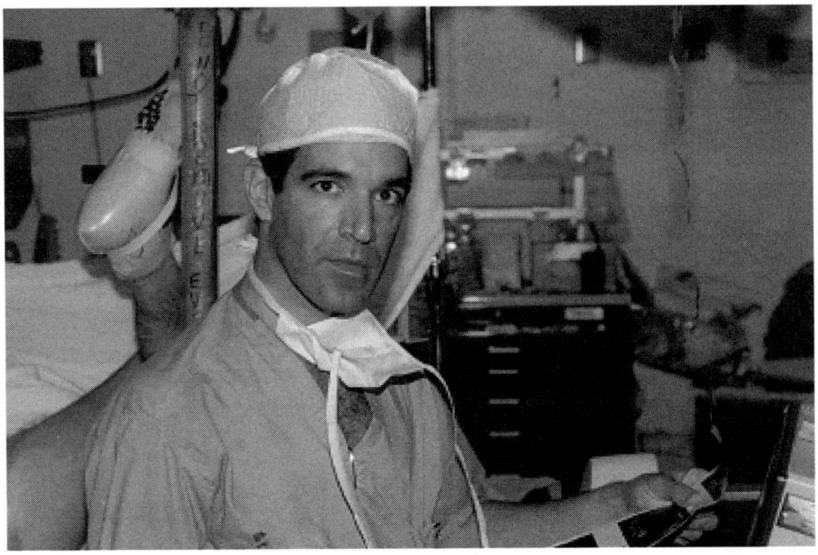

Michael J. Dattoli

Chapter 2

1895-1997

THE EARLY DAYS

Prostate brachytherapy in various forms has fluctuated in popularity for almost 100 years (**Figure 2-1**). During most of that time, it was more of a curiosity than a generally accepted method of treatment. It has never been widely accepted by the medical community for a variety of reasons. The history of prostate brachytherapy is punctuated by a few basic ideas, re-implemented in various ways depending on the technology available.

Benjamin S. Barringer, chief of urology at what is now Memorial Sloan-Kettering Cancer Center in New York (MSKCC), was among the first to espouse the use of transperineal radium needles for prostate brachytherapy.(Barringer 1917)

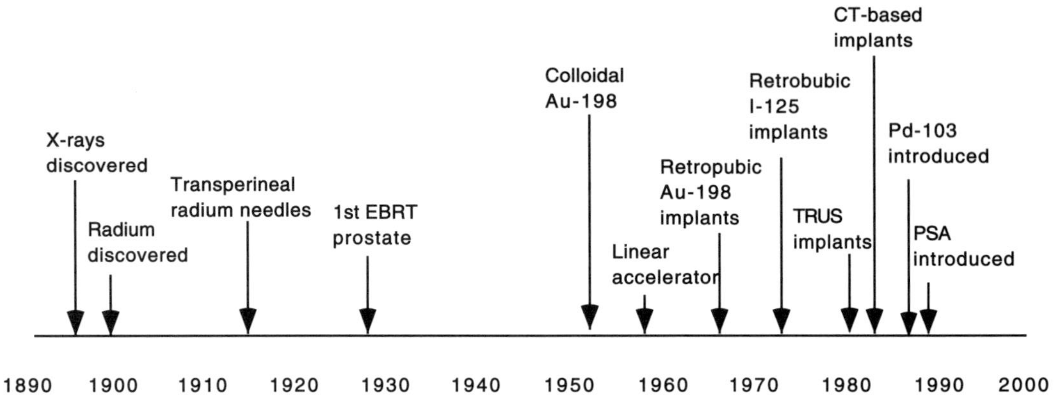

Figure 2-1. Time line showing major developments in prostate brachytherapy and EBRT from 1895 through 1990.

He was impressed with the results. He concluded his 1917 report in the Journal of the American Medical Association (JAMA) with...

> *"...because of the initial success of radium treatment, I now take the stand that no patient with prostate cancer should be operated on.."*

RETROPUBIC IMPLANTS

The first widespread adoption of prostate brachytherapy occurred in the 1970s, when the retropubic method was popularized by Basil Hilaris and Willett Whitmore at MSKCC.(Whitmore 1972) Early reports appeared favorable, but subsequent reports with longer follow-up were not.(Fuks 1991)(Schellhammer 1993) In retrospect, the introduction of retropubic methods was probably a step backward from Barringer's use of transperineal needle placement. The technical quality of retropubic implants was terrible (**Figure 2-2**). Their poor quality was not due to incompetence of the physicians involved, but to technical difficulty in performing the implants and lack of dosimetric analysis.

Although it sounds simple enough to place an implant under direct visualization of the exposed prostate, it was not. The prostate is not well exposed, the operative field is bloody, and without transrectal ultrasound (TRUS) it was not possible to visualize the source location within the prostate. The brachytherapist would have had little idea of whether or not the procedure was proceeding well.

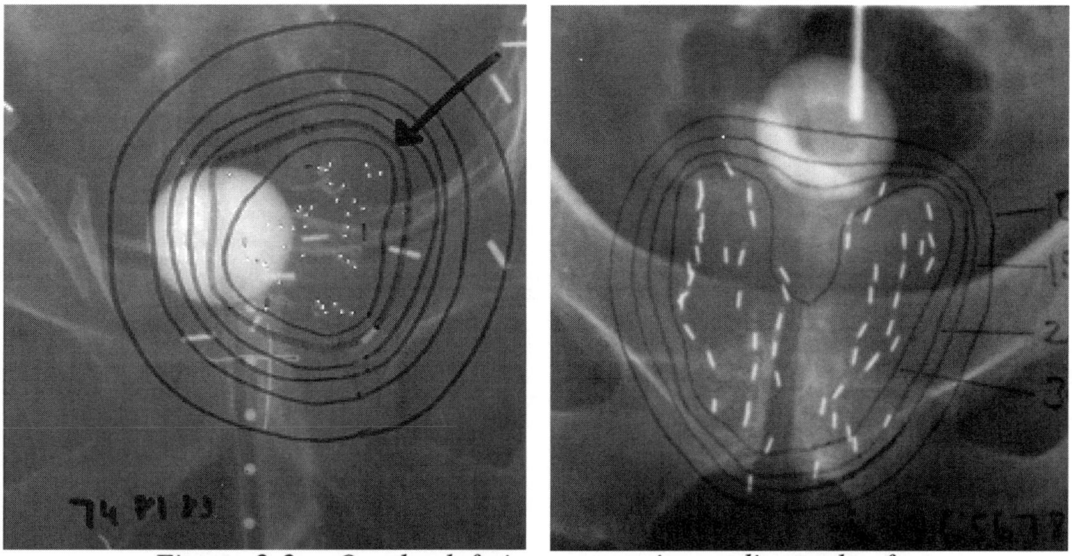

Figure 2-2. On the left is an anterior radiograph of a retropubic implant, performed at MSKCC in 1978. You don't need a Ph.D. in physics to recognize that the I-125 sources could not possibly be distributed throughout the prostate. The implant on the right was performed with modern transperineal techniques, also at MSKCC (1994). The implant on the left is included in previous reports of retropubic implant results at MSKCC.(Fuks 1991) *Such poor technical quality is not representative of what can be achieved today. Unfavorable tumor control rates resulting from poor quality implants should not dim enthusiasm for modern implant techniques.*

To compound the technical difficulties, there was limited quality assurance. Post-implant radiation doses were calculated from plain x-rays, without the ability to determine the relationship between radiation dose and the prostatic margins (see Chapter 9). Without a system of quality assurance, good or bad implant techniques could not have been accurately documented.

THE BABY AND THE BATH WATER

Understandably, when unfavorable long-term follow-up reports for retropubic implants were published, the urological oncology community went from enthusiastic about to suspicious of the use of brachytherapy. With the introduction of nerve-sparing surgery and the widespread availability of linear accelerators, interest in prostate brachytherapy fell substantially in the 1980s. Less understandable is that unfavorable reports of retropubic implants are still used today to downplay the potential of modern prostate brachytherapy. We are often reminded that the results of I-125 prostate brachytherapy, even at its birthplace (MSKCC), were suboptimal. Using these past results as an argument against brachytherapy today is misleading. The retropubic implants performed in the 1970s were so bad technically that the clinical results are irrelevant in light of today's technology.

It is also commonly remarked that the failures with retropubic implants became evident only with a 10 to 15 year follow-up, and that current follow-up with modern techniques is too short to be encouraging. Only partly true. While long follow-up is necessary to assess the curative potential of any modality, the shortcomings of retropubic implants would have been apparent much earlier in their history if prostatic specific antigen (PSA) had been available to detect biochemical evidence of tumor persistence. The need for long follow-up is no different for brachytherapy than it is for prostatectomy or external beam radiation (EBRT).

IR-192 BRACHYTHERAPY

While the rise and fall of retropubic implants was playing out, a limited number of brachytherapists took up temporary implants. The most influential and innovative were Nisar Syed and Ajmel Puthawala. In the 1970s and 80s, They treated patients with 30-40 Gy EBRT plus a temporary "intermediate dose rate" (40 cGy/hour) Ir-192 boost of an additional 30-35 Gy. Their treatment system was better tailored to the prostatic anatomy: source loading was based on CT scan reconstruction of the prostate after the source guides were in place, allowing the radiation dose to be conformed to the geometry of the prostate. It most likely was as accurate a system for dose delivery as current TRUS-guided transperineal methods. Nine year clinical follow-up results were comparable or better than those of any other modality. (Syed 1992)

Despite the favorable results of Syed and colleagues, the popularity of Ir-192 implants has declined substantially, partly due to the potential for radiation exposure to medical personnel, the need for specialized treatment rooms, and higher morbidity in some series. Like retropubic implants, temporary ones have been eclipsed by the "nerve-sparing" prostatectomy, three dimensional conformal radiation (3DCRT), and now by permanent transperineal implants. The demise of Ir-192 prostate brachytherapy has probably been hastened by the fact that its proponents were slow to publish their results using PSA-based tumor control parameters. In the absence of PSA-based follow-up, skepticism will build toward any modality.

PSA WAS A WAKE-UP CALL

Widespread adoption of improved surgical techniques and of computer-aided EBRT generated renewed enthusiasm for treatment of early stage prostate

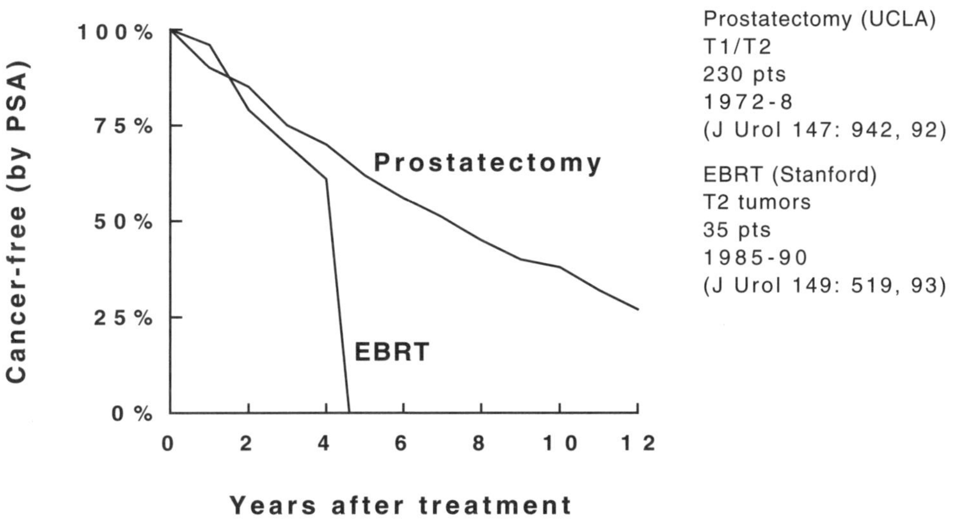

Figure 2-3. First PSA-based tumor control rates with conventional EBRT or prostatectomy, reported in early 1990s: the results, even from highly respected institutions, were dismal. With no plateau on the cancer-free curves, the question was raised as to whether any patients could be cured with conventional techniques. These results were a shocking revelation at the time.

cancer. Using survival as the endpoint, the 5 and 10 year results looked good. Then, the introduction of PSA follow-up in the late 1980s showed us how ineffective conventional EBRT and surgery were for eradicating even early stage cancers. It forced a re-assessment of the various treatment modalities (**Figure 2-3**).(Stein 1992)(Zietman 1994) Combined with the introduction of TRUS-based and CT-based transperineal implant techniques, renewed interest in prostate brachytherapy mounted, at least in some quarters.

THE LAST 10 YEARS

Prostate brachytherapy has been reborn over the last 10 years (**Figure 2-4**). CT scanners were introduced in the mid-1970's and TRUS scanning in the early 1980s. Computer-based treatment planning became widely available in the late 1970s. By the mid-1980's, these technologies had been combined with the old idea of transperineal implantation, to allow high-quality prostate brachytherapy.(Holm 1983)(Blasko 1987)(Osian 1989)

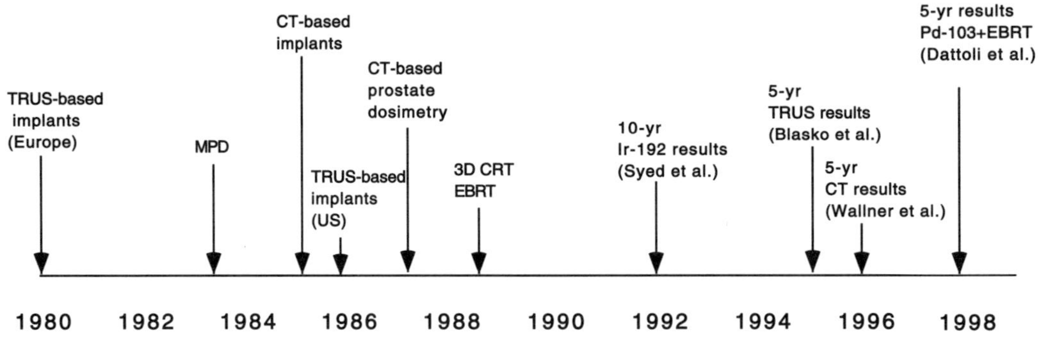

Figure 2-4. Time line showing some of the major developments in prostate brachytherapy from 1980-1998.

WHERE THE CONTROVERSY LIES

Brachytherapy has a number of advantages over prostatectomy or EBRT, including patient convenience, better potency preservation and lower costs. The veracity of these advantages has not been controversial. There is intense controversy, however, as to how the cancer control rates with brachytherapy compare with those of the other modalities.

Several groups are approaching 10-year follow-up for transperineal methods, with biochemical-based cancer-free rates that compare favorably with surgery. Favorable biochemical tumor control rates, combined with the practical advantages of brachytherapy are fueling an incredible resurgence of interest in this treatment modality.

BRACHYTHERAPY HAS BEEN AROUND LONGER

Transperineal prostate brachytherapy predates EBRT by approximately 15 years (**Figure 2-1**). Modern transperineal implants predate 3DCRT by approximately two years. Given the longer follow-up for modern brachytherapy, it is surprising that some prominent, otherwise rational radiation oncologists are already hailing 3DCRT as a major advance, but still caution that follow-up for transperineal implants is too short to justify its emergence from the "experimental" stage.

FRINGE PHYSICIANS AND PATIENT ACTIVISM

The emergence of prostate brachytherapy is largely due to a handful of individual physicians and their determination to proceed despite the admonitions

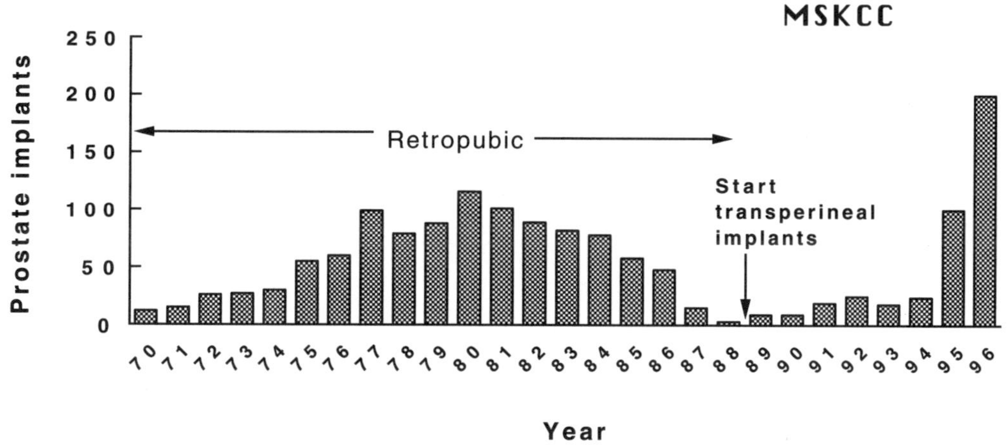

Figure 2-5. Number of retropubic and transperineal I-125 implants performed per year at MSKCC from 1970 through 1996.

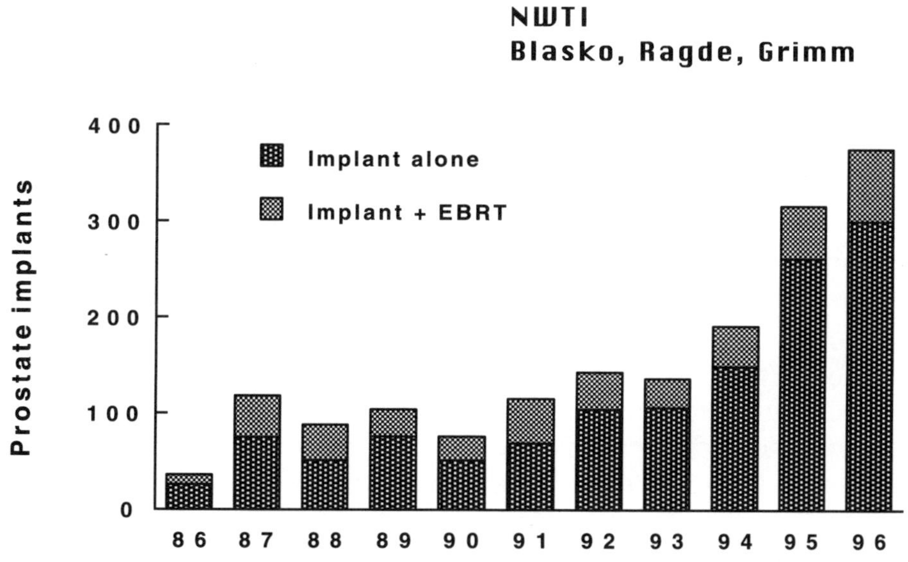

Figure 2-6. Number of prostate implants per year (I-125 & Pd-103) at Northwest Tumor Institute (NWTI), since the start of their brachytherapy program in 1986.

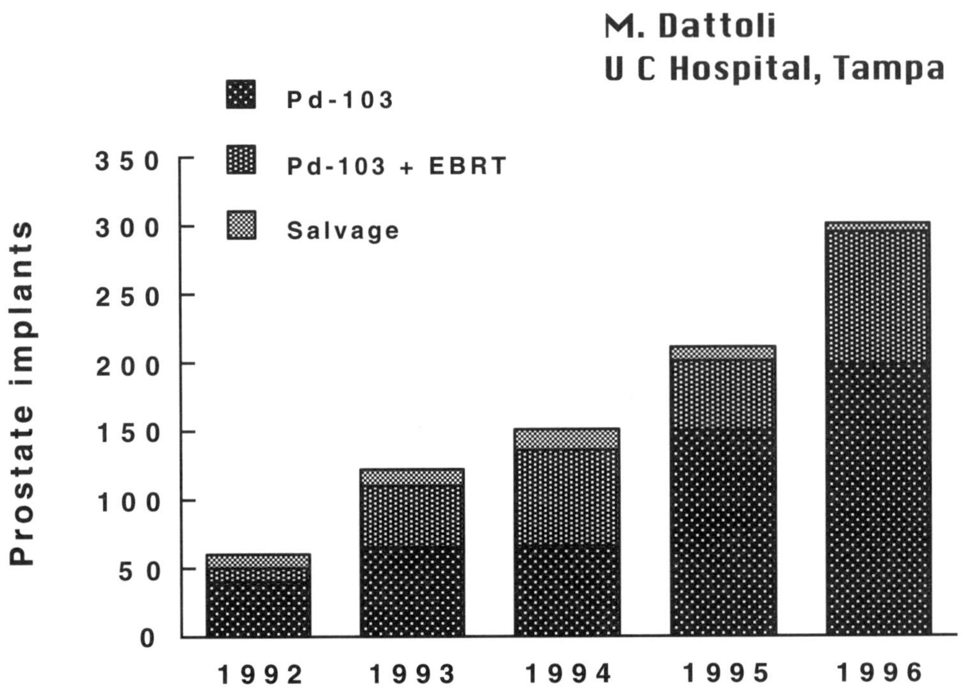

Figure 2-7. Number of prostate implants per year by M. Dattoli at University Community Hospital, Tampa since the start of the brachytherapy program in 1991.

of much of the medical establishment. Until recently, relatively few physicians were involved in transperineal brachytherapy. John Blasko, Haakon Ragde and Peter Grimm were the first to achieve prominence as advocates in the United States. They were considered to be far out of the mainstream. The medical and lay community are becoming increasingly impressed by the reported results.[Blasko 1995] The dramatic increase in the number of implants performed at Northwest Tumor Institute (NWTI) at Northwest Hospital, MSKCC and University Community Hospital, Tampa (UCH, Tampa) reflects the increasing interest in brachytherapy (**Figures 2-5, 2-6 and 2-7**).

The resurgent interest in prostate brachytherapy is also due to direct patient involvement. In the 1990s, patients increasingly began investigating less conventional options and spreading the word among prospective patients through formal channels (support groups, news articles) and informal ones (the Internet, personal contact). These efforts have had a substantial impact and made many potential patients aware of brachytherapy.

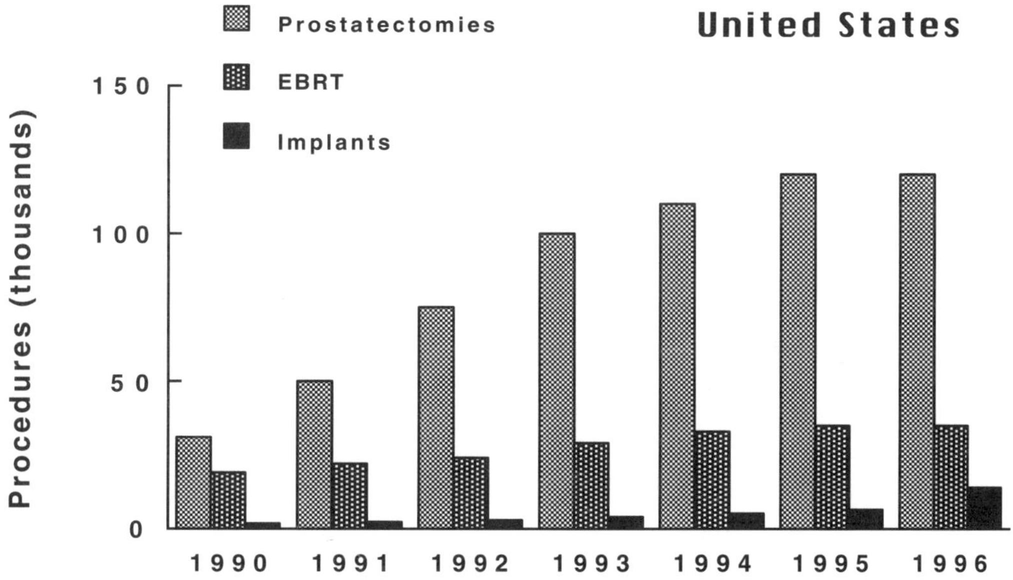

Figure 2-8. Approximate number of prostatectomies, EBRT and implants per year in the United States, from 1990 through 1996. The general increase is largely due to increased detection with PSA. The use of brachytherapy is growing faster than surgery or EBRT, but it is still a small fraction of the overall treatments. However, the growth of brachytherapy is accelerating, and it will likely reach parity (or more) with other modalities soon.

MIXED EMOTIONS

As a result of the technological developments that have taken place over the past 10 years, brachytherapy is gaining an increasingly prominent role in the fight against prostate cancer (**Figure 2-8**). As in the past, there is both great excitement and great skepticism about prostate brachytherapy.

REFERENCES

1. Barringer BS. Radium in the Treatment of Carcinoma of the Bladder and Prostate. JAMA 1917; 68:1227-1230.

2. Blasko J C, Ragde H, Schumacher D. Transperineal percutaneous iodine-125 implantation for prostatic carcinoma using transrectal ultrasound and template guidance. Endo/Hypertherm 1987; 3:131-139.

3. Blasko JC, Wallner KE, Grimm PD, Ragde H. PSA-based disease control following ultrasound-guided I-125 implantation for stage T1/T2 prostatic carcinoma. J Urol 1995; 154:1096-1099.

4. Fuks Z, Leibel SA, Wallner KE, et al. The Effect of Local Control on Metastatic Dissemination in Carcinoma of the Prostate: Long Term Results in Patients Treated with 125-I Implantation. Int J Radiat Oncol Biol Phys 1991; 21:337-347.

5. Holm HH, Juul N, Pederson JF, Hansen H, Stroyer I. Transperineal 125-Iodine Seed Implantation in Prostatic Cancer Guided by Transrectal Ultrasonography. J Urol 1983; 130:283-286.

6. Osian AD, Anderson LL, Linares LA, Nori D, Hilaris BS. Treatment planning for permanent and temporary percutaneous implants with custom made templates. Int J Radiat Oncol Biol Phys 1989; 16:219-223.

7. Schellhammer PF, El-Mahdi AM, Wright GL, Kolm P, Ragle R. Prostate-specific antigen to determine progression-free survival after radiation therapy for localized carcinoma of prostate. Urology 1993; 42:13-20.

8. Stein A, deKernion JB, Smith RB, Dorey F, Patel H. Prostate specific antigen levels after radical prostatectomy in patients with organ confined and locally extensive prostate cancer. J Urol 1992; 147:942-946.

9. Syed AM, Puthawala A, Austin P, Cherlow J. Temporary iridium-192 implant in the management of carcinoma of the prostate. Cancer 1992; 69:2515-2524.

10. Whitmore WF, Hilaris B, Grabstald H. Retropubic Implantation of Iodine 125 in the Treatment of Prostatic Cancer. J Urol 1972; 108:918-920.

11. Zietman AL, Coen JJ, Shipley WU, Willett CG, Efird JT. Radical radiation therapy in the management of prostatic adenocarcinoma: The initial prostate specific antigen value as a predictor of treatment outcome. J Urol 1994; 151:640-645.

Chapter 3

Radiobiology

VERY FEW FACTS STRETCHED VERY THIN

Radiobiology is a fascinating area of study. Unfortunately, its usefulness in clinical decision-making is tenuous. Most radiobiological data is based on theoretical in vitro experiments. In vivo work, which should be closer to the clinical situation, has nearly all been derived from transplantable mouse (murine) tumors, which probably behave far differently than spontaneous human tumors.

The radiobiological rationale most often quoted regarding prostate brachytherapy is purely theoretical.(Ling 1992) While the theoretical work of Clifton Ling and others is important if we are to make advances beyond what has been learned by clinical trial and error, its practical relevance to current medical practice is questionable. The point here is not to belittle such theoretical efforts, but to keep them in perspective.

BRACHYTHERAPY VERSUS EBRT

There are three principal differences between brachytherapy and external beam irradiation (EBRT):

1. dose distribution
2. total dose
3. dose rate

All three factors may be advantages of brachytherapy over EBRT for eradicating prostatic carcinoma. There is much that is still not known biologically about these factors, especially about dose rate.

DOSE LOCALIZATION-RECTUM

The rectum is relatively sensitive to radiation, the anterior rectal wall being the principal dose-limiting structure for EBRT.(Lee 1996) A small rectal area can tolerate a large dose, but as the area irradiated increases so does the risk of complications.(Wallner 1995)

Even with conformal EBRT, the potential for prostate motion (typically 0.5 cm in the anterior-posterior direction) requires that a relatively large portion of the anterior rectal wall be included in the target volume to avoid underdosing the posterior prostate.

With brachytherapy, a higher radiation dose can be given to the prostate without undo risk of rectal ulceration or fistula because of the rapid dose fall-off at the prostatic margins. The rapid radiation dose fall-off with an implant limits the area of rectum that receives the prescription dose or higher (**Figure 3-1**). With an I-125 implant, only approximately 50 mm^2 of rectal surface area receives the prescription dose or higher. In contrast, in a typical conformal EBRT at MSKCC, approximately 1000 mm^2 of anterior rectal wall will receive the prescription dose or higher (**Figure 3-2**).

DOSE LOCALIZATION-BLADDER

Bladder tolerance is not a dose-limiting concern with prostate brachytherapy or conformal EBRT. Because of rapid dose fall-off, no more than a one centimeter (cm) margin of bladder receives the prescription dose or higher from an I-125 or Pd-103 implant. Even with combined EBRT plus brachytherapy boost, radiation to the bladder is probably of little consequence because the dose that the whole bladder receives would be no higher than 50 Gy, even if the whole pelvis were included in the supplemental EBRT field. In practice, very few radiation

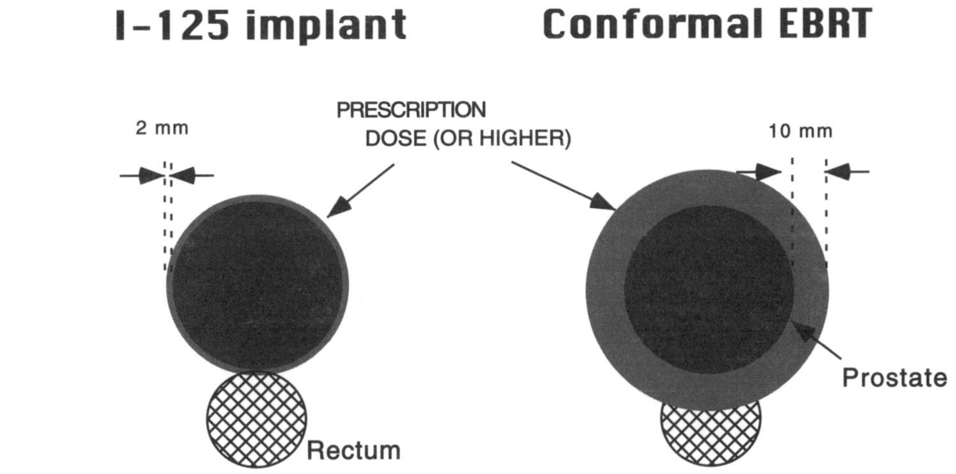

Figure 3-1a. Prescription dose in relation to the prostate and rectum, for brachytherapy versus EBRT. Much more rectal surface is included in the high dose region with EBRT compared to brachytherapy.

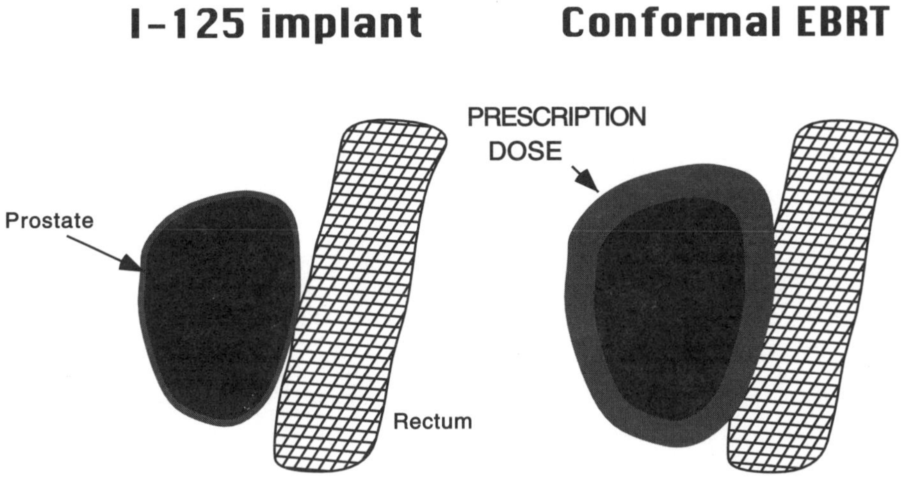

Figure 3-1b. Lateral view of dose localization to the prostate and rectum with brachytherapy versus EBRT. With brachytherapy, only a minimal portion of the rectum receives the prescription dose because of rapid dose fall-off and the fact that no allowance need be made for prostate motion.

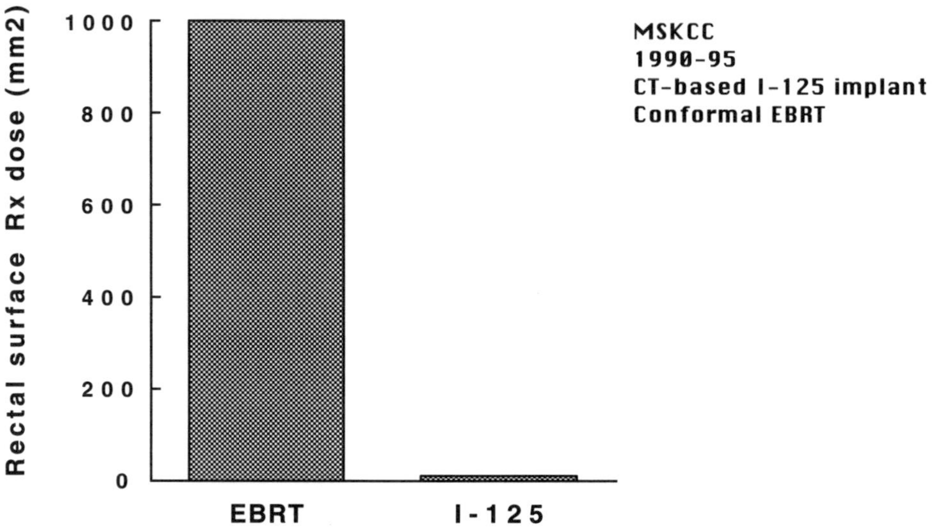

Figure 3-2. Approximate area of anterior rectal wall treated to prescription dose or higher with conformal EBRT versus I-125 brachytherapy. With a well-executed implant, an average of 50 mm^2 of the anterior rectal surface receives greater than the prescription dose. With EBRT, approximately 20 times as much rectal wall receives the prescription dose or higher.

oncologists still radiate the whole pelvis routinely, so that only a portion of the bladder is included in the EBRT fields. Brachytherapy-related urinary morbidity is probably predominantly due to urethral inflammation, not bladder irritation.

TOTAL DOSES

The total brachytherapy radiation dose is approximately twice that given with EBRT (**Figure 3-3**). Total doses of 70 Gy for EBRT, 160 Gy with I-125 and 115 Gy with Pd-103 are apparently roughly clinically equivalent in regards to tumor eradication, at least for patients with pre-treatment PSA below 10 ng/ml.

A modification of the TDF tables has been made to allow interconvertability between EBRT and low dose rate brachytherapy.(Orton 1977) While the modification reflects currently used prescription doses, its clinical applicability is unclear.

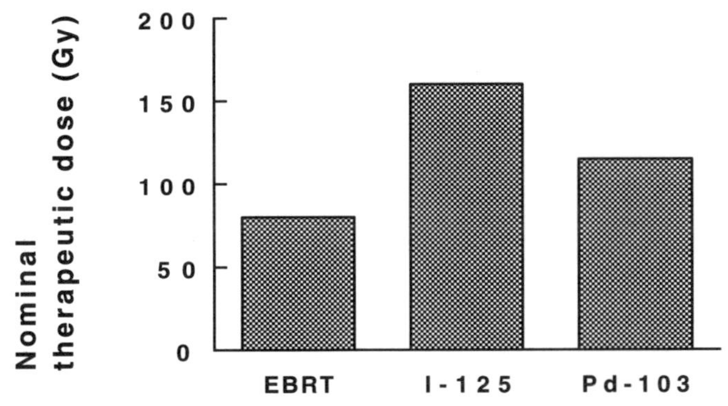

Figure 3-3. Typical prescription dose of EBRT, I-125 and Pd-103. The total dose delivered with low dose rate brachytherapy is approximately twice that delivered with EBRT.

DOSE RATE

The most dramatic difference between EBRT and I-125/Pd-103 brachytherapy is one of dose rates. The typical initial dose rate of an I-125 or Pd-103 implant is less than 1% of that of a linear accelerator (**Figure 3-4**). The dose rate of a linear accelerator is approximately 2 Gy/minute. In contrast, the initial dose rate of an I-125 implant is 0.0013 Gy/minute. The marked difference in dose rates dwarfs the moderate difference in total doses, and may lead to marked differences in radiation damage repair, reassortment, reoxygenation and redistribution in the cell cycle.

With very few exceptions, lower dose rates yield lower cell killing, given the same total dose. As the dose rate gets low enough, the dose rate effect diminishes, presumably because of the dominance of single hit cell killing at low dose rates. In fact, very little work has been done with dose rates as low as those of I-125/Pd-103 brachytherapy.[Ling 1995] The comparability of high and low dose rate radiation against human tumors specifically is unknown.

We do not even know over what time interval the dose rates should be compared. The stated dose rate for any modality is markedly different, depending on the time interval chosen for the denominator. The initial dose rates for EBRT and I-125/Pd-103 brachytherapy are markedly different, but the dose rates are similar when compared over a longer time interval. For instance, the dose per week with EBRT is approximately 10 Gy/week, versus 13 Gy/week for an I-125 implant (**Figure 3-4**).

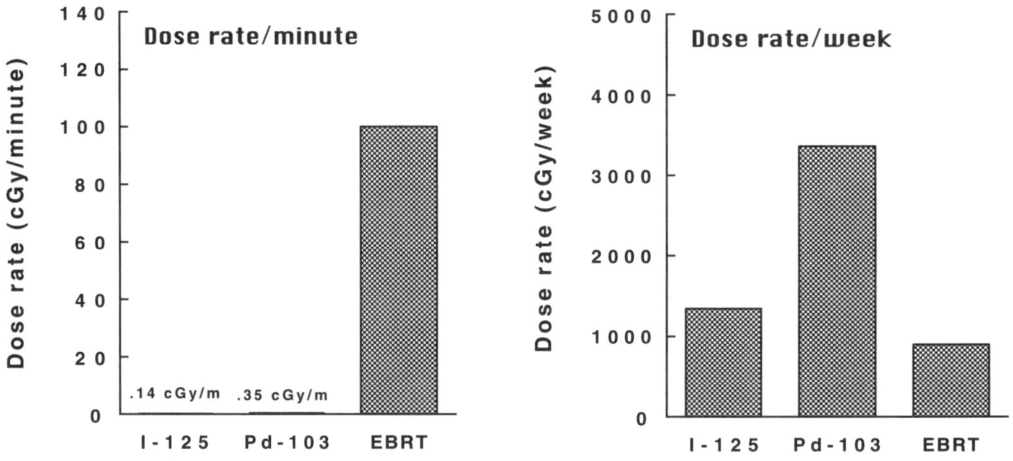

Figure 3-4. The pulse dose rate of a linear accelerator is far higher than the dose rate at the periphery of a I-125 or Pd-103 implant (left). However, the brachytherapy dose rates, when considered over a longer time interval, are similar or greater than that of EBRT (right). The clinical relevance of these differences is not understood.

OXYGEN ENHANCEMENT RATIO (OER)

Sterilizing poorly oxygenated (hypoxic) tumors requires 2.5 to 4 times as much radiation as that needed for fully oxygenated tumors. Low dose rate radiation of I-125/Pd-103 brachytherapy may decrease hypoxia-related radiation resistance.(Hall 1974) However, the relationship between the OER and dose rate is complicated, being dependent on cell type and the dose rate.(Ling 1985)

While brachytherapy might offer an advantage in the eradication of hypoxic tumors, it is not known how the OER with low dose rate brachytherapy compares with EBRT in human tumors. There are no published data regarding oxygen tension in human prostate tumors. Judging from the generally viable appearance of prostate tumors on microscopy, it is unlikely that substantial areas of hypoxia exist. Therefore, the OER may have little relevance in early stage prostate cancer.

HORMONAL MANIPULATION

There is increasing interest in the use of hormonal deprivation as an adjunct to EBRT and to brachytherapy and prostate cancer patients commonly receive adjunctive hormonal therapy. There are two rationales for combining androgen deprivation radiation: physical and radiobiological.

Physical

Decreasing the prostate size decreases the integral dose to adjacent rectum, bladder and small bowel.(Zelefsky 1994)(Forman 1995) While this has been demonstrated only for EBRT, the same should hold true for brachytherapy. Additionally, a smaller prostate volume facilitates implantation of the anterior prostate in patients for whom pubic arch interference is likely.

Biological

Hormonal deprivation may enhance radiation sensitivity. However, to date, there is minimal data in regard to how hormonal status affects radiation sensitivity. Zietman and colleagues showed that hormonal deprivation increases the

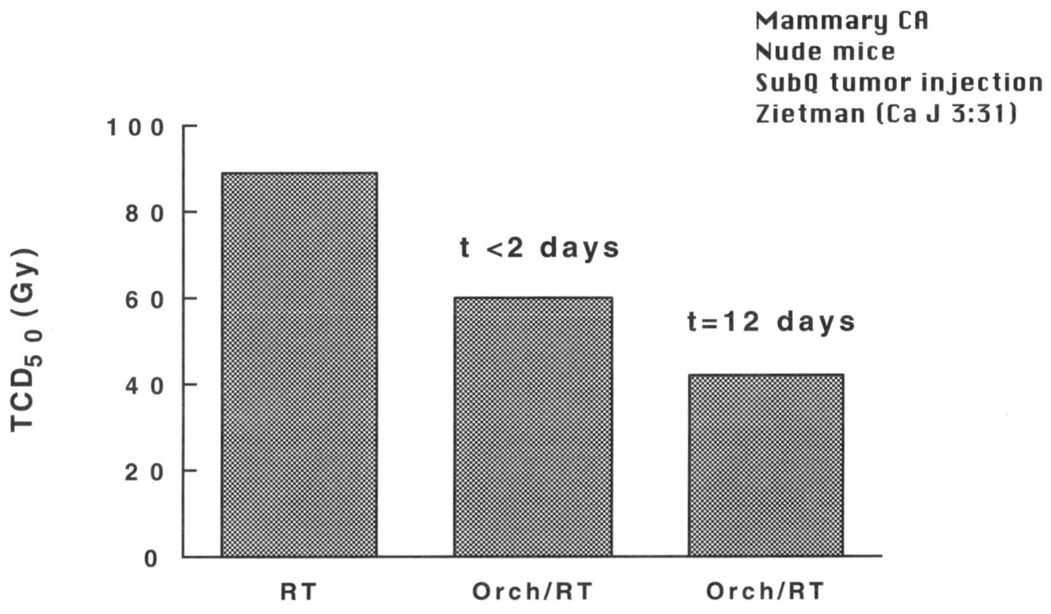

Figure 3-5. Radiation dose required to control 50% of androgen-dependent mammary tumors in mice. The hormonal sensitizing effect was greater if more time elapsed between orchiectomy and radiation, possibly due to more tumor shrinkage with longer anti-androgen effect.

radiation sensitivity of androgen dependent mammary tumors carried in nude mice.(Zietman 1997) The radiation sensitivity enhancement was most marked if hormonal deprivation was completed greater than 48 hours prior to radiation, possibly due to greater volume reduction (**Figure 3-5**). While Dr. Zietman and colleagues are to be congratulated for their attempt to add some rationale to clinical practice, the applicability of their findings about subcutaneous, transplantable mouse mammary tumors to human prostate cancer is dubious.

Two large randomized clinical trials of hormonal ablation combined with radiation have shown a benefit in terms of suppressing overt metastases, but have shown no difference in survival rates (**Figure 3-6**).(Pilepich 1997)(Pilepich 1995) The most likely explanation is that androgen ablation suppresses the clinical, biochemical and pathological evidence of cancer after EBRT, but does not enhance tumor eradication. This explanation would be consistent with multiple negative surgical trials demonstrating a similar phenomenon with pre-surgical hormonal ablation.

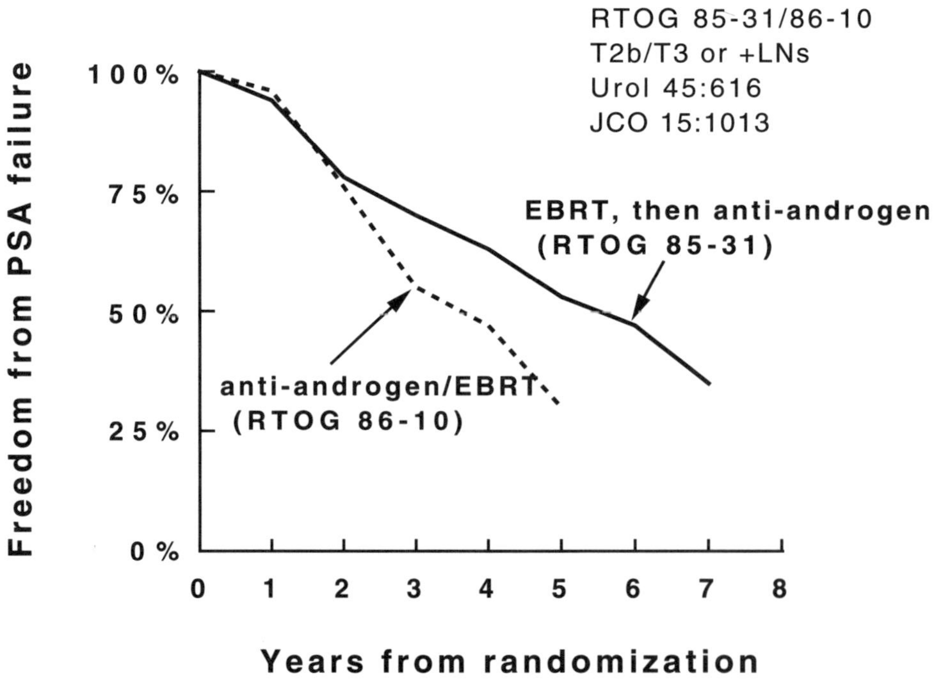

Figure 3-6. Although clinically evident tumor recurrence is delayed with hormonal deprivation, there is still no evidence of a plateau on the disease-free survival curve, whether hormonal ablation preceded (RTOG 86-10) or followed (RTOG 85-31) EBRT.

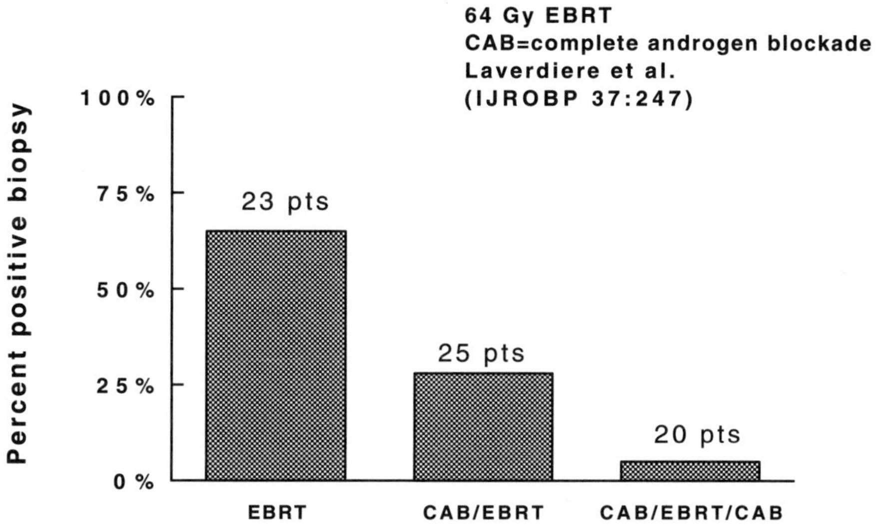

Figure 3-7. Positive biopsy rates after 64 Gy EBRT alone, EBRT preceded by 3 months androgen blockade, or EBRT preceded (3 months) and followed (6 months) by androgen blockade.

Laverdiere and colleagues reported that androgen blockade decreases the likelihood of a positive biopsy after conventional dose EBRT.(Laverdiere 1997) The effect was most marked if androgen blockade was continued for six months after completion of EBRT (**Figure 3-7**). The findings are compelling, but could easily be explained as another example of cancer masking, without a real change in the cure rate. Longer biochemical follow-up will address this issue. Unfortunately, the laudable efforts of Laverdiere and colleagues will be hampered by their small patient numbers and incomplete follow-up biopsies.

There are currently no *in vitro*, *in vivo,* or controlled clinical studies regarding the effect of hormonal ablation on brachytherapy radiation sensitivity. Work in this area would be welcome.

APOPTOSIS

Apoptosis is "signal-induced, programmed" cell death, seemingly distinct from mitotic death due to indiscriminate DNA damage. It occurs as a natural involution process in lymphocytes, and to some extent in other tissues. It is probably the mechanism of prostate cell death following androgen-deprivation.(McDonnell 1992)

The role of apoptosis in radiation-related death of prostate cancer is unclear. It accounts for only a small percent of radiation cell killing in most human cell types, and there is no good evidence that it is important in prostate cancer.(Algan 1996)

HYPERTHERMIA

Hyperthermia is the use of elevated temperatures to enhance the cytotoxic effect of radiation. Hyperthermia may act primarily by suppressing sublethal damage repair.(BenHur 1974) The thermal enhancement ratio varies from one to five, depending on the temperature and time the hyperthermia is given. Temperatures of 41° to 42°C for 30-90 minutes are most practical with the technology currently available.

Hyperthermia generated substantial enthusiasm in the 1980's, when a variety of external and interstitial heating devices were designed for clinical use. Prostate cancer was studied widely, due to accessibility to interstitial heating with radiofrequency antennae. Unfortunately, only locally advanced or recurrent tumors were studied.(Prionas 1993) Patients with locally advanced tumors are generally not curable with any local modality, and the chance of showing a benefit from hyperthermia would have been miniscule.

While there were anecdotal reports of good local response, patients did poorly overall, as would be expected. It is still unclear whether hyperthermia would add to local control. In the meantime, it has generally fallen out of favor due to technical difficulties in achieving homogeneous hyperthermia with the available technology.

I-125 VERSUS PD-103

There has been a long-running controversy about which is the best radionuclide for prostate brachytherapy. Much has been written about the advantages and disadvantages of I-125 versus Pd-103. It has been argued that inferior results with the implants done with I-125 in the 1970s were due to suboptimal radiobiologic properties. Probably not. Technically, retropubic implants were embarrassingly poor (see Chapter 2). Their high long-term failure rates probably had little or nothing to do with the type of radionuclide used.

In vitro

Low energy photons have a higher linear energy transfer (LET), leading to higher radiobiologic effect (RBE). The higher RBE presumably results from more energy deposition per cell that the photon traverses. The average energy of Pd-103 photons is 21 keV versus 30 keV of I-125, so that Pd-103 would be expected to have a slightly higher LET and RBE.

The RBE of I-125 versus Pd-103 has been compared in only one system - rat embryo cells transfected with Ha-ras oncogene.(Ling 1995) Using this system, Ling and colleagues found that the RBE of I-125 was 1.4, compared to 1.9 for Pd-103. A difference of this magnitude is numerically substantial, and may justify a reduction in total dose by approximately 30%. Unfortunately, it has been studied in only one system, and may have little relevance to human prostate tumors.

There are no *in vitro* studies comparing the use of I-125 to Pd-103 against prostate cancer specifically. This is due in part to the limited number of cell lines available. There are several rodent models, but only a handful of human models. The applicability of laboratory grown immortal murine cancer cell lines to the clinic is questionable.

In vivo

Nag and colleagues studied the effect of I-125 versus Pd-103 in transplantable Nb AI-1 prostate tumors in Noble rats.(Nag 1993) At similar doses, tumor growth delay and tumor eradication rates were increased by a factor of two or more with Pd-103 versus I-125. The increased tumorcidal effect of Pd-103 was higher than what would be expected by its higher RBE alone, and suggests an enhanced therapeutic ratio.(Ling 1995)

The results of Nag and colleagues are intriguing, but were based on a limited number of animals (five per group). Large inter-animal differences in tumor response to identical treatment require that experiments be repeated multiple times, to allow more confidence in the findings. Their findings should also be viewed skeptically because of inconsistencies within their data, such as tumor control rates not increasing with increasing dose. Also, their dosimetry was presumably even less precise than that used clinically. More in vivo work is needed, using larger numbers of animals and a variety of prostate tumor types, to determine the generalizability of such findings.

Theoretical arguments

Ling has written about the relative efficacy of I-125 and Pd-103, based on theoretical calculations. Based on the biologically effective dose (BED) formula, he has shown that Pd-103 is more likely to be effective against faster-growing tumors -- those with a shorter doubling time (**Figure 3-8**).(Ling 1992) While interesting and potentially valuable work, its applicability to the clinic is questionable, due to the highly theoretical nature of the data. For instance, a tumor doubling time of less than 10 days is found to be a criteria for better tumor control with Pd-103, while probably all prostate cancers have doubling times far in excess of 10 days.

Figure 3-9 summarizes the core equation used by Ling to calculate the surviving fraction with various radionuclides. The equation includes five variables of

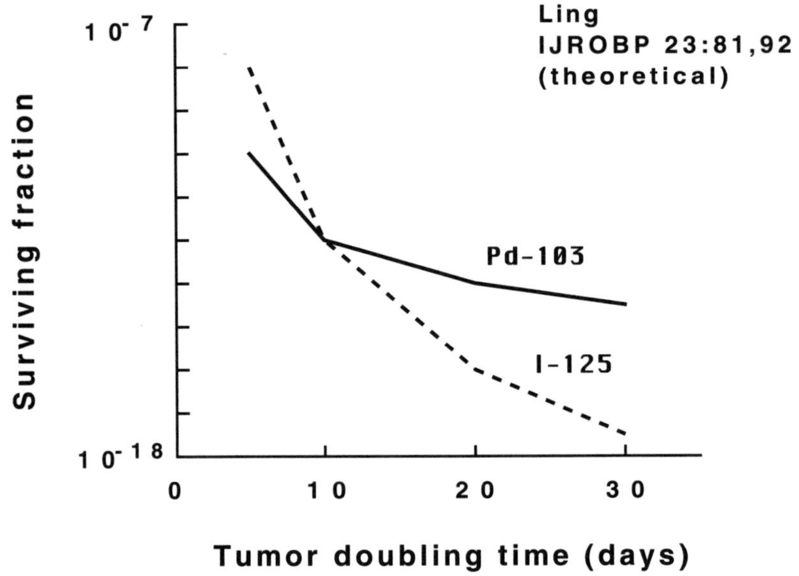

Figure 3-8. Surviving cell fractions following I-125 or Pd-103 versus tumor doubling times. Numbers are theoretical, based on biological equivalent dose calculations.

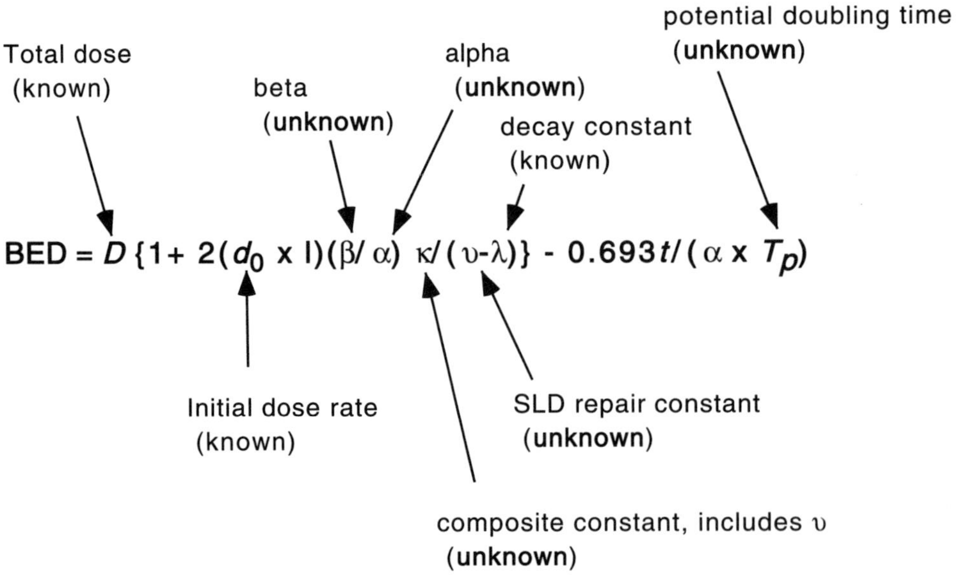

Figure 3-9. Equation used for graph in Figure 3-8 to determine cell survival levels comparing I-125 and Pd-103. There are five variables in the equation, the values of which are unknown.

Table 3-1. Factors that may affect the degree of cell killing, and how much is known about each factor, for human prostate cancers.

Factor	Quantifiable in vivo?
Dose	Roughly*
Dose rate	Roughly*
Damage repair	No
Oxygen enhancement ratio	No
RBE	No
Apoptosis	No
Repopulation	No
Reassortment	No

*Even the precise dose and dose rate are difficult to quantify, due to rapid fall-off near the sources of an implant

which virtually nothing is known for prostate cancer in humans (**Table 3-1**). Although the variables would presumably be equivalent for different patients, and should essentially "cancel out" in the comparisons between radionuclides, the use of equations with so little basis in reality should raise skepticism about their relevance. This work is of theoretical importance and a good starting point for planning in vitro and in vivo experiments. Basing clinical decisions on it, however, is absurd.

I-125 versus Pd-103: Tpot

Potential tumor doubling time (Tpot) is a balance between the cell proliferation rate and the cell loss rate. If the proliferation rate increases, or the loss rate decreases, Tpot decreases and the tumor grows faster. Tpot can be estimated by the ratio of DNA synthetic phase (S-phase) and the labeling index.[Begg 1985]

Tpot variability could substantially affect time-related radiation effects, such as radiation damage repair. It has been argued that tumors with a more rapid proliferation rate, or shorter Tpot, should be treated with a shorter acting radionuclide to allow less time for cell repopulation during the radiation interval.[Ling 1992]

The determination of tumor doubling times is work that is still in its infancy. Results with human tumors in general, have been mixed.[Bourhis 1996] Using an anti-bromodeoxyuridine monoclonal antibody, researchers have correlated the percent of S-phase cells with Gleason score.[Nemoto 1989] Using bromodeoxuridine administered prior to needle biopsy, Scrivner and colleagues showed that the labeling index correlated with Gleason score.(Scrivner 1989) It is possible that such indices of tumor growth rates could be used to guide radionuclide choice. Use of such tests, however, is clouded by tumor heterogeneity, by which different parts of a tumor have different S-phase fractions, just as there is heterogeneity of the Gleason score within a tumor. To date, there are no clinical reports regarding Tpot and radiation response in human prostate cancer.

We just don't know

Theoretical arguments can be made for any radionuclide and the ultimate answer may well be that none is clearly superior. But the choice may be important, and resolving the controversy will require large, well-designed human trials.

DO WE NEED A RADIATION SENSITIZER?

Much effort has been expended to develop chemical radiation sensitizers (enhancers), without success. In fact, radiation sensitizers may be of limited value for prostate cancer, given the high negative biopsy rates after brachytherapy.(Prestidge 1997) It appears that local control can be achieved in most cases. The remaining impediment to increased cure rates will be the presence of micrometastases at the time of diagnosis. A better systemic, cytotoxic drug would be more helpful than a radiation sensitizer.

HUMAN TUMORS - THE GREAT UNKNOWN

Almost nothing is known about radiobiology of brachytherapy against prostate human tumors specifically. Existing *in vivo* and *in vitro* work has been done primarily with rodent-derived cell lines, with questionable applicability to human prostate cancers. Work with more closely-related tumor models might offer some insight on how to best use the radionuclides available, and perhaps on how to best combine them with EBRT. This is an opportunity for the radiation oncology community to revive radiobiology, an area which has been hard hit by cynicism and budgetary constraints.

REFERENCES

1. Algan O, Stobbe CC, Helt AM, Hanks GE. Radiation inactivation of human prostate cancer cells: the role of apoptosis. Radiat Res 1996; 146:267-275.

2. Begg AC, McNally NJ. A method to measure the duration of DNA synthesis and the potential doubling time from a single sample. Cytometry 1997; 6:620-623.

3. BenHur E, Elkind MM, Bronk BV. Thermally enhanced radioresponse of cultured Chinese hamster cells: inhibition of repair of sublethal damage and enhancement of lethal damage. Radiat Res 1974; 58:38-51.

4. Bourhis J, Dendale R, Hill C, Bosq J. Potential doubling time and clinical outcome in head and neck squamous cell carcinoma treated with 70 Gy in 7 weeks. Int J Radiat Oncol Biol Phys 1996; 35:471-476.

5. Forman JD, Kumar R, Haas G, Montie J. Neoadjuvant hormonal downsizing of localized carcinoma of the prostate: Effects on the volume of normal tissue irradiation. Ca Invest 1995; 13:8-15.

6. Hall EJ, Roizin-Towle LA, Colvett RD. RBE and OER determinations for Radium and Californium-252. Radiol 1974; 112:425-430.

7. Laverdiere J, Gomez JL, Cusan L, Suburu ER. Beneficial effect of combination hormonal therapy administered prior and following external beam radiation therapy in localized prostate cancer. Int J Radiat Oncol Biol Phys 1997; 37:247-252.

8. Lee WR, Hanks GE, Hanlon AL, Schultheiss TE. Lateral rectal shielding reduces late rectal morbidity following high dose three-dimensional conformal radiation therapy for clinically localized prostate cancer: Further evidence for a significant dose effect. Int J Radiat Oncol Biol Phys 1996; 31:251-257.

9. Ling CC. Permanent implants using Au-198, Pd-103 and I-125: radiobiological considerations based on the linear quadratic model. Int J Radiat Oncol Biol Phys 1992; 23:81-87.

10. Ling CC, Li WX, Anderson LL. The relative biological effectiveness of I-125 and Pd-103. Int J Radiat Oncol Biol Phys 1995; 32:373-378.

11. Ling CC, Spiro IJ, Mitchell J, Stickler R. The variation of OER with dose rate. Int J Radiat Oncol Biol Phys 1985; 11:1367-1373.

12. McDonnell TJ, Troncoso P, Brisbay SM, Logothetis C. Expression of the protooncogene bel-2 in the prostate and its association with emergence of androgen-independent prostate cancer. Ca Res 1992; 52:6940-6944.

13. Nag S, Sweeney PJ, Wienthjes MG. Dose-response study of Iodinc-125 and Palladium-103 brachytherapy in a rat prostate tumor (Nb-AI-1). Endocur/Hypertherm 1997; 9:97-104.

14. Nemoto R, Uchida K, Shiimazui T, Hattori K. Immunocytochemical demonstration of S phase cells by anti-bromodeoyuridine monoclonal antibody in human prostate adenocarcinoma. J Urol 1989; 141:337-340.

15. Orton CG, Webber BM. Time-dose factor (TDF) analysis of dose rate effects in permanent implant dosimetry. Int J Radiat Oncol Biol Phys 1977; 2:55-60.

16. Pilepich MV, Caplan R, Byhardt RW, Lawton CA. Phase III trial of androgen suppression using goserelin in unfavorable-prognosis carcinoma of the prostate treated with definitive radiotherapy: Report of Radiation Therapy Oncology Group Protocol 85-31. J Clin Oncol 1997; 15:1013-1021.

17. Prionas SD, Kapp DS, Goffinet DR, Ben-Yosef R. Thermometry of interstitial hyperthermia given as an adjuvant to brachytherapy for the treatment of carcinoma of the prostate. Int J Radiat Oncol Biol Phys 1993; 28:151-162.

18. Scrivner DL, Meyer JS, Rujanavech N, Fathman A. Cell kinetics by bromodeoxyuridine labeling and deoxyribonucleic acid ploidy in prostatic carcinoma needle biopsies. J Urol 1991; 146:1034-1039.

19. Wallner KE, Roy J, Harrison L. Dosimetry guidelines to minimize urethral and rectal morbidity following transperineal I-125 prostate brachytherapy. Int J Radiat Oncol Biol Phys 1995; 32:465-471.

20. Zelefsky MJ, Leibel SA, Burman CM, Kutcher GJ. Neoadjuvant hormonal therapy improves the therapeutic ratio in patients with bulky prostatic cancer treated with three-dimensional conformal radiation therapy. Int J Radiat Oncol Biol Phys 1994; 29:755-761.

21. Zietman AL, Nakfoor BM, Prince EA, Gerweck LE. The effect of androgen deprivation and radiation therapy on an androgen-sensitive murine tumor: An in vitro and in vivo study. Ca J 1997; 3:31-36.

Chapter 4

TRUS, CT or MR?

The primary advantage of modern prostate brachytherapy is the ability to image the prostate, in order to plan the activity needed and to guide source placement during the procedure. Prostate imaging is not necessarily simple or reproducible.

Prostate volumes can be derived from TRUS, CT or magnetic resonance (MR) images. Each modality has it advantages and disadvantages. Nearly all brachytherapists currently use TRUS images. CT images are used at a limited number of institutions. To date, no reports on the use of MR imaging have appeared, but there is some interest in its use.

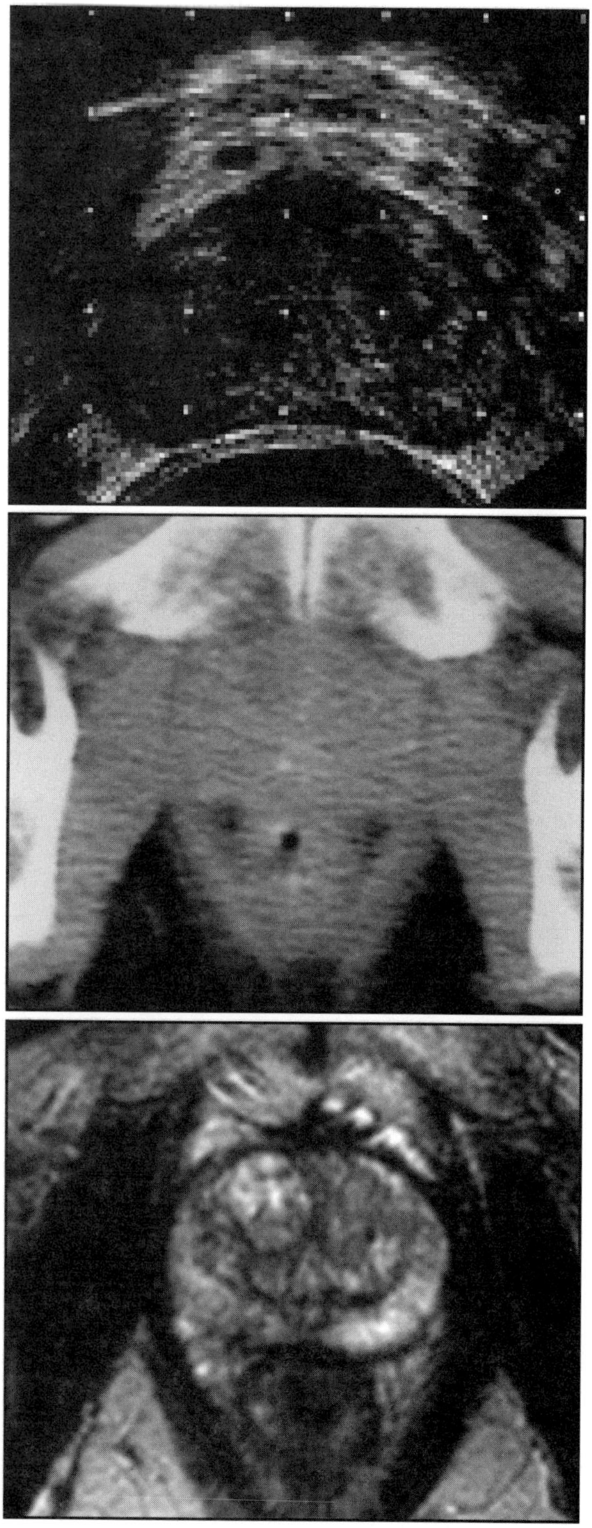

Figure 4-1. Cross section at mid prostate, viewed by TRUS (top), CT and MR (bottom). TRUS usually gives a sharper image of the prostate contour, while MR gives a better image of internal architecture. CT gives the least sharp image of internal architecture and outer contour, but is better at showing the spatial relationship between the prostate gland and the pubic bones.

The prostate's appearance differs markedly with different imaging modalities (**Figure 4-1**). Images of the prostate's shape and volume are influenced by the imaging modality, the vagaries of the specific equipment manufacturer, and the way the images are interpreted by a particular physician. Variability in the target definition arising from differences in imaging techniques can markedly affect the degree of prostate coverage by the prescription dose (see Chapter 6).

ADVANTAGES OF TRUS

Real-time imaging

The ability for real-time imaging is the most compelling aspect of TRUS - it allows visualization of the prostate and the needles within the prostate during the procedure. Correct needle placement can be verified before sources are placed.

Sharp prostate contour

The prostate's shape and volume, determined by the contour, is the primary determinant of the radioactivity needed and how it is placed. Obtaining a sharp contour image should minimize dosimetric inconsistencies. With TRUS, the posterior prostate contour is sharply delineated and is not highly dependent on image interpretation. The margins of the anterior portion of the prostate are more difficult to define, due to edge effect and increased distance from the ultrasound transducer.

Rectal wall can be imaged

By visualizing the rectal wall and the posterior prostate simultaneously, TRUS helps insure against needle placement in the rectal wall, minimizing the likelihood of rectal complications.

Biplanar capabilities

Newer TRUS units incorporate biplanar imaging which helps visualize spatial orientation of needles within the prostate (see Chapter 10).

DISADVANTAGES OF TRUS

Imprecise correlation with true prostate volume

Although real-time TRUS images show a fairly sharp prostatic margin, the images may underestimate the true prostatic size. Several conflicting reports describe the relation between the TRUS prostate volume and that determined from the prostatectomy specimen.

Rahmouni and colleagues, from Johns Hopkins University (JHU) compared the preoperative TRUS and MR prostate volume with that of the surgically resected gland.(Rahmouni 1992) The prostatic volume taken from the TRUS images was only 65 to 70% of that measured at the time of prostatectomy (**Figure 4-2**).

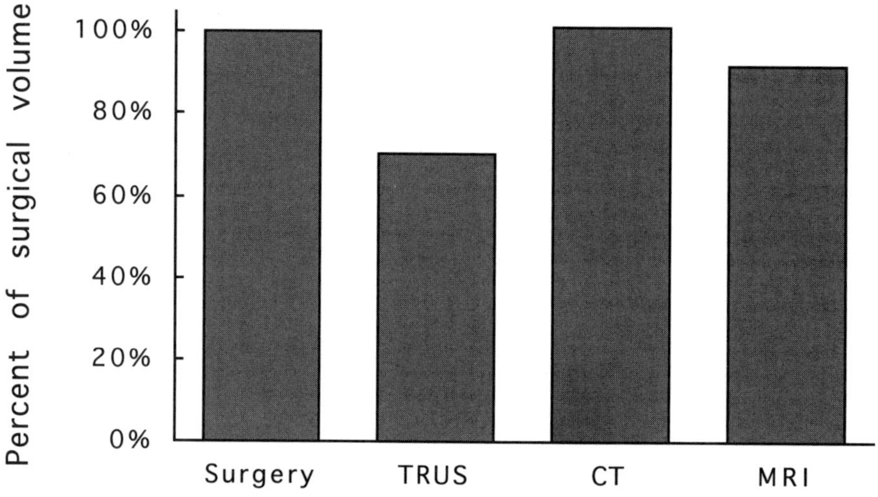

Figure 4-2. Prostate volume measured at time of surgery versus that determined from CT, TRUS or MR. MR and TRUS values are taken from Rahmouni and colleagues. CT data was extrapolated by comparing CT and MR scans on patients treated by K. Wallner.

The finding of the JHU investigators might be criticized on the grounds that the prostatic volumes were calculated by the elliptical volume formula (.525 x D1 x D2 x D3) rather than step-section planimetry, which may be more accurate. However, several investigators have reported that prostate volumes are similar, on average, when determined by step-section planimetry or elliptical volume estimation.(Terris 1991) Stone and colleagues, for instance, showed that prostate volumes are generally smaller with step-section planimetry than with an elliptical volume approximation. If so, underestimation of the prostate volume would be even more marked than that reported from JHU.(Stone 1995)

Other investigators have found less discrepancy between TRUS volume and the volume of the resected prostate.(Kim 1984)(Bartsch 1982) Differences among investigators might be explained by the disparity in how TRUS images are interpreted, the formulas used to approximate the volume, or by differences in the equipment.

Underestimation of prostate volume by TRUS could lead to a substantial underdose of the prostatic periphery. Volume underestimation may be fortuitously adjusted for by the dose scheme currently in place, in that the prescribed dose of 160 Gy may be greater than that needed to eradicate cancer. For instance, it may be that only 120 Gy is needed to eradicate cancer, and the prostate periphery may receive 120 Gy when 160 Gy is prescribed to an erroneously small TRUS-based prostate volume.[Stock 1996]

One way to account for what might be artificially small prostatic volumes determined by TRUS would be simply to draw the target volumes outside of the visualized prostatic margins. In practice, this is commonly done (See Chapter 6). While over-drawing the prostatic contour may be effective, it adds a degree of uncertainty to target definition.

Lack of reproducibility

There are conflicting reports regarding TRUS reproducibility. Suboptimal reproducibility can occur between interpreting physicians and from one scan to the next, performed by the same physician. There can be a 1 to 25% variability in the prostate volume when a patient is re-scanned by the same ultrasonographer on the same day.[Bazinet 1996] If a scan is performed in succession by two different observers, there will be approximately 10% variability. The lack of reproducibility is not explained by image interpretation, because computer-assisted interpretation does not diminish the inter or intra observer variability.[Nathan 1996] The degree of variability may be less if planimetry, rather than dimension-estimated volumes, are used.[Aarnink 1996]

Some lack of reproducibility may be explained by real physiologic variation. Prostate volume, measured by TRUS or MR, changes by approximately 10% from day to day.[Al-rimawi 1994] This variation is consistent between TRUS and MR, so that it probably reflects real changes in volume rather than an inconsistency of TRUS. Lack of reproducibility due to physiological changes would vex all imaging modalities, including MR and CT.

Variability in prostate volume determinations is partly explained by differences in ultrasound probe angulation, which can lead to 2 to 4% volume changes.[Nathan 1996] Prostate volume and shape changes are also common in fully awake versus anesthetized patients, though this has not been quantified (M. Dattoli observation).

TRUS reproducibility or lack thereof is not fully understood or quantified. Like volume determinations, it adds some degree of uncertainty to target definition.

Inability to visualize cancer

An ideal imaging modality would allow visualization of the malignant portion of the prostate, so that a higher dose might be delivered to it. Like CT and MR, TRUS cannot reliably image the presence or extent of intraprostatic cancers.

Image deterioration

Another disadvantage of TRUS is its limited ability to identify individual sources in the prostate, especially after several needles and sources have been placed. Sources and needles within the prostate create artifact that interferes with the image, so that identification of the target and of individual sources becomes difficult as more sources and needles are inserted (see Chapter 10). This can be overcome to some degree by starting with anterior sources, so that more posterior sources can still be seen. Another solution to image deterioration as sources are placed is the use of fluoroscopy during the procedure to monitor source placement. Methodology to improve source visualization by TRUS may be developed in the future.

Inability to visualize the pubic bones

Pubic arch interference can prevent adequate implantation of the anterior and lateral portions of the prostate. Use of the extended lithotomy position or posterior probe angulation can usually circumvent the problem (see Chapter 10). However, it may be difficult to implant the entire prostate of patients who have large prostate volumes or small pubic arches. In these cases, it would be helpful to be able to image the pubic arch ahead of time and plan needle angulation as needed. TRUS is not capable of imaging the pubic bones well, primarily because of their distance from the probe. Consequently it is not practical to use TRUS images to plan for possible pubic arch interference, at least with current ultrasound technology.

ADVANTAGES OF CT-BASED IMPLANTS

Lack of operator dependence

Planning CT scans are easy to perform and require minimal preparation. CT scans are not dependent on the skill of the person taking the scan, and are less subject to technical error in obtaining the scan. Rectal markers and the necessity for special attention to leg placement, described in earlier publications, are unnecessary (See Chapter 9).

More accurate volumes (?)

Like TRUS, the accuracy of CT prostate volume determination is unclear. Most investigators agree that CT volumes are larger than those determined by TRUS. M. Roach and colleagues reported that CT volumes were approximately 30% larger than those determined by MR, and presumably even larger in comparison to TRUS volumes.[Roach 1996] The volumes determined by the University of California, San Francisco (UCSF) investigators, however, would be larger than those determined by K. Wallner and colleagues (see Chapter 6). Judging from the

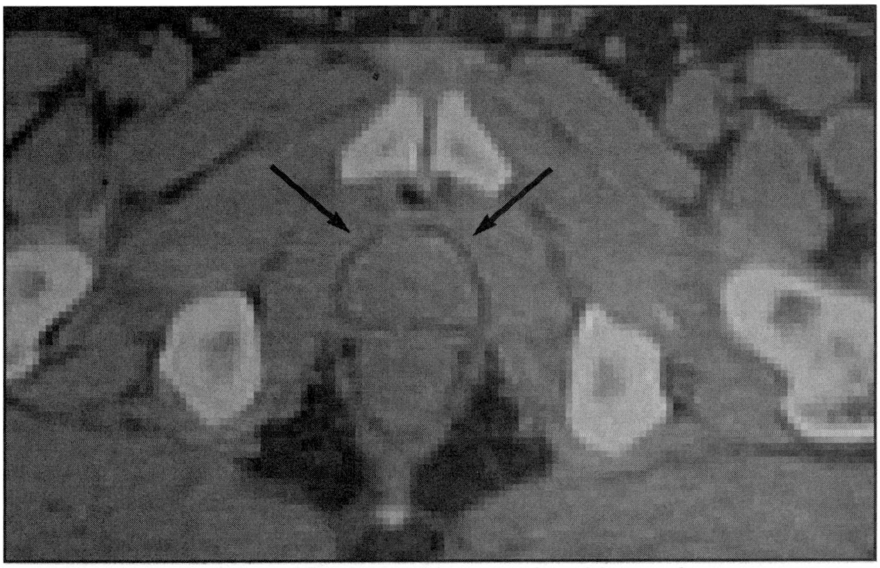

Figure 4-3. Magnification of example of how the prostatic margins were drawn by Roach and colleagues at UCSF, to compare prostate volumes by CT versus MR.(Roach 1996) *In this example, the puborectalis muscles are included in the target volume (arrows), giving an artificially large prostate volume on CT. Only the prostatic margins should be traced, not including the puborectalis muscles (See Chapter 6). Excluding non-prostatic tissue should lead to a more accurate prostate volume determination. Dr. Roach agrees (personal communication)*

representative case shown in Dr. Roach's paper, the puborectalis muscle was included within the target volume (**Figure 4-3**). As a result, the prostatic volume would be erroneously increased.

With the method of CT target volume illustrated in Chapter 6 (used routinely by Wallner and colleagues), CT scans give prostatic volumes that are slightly larger than those of MR scans, and perhaps as much as 30% larger than those of TRUS. This would place the CT volume very close to that of measured prostatectomy specimens at least, extrapolating between MR and TRUS, as reported from Johns Hopkins University (**Figure 4-2**).(Rahmouni 1992) If CT measures the prostatic volume more accurately, one is more likely to treat the prostate to the prescription dose, if no adjustments were made when drawing the target volumes.

Visualization of the pubic bones

The pubic bones are well visualized on CT scan, and their potential interference implanting the anterior portion of the prostate can be anticipated. For patients with potential pubic arch interference, the needles can be sharply angulated (see Chapter 9). To do so may require some modification of commercial treatment planning software systems, but this is feasible and has been done with custom written software.(Wallner 1991)

DISADVANTAGES OF CT-BASED IMPLANTS

Lack of real-time imaging

The primary limitation of CT-based implants is the lack of real-time imaging. Although CT might show a more accurate prostate volume, there is currently no widely available way to verify correct needle placement with CT scan during the procedure. The CT-based method described in Chapter 8 does not require real-time CT imaging, as all volumes and needle placement positions are transferred to a coordinate system that can be verified by anterior and lateral fluoroscopy. Nevertheless, real-time CT imaging would add a degree of certainty that the sources are placed as intended. With wider availability of faster scan reconstruction capability and smaller, portable scanners, real-time intra-operative CT scanning may become widely available.

Fuzzy margin

Another disadvantage of CT scan as a treatment planning modality is its inability to produce well-defined images of the prostatic margins. There is considerable subjectivity when drawing the prostatic margins, probably more so than with TRUS. CT-based prostate implants could vary substantially, depending on how a particular brachytherapist outlines the target on the scan.

Inability to visualizc cancer

CT scans give the least information regarding internal prostate architecture. The significance of this shortcoming is probably minimal because the entire prostate is treated to the prescription dose, due to the high likelihood of multifocal disease.

ADVANTAGES OF MR

More accurate prostatic volume (?)

Like CT scanning, MR shows a larger prostatic volume than TRUS (**Figure 4-2**). As with CT, however, it is unclear which modality is more accurate. If the MR volume were more accurate, it would lead to a better fit between the prescription dose and the prostate.

Can visualize internal architecture

MR shows the most detailed image of the internal architecture of the prostate. While the images are striking in their degree of detail, their usefulness is questionable, because the entire prostate should be treated to prescription dose to treat all areas of potential microscopic disease.

MR's ability to image the internal architecture probably makes identification of the prostatic apex more accurate.

SHARP MARGINS

MR images show a sharper prostatic margin than do CT or TRUS. Sharp margins should leave less subjectivity when drawing the target, and should make the planning process more reproducible.

DISADVANTAGES OF MR

Not real time

Like CT scanning, real-time MR is not readily available. Like the CT-based method described in Chapter 5, MR could be used to determine prostatic shape and volume for planning purposes, and the prostate and seed coordinates could be transferred to a system that can be verified intra-operatively with fluoroscopy, using a urethral marker as a landmark for verification of proper needle placement. MR-based methodology has not yet been reported on, but it would be easy to do.

Cost/price

Perhaps the biggest disadvantage of MR is its price. The price of a diagnostic pelvic MR is two to three times that of a TRUS or CT (**Figure 4-4**). The higher price of MR reflects primarily the higher cost of the hardware. The price could vary substantially, depending on how billing was designed. It could probably be substantially less for a limited pelvic scan that included only the prostate and pubic bones.

DOES IT MATTER?

There is substantial uncertainty as to the relative accuracy and reproducibility of the different prostate imaging modalities. That the clinical results with modern transperineal brachytherapy appear favorable even with widely varying techniques probably means that the differences described above are of little practical consequence. Operator skill is probably far more important to achieving satisfactory results than the particular equipment used to get there.

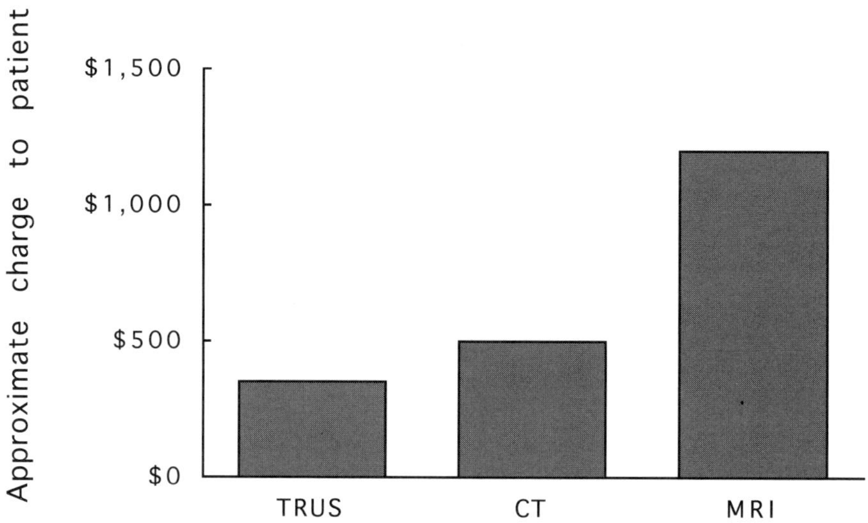

Figure 4-4. Approximate charge for diagnostic TRUS , CT or MR.

REFERENCES

1. Aarnink RG, De La Rosetter JJ, Debruyne FMJ, Wijkstra H. Reproducibility of prostate volume measurements from transrectal ultrasonography by an automated and a manual technique. Br J Urol 1996; 78:219-223.

2. Al-rimawi M, Griffiths DJ, Boake RC, Mador DR. Transrectal ultrasound versus magnetic resonance imaging in the estimation of prostatic volume. Br J Urol 1994; 74:596-600.

3. Bartsch G, Egender G, Hubscher H, Rohr H. Sonometrics of the prostate. J Urol 1982; 127:1119-1121.

4. Bazinet M, Karakiewicz PI, Aprikian A, Trudel C. Reassessment of nonplanimetric transrectal ultrasound prostate volume estimates. Urol 1996; 47:857-862.

5. Kim RY, Brascho DJ, Wilson EE. Use of ultrasound scan in prostatic I-125 implantation. Int J Radiat Oncol Biol Phys 1984; 10:1971-1973.

6. Nathan MS, Seenivasagam K, Mei Q, Wickham JEA. Transrectal ultrasonography: why are estimates of prostate volume and dimension so inaccurate? Br J Urol 1996; 77:401-407.

7. Rahmouni A, Yang A, Tempany C, Frenkel T. Accuracy of in-vivo assessment of prostatic volume by MRI and transrectal ultrasonography. J Comp Assist Tomo 1992; 16:935-940.

8. Roach M, Faillace-akazawa P, Malfatti C, Holland J. Prostate volumes defined by magnetic resonance imaging and computerized tomographic scans for three-dimensional conformal radiotherapy. Int J Radiat Oncol Biol Phys 1997; 35:1011-1018.

9. Stone NN, Stock RG, DeWyngaert JK, Tabert A. Prostate brachytherapy: Improvements in prostate volume measurements and dose distribution using interactive ultrasound guided implantation and three-dimensional dosimetry. Radiat Oncol Invest 1995; 3:185-195.

10. Terris MK, Stamey TA. Determination of prostate volume by transrectal ultrasound. J Urol 1991; 145:984-987.

11. Wallner KE, Chiu-Tsao S, Roy J, et al. An Improved Method for Transperineal Prostate Implants. J Urol 1991; 146:90-95.

Chapter 5

Radionuclides

There are many radionuclides that could be used for prostate brachytherapy. Only I-125, Pd-103 and Ir-192 are commonly used at present.

TEMPORARY VS PERMANENT IMPLANTS

Prostate brachytherapy can be done with permanent or temporary sources. Temporary implants are done with Ir-192 placed in plastic hollow catheters. The technique is termed "temporary" because the sources are removed after the dose is delivered.

Traditionally, Ir-192 sources were left in place for 2 to 4 days to deliver a 20 to 30 Gy boost to an abbreviated course of EBRT (40 to 60 Gy). There is growing interest in high dose rate temporary Ir-192 implants, which can deliver 20 to 60 Gy within an hour.

The dose rates for Ir-192 implants are far higher than those for I-125 or Pd-103 permanent implants (**Figure 5-1**). Ir-192 implants can be either intermediate or high dose rate. The benefits of different dose rates are unclear (see Chapter 3).

Advantages of temporary implants

A major advantage of temporary implants or 'afterloading' techniques is that after the sources are removed, no radioactivity remains and no radioprotection precautions are needed. A second advantage is that source activity or insertion time can be modified to adjust for less than ideal needle placement, determined from plain films or CT scan. Dosimetry can also be calculated using TRUS images at the time of needle placement, which should help minimize any adverse effect of needle motion.(Edmundson 1995)

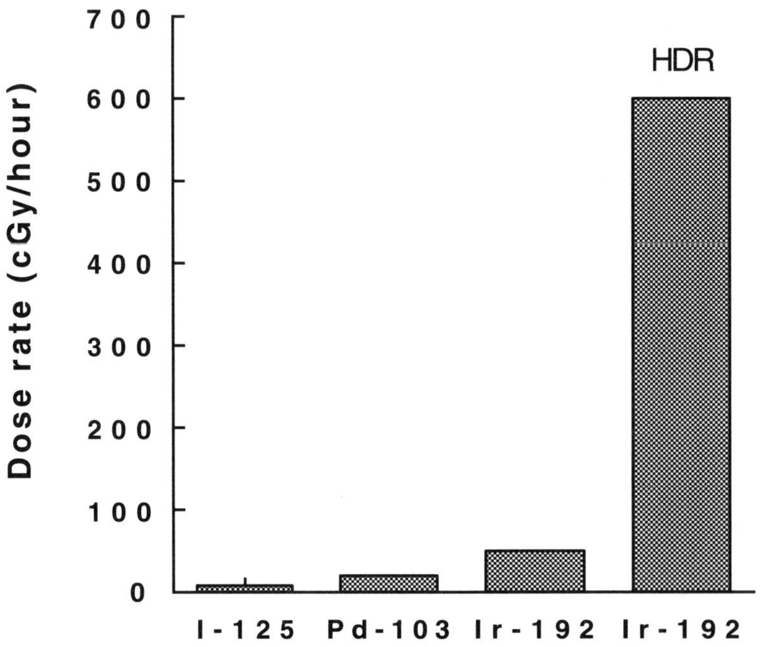

Figure 5-1. Initial dose rate to the prostate periphery with I-125 or Pd-103 permanent implants versus temporary Ir-192 implants.

The option to change the loading time is appealing because it allows modification of the implant dosimetry after needle placement. With permanent implants, the only way to modify dosimetry after the sources are placed is to take the patient back to the operating room to place more sources. If too many permanent sources are placed they cannot be removed, short of doing a prostatectomy. Such corrective options could be a major source of embarrassment, or worse.

Disadvantages of temporary implants

The major shortcoming of temporary implants is the need for hospitalization during the radiation delivery, for the purpose of radiation protection. The patient is confined to bed for the duration of the implant (1 to 3 days), to prevent displacement of the catheters. Hospital confinement is expensive and carries a risk of venous thrombosis, infectious complications, and high hospital bills. For high dose rate Ir-192 temporary implants, overnight hospitalization could be avoided by repeated needle placement on different days, but this is asking a lot of the patient and is time-consuming for the physician and physicist. Giving a substantial dose (greater than 8 Gy) in a single day, without overnight hospitalization, would probably invite complications.

Results with Ir-192 are probably comparable to permanent implants...

Favorable results have been reported for temporary Ir-192 implants by several authors.[(Syed 1992)(Khan 1992)] Results with Ir-192 are probably comparable to those with permanent implants, but high-quality, peer-reviewed PSA-based follow-up is scarce.

...but the convenience of permanent implants is appealing

The use of temporary implants has fallen in popularity, relative to permanent implants. In contrast to Ir-192 brachytherapy, permanent implants are a brief outpatient procedure. There is no need for overnight hospitalization or repeated needle insertion (**Table 5-1**).

Table 5-1. Pros and cons of permanent vs temporary implants.

	Pros	Cons
Permanent	Convenient Substantial PSA-based data	Can't alter source loading
Temporary	Can alter source loading	Minimal PSA-based data Inconvenient (for patient & doctor)

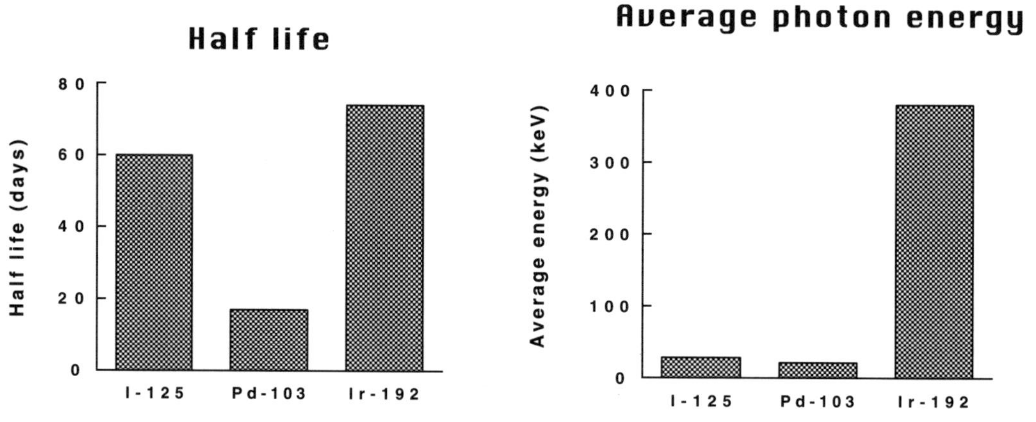

Figure 5-2. Physical characteristics of the radionuclides used for prostate brachytherapy (HVL=half value layer).

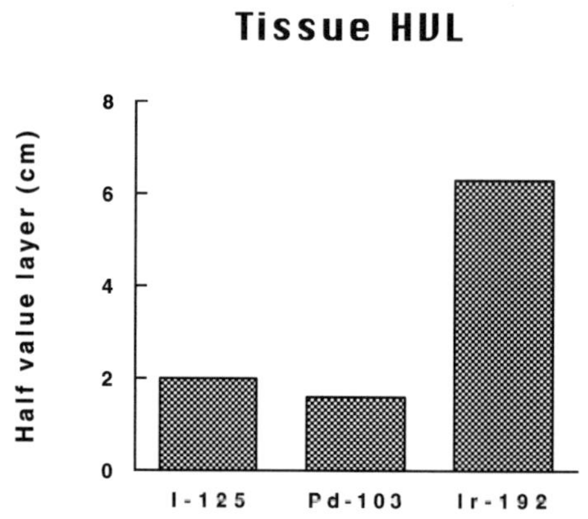

RADIONUCLIDES FOR PERMANENT IMPLANTS

I-125 and Pd-103 are the only commonly used radionuclides for permanent prostatic implants. They differ in their half life and photon energy, factors which probably influence their biological effects (**Figure 5-2**).

I-125

I-125 is produced in a nuclear reactor, from Xe-124. I-125 decays by electron capture and internal conversion to Te-125. In the process, it emits photons of 27, 31 and 35 keV, for an average energy of 29 keV. I-125's low average energy of 29 keV minimizes shielding requirements. The half value layer thickness of lead is only 0.02 mm.

The I-125 is absorbed on a silver rod, and encased in a 0.05 mm titanium capsule. It is the silver rod that is visible on a radiograph (**Figure 5-3**). The outside dimensions of the source are 4.5 x .8 mm.

I-125 has been the most widely used radionuclide. Its relatively long half life of 60 days is a practical advantage in that it can be held for several weeks prior to use.

In recent years, Amersham™ has been the only company to manufacture I-125 sources. Best Industries may introduce another I-125 source, designed to have less anisotropy (**Figure 5-3**). Other companies will likely be marketing competing sources soon.

A bad rap for I-125

Some authors have attributed the inferior results with retropubic implants performed in the 1970s to the choice of I-125 as the radionuclide. Probably not. Current 5 to 10 year results with good quality I-125 implants support the contention that poor results in some retropubic series were due to poor source placement, not the source itself.

Pd-103

Pd-103 is the second commonly used isotope for permanent implants. It was initially produced in a nuclear reactor, from Pd-102 absorbing a neutron.

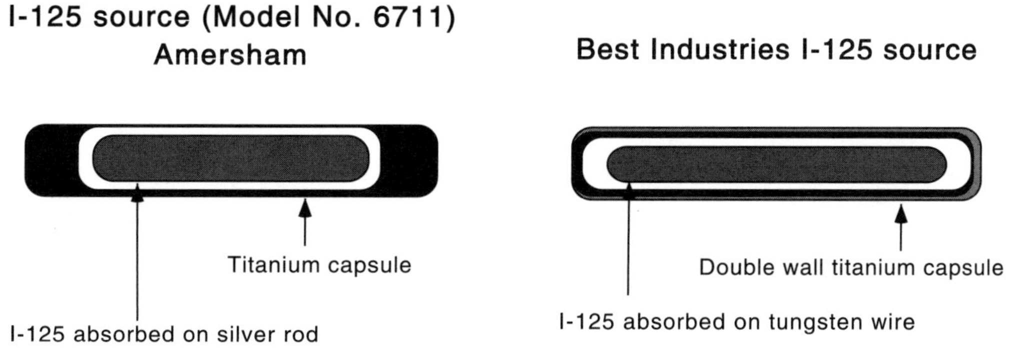

Figure 5-3. Construction of Amersham I-125 source and new (Best Industries) I-125 source, which has less anisotropy due to thinner capsule at ends of source.

Currently, it is produced in a cyclotron, within which rhodium is bombarded with protons. It decays by electron capture and internal conversion to Rhodium-103. Photons of 20, 23, 40 and 357keV are emitted, with an average energy of 21 keV. Pd-103 sources are the same size as I-125 sources (4.5 x .8 mm), but Pd-103 sources appear differently on radiographs, because the activity is absorbed on radiolucent graphite cylinders at each end of the source (**Figures 5-4 and 5-5**). A lead wire is added to the center of the source to make it visible on x-ray films.

Pd-103's shorter half-life of 17 days may be a radiobiological advantage for high grade tumors (**Table 5-2**). Radiobiological arguments for Pd-103 are conceptually appealing, but are not based on clinical data (see Chapter 3).

Another potential advantage of Pd-103 could be a shorter duration of radiation prostatitis, though there are no objective published data in this regard.

The decreased average energy and more rapid dose fall-off of Pd-103 should decrease radiation to the rectal wall and might lower the likelihood of rectal complications. However, it is also more likely to lead to cold spots in the prostate, if sources are placed farther apart than intended.

The biggest disadvantage of Pd-103 compared to I-125 is its short shelf life. Because of the short half life, Pd-103 realistically can be held only for about 6 days before the activity is too low to be practical (too many sources would be required).

Because of the lower specific activity, more sources are required than with I-125 and as a result, larger prostates are more time consuming to implant due to the large number of sources required.

COST OF I-125 VERSUS PD-103

As of 1997, I-125 sources cost $32 each, versus $46 for Pd-103. Combined with the need for more sources, a full dose Pd-103 implant will cost about $1500

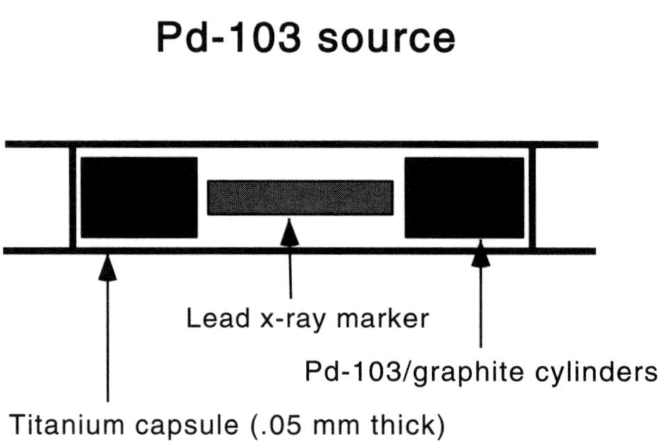

Figure 5-4 Construction of Pd-103 sources (Theragenics Corporation).

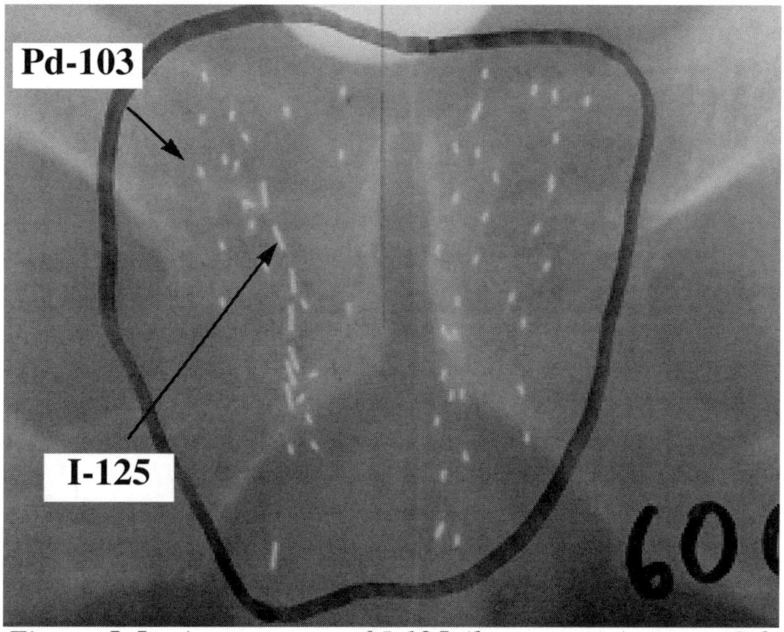

Figure 5-5. Appearance of I-125 (long arrow) versus Pd-103 sources (short arrow) on plain radiograph. Several I-125 sources were mistakenly implanted in this patient, who was intended to have a 60 Gy Pd-103 implant. (Name of patient, physician, physicist and institution withheld)

Table 5-2 Pros and cons of I-125 versus Pd-103.

	Pros	Cons
I-125	Longer shelf-life	Low dose rate (?)
	Less expensive	Side effects last longer(?)
	Radiobiological advantage(?)	
Pd-103	Radiobiological advantage(?)	More expensive
	Shorter time side effects(?)	Short shelf-life (6 days)
	More rectal sparing (?)	

more than a full dose I-125 implant (**Table 5-3**). Suture mounted I-125 sources cost more than loose I-125 sources, and bring the price closer to that of unmounted Pd-103 sources.

> ***I-125 versus Pd-103: Where we stand***
>
> There is continued controversy regarding the choice of I-125 versus Pd-103. Recommendations have been made to base the choice on Gleason score. It is safe to say that we currently do not know when to use one source over the other. Favorable reports have appeared about each source, and there is currently no clear evidence that one is superior to the other, regardless of tumor stage or Gleason score. We are probably many years from having good quality data to guide radionuclide choice.

ANISOTROPY (ISODOSE SHAPE)

Both I-125 and Pd-103 sources have more dose attenuation at the ends of the sources than at the central plane due to absorption at the thick ends of the metal capsule, and due to some absorption by the silver or aluminum carrier itself (**Figure 5-6**). Decreased dose at the ends of the source could significantly affect the dose distribution of the implant itself. This effect would be greatest if the sources were uniformly aligned.

Most commercial planning programs allow for this decreased dose at the source ends to be taken into account when calculating doses. However, the programs assume that sources will be uniformly oriented in the longitudinal axis. In fact, sources often tilt to some degree.

The actual orientation is not generally taken into account for implant evaluation because it would be technically difficult to enter precise orientation data. For retropubic implants, this would probably not have lead to important errors because the source orientation was more random than with transperineal implants.

Table 5-3. Cost of I-125 vs Pd-103 for a typical full dose implant of a 45 cc prostate.

	I-125 (160 Gy) (loose sources)	I-125 (160 Gy) (RAPIDStrand™)	Pd-103 (115 Gy)
Activity/source	0.5 mCi	0.5 mCi	1.4 mCi
Number sources	80	80	90
Cost/source	$32	$42	$46
Total cost	**$2560**	**$3360**	**$4140**

However, with modern transperineal implants ignoring anisotropy could lead to some underdose in the longitudinal direction, because of more uniform source orientation. Calculating the anisotropy effect would add a substantial degree of complexity to planning and evaluation of the dose distribution, but it could be automated with the proper software.

SOURCE INSERTION

Mick Applicator

Probably the most commonly used device to place sources is the Mick Applicator™. It has been manufactured in various models since 1972. It has a needle retraction mechanism, in which sources are fed from a cartridge (**Figure 5-7**). The primary advantages of the Mick Applicator™ are that many brachytherapists are familiar with it from use in other sites, and that when using it there is maximal flexibility to change source spacing at the time of the implant to adjust for source sliding along the needle path, or adding extra sources ad hoc. One lim-

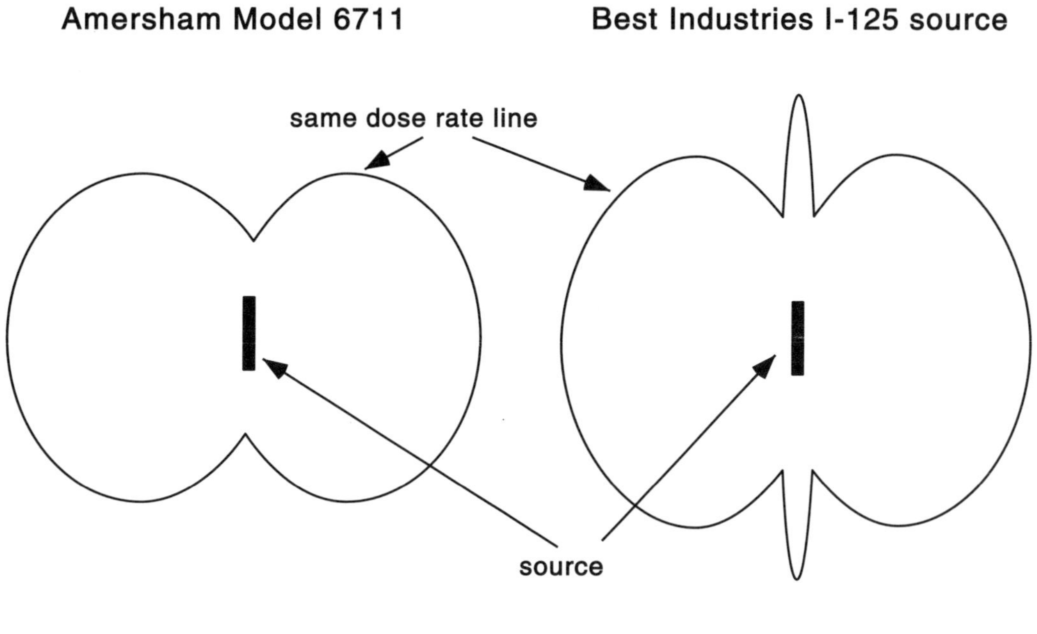

Figure 5-6. Effect of source orientation on dose distribution. The isodose lines are constricted at the source ends (anisotropy). Anisotropy could cause underdosage in the longitudinal axis of an implant, when all sources are closely aligned in the longitudinal direction.

itation of the Mick Applicator™ is that it occasionally jams, but jams are relatively easy to correct. Also, effective use of its flexibility requires some experience, perhaps more so than for pre-loaded needles.

Pre-loaded needles

Probably the method of source placement that leaves the least room for operator error is the use of pre-loaded needles. 18-gauge needles are loaded with sources. To provide gaps where needed, absorbable spacers (No. 3 absorbable gut suture material) of appropriate multiples of 5 mm are placed between the sources (**Figure 5-8**).

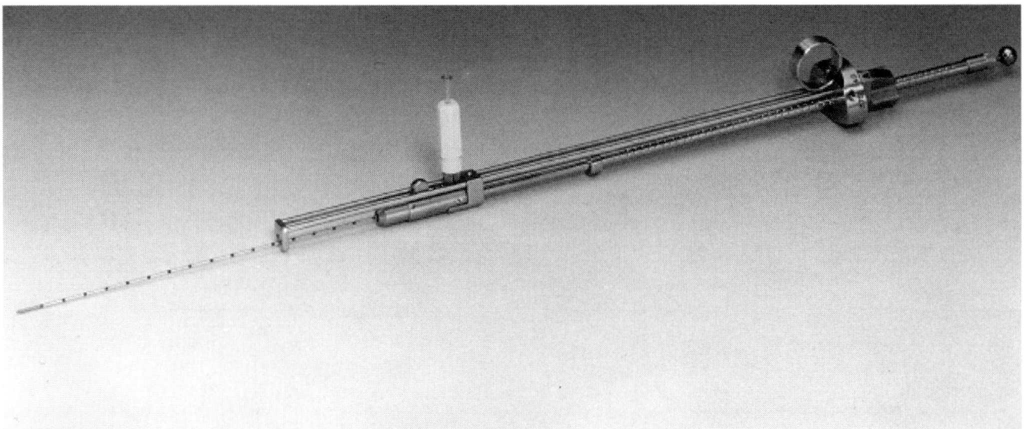

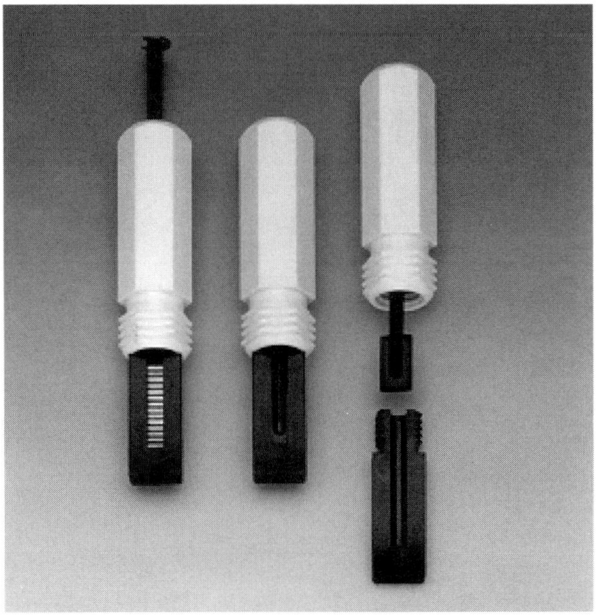

Figure 5-7. Mick Applicator™ (top). Sources are fed into the retracting needle by cartridges which usually are loaded with 10 sources per cartridge (left).

The disadvantages of pre-loaded needles are that they are tedious to set-up, they offer less flexibility for adding sources ad hoc at the time of the procedure, and if a mistake is made at the time of the procedure, the entire row of sources may be off.

Suture mounted sources

Suture-mounted I-125 sources (125 RAPID Strand™, by Amersham Healthcare) are mounted in #1 Vicryl™ (polyglactin 910). The suture has been stiffened, and sterilized with ethylene oxide gas prior to shipment. They are shipped inside a plastic spacing jig, inside a stainless steel shielding tube (**Figure 5-9**). Suture-mounted sources are more likely to maintain their position, and should not migrate if one or two sources of the suture are protruding partly out of the prostate. The ultimate advantage of suture mounting in regard to extraprostatic sources is unclear, because some of those sources might still migrate in 10 to 20 days when the suture begins to dissolve. Longer-term spatial stability of source-mounted sources has not been studied.

Because of their suture mounting, RAPIDStrand sources should stay aligned better than those deposited with a Mick Applicator™. Whether the decreased likelihood of source migration or better source alignment is truly advantageous is unclear, but suture-mounted sources may facilitate better implants.

While proper placement at one cm intervals is assured with 125 RAPID Strand™, one cm spacing may not be the best way to achieve coverage of parts of the prostate. If more flexibility in source placement is desired, it is necessary to place some additional sources with a Mick Applicator™ or pre-loaded needles.

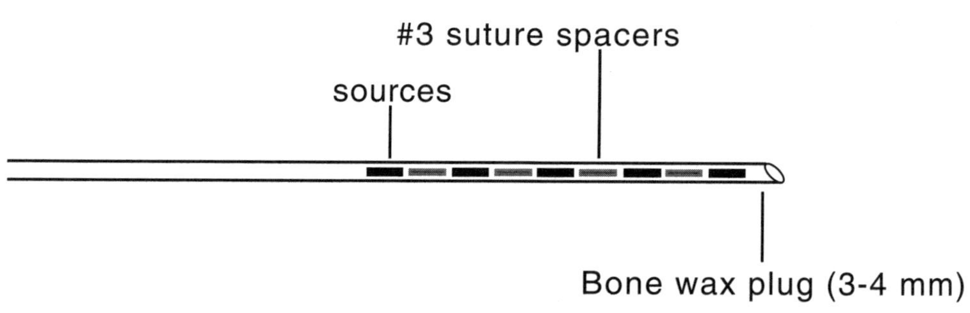

Figure 5-8. Schematic view of pre-loaded needles.

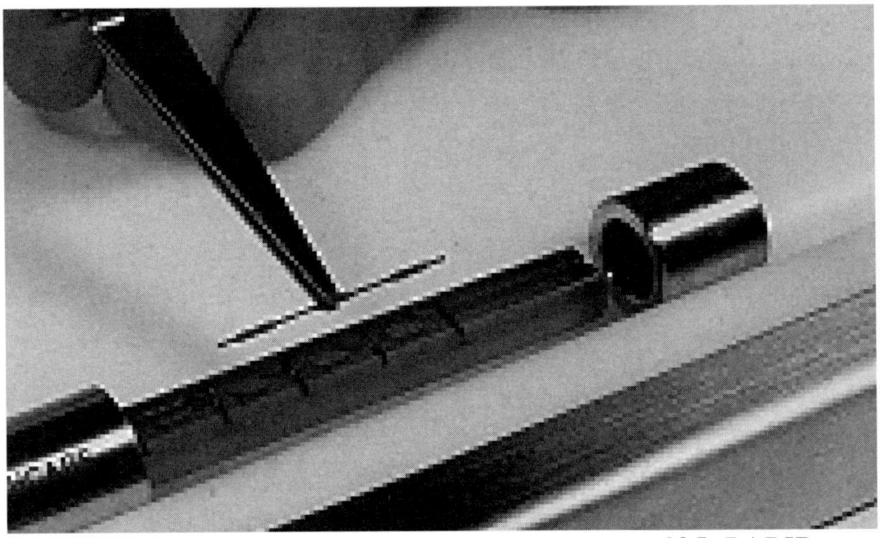

Figure 5-9. Suture-mounted I-125 sources (125 RAPID Strand™). The strand should be picked up with tweezers, grasping only the portion that holds a source.

The primary disadvantage of suture-mounted sources has been their tendency to stick inside the needles. Plugging the needle tips with heated Anusol-HC™ provides lubrication and helps prevent needle jamming problems. Jamming may be minimized by loading the needles immediately prior to the procedure. Using larger bore needles may help. There is clearly an "art" to the proper use of RAPID Strand™. If they are to be used, it would be wise to first spend some time observing a skilled brachytherapist who is comfortable with their use.(Butler 1996)

SO MANY WAYS...

There are a variety of source placement techniques, and different equipment to carry them out. As prostate brachytherapy continues to gain widespread acceptance, more manufacturers will get involved, and offer a larger variety of equipment. This is to be applauded. There must be better ways to insert sources, ways which are less prone to human error.

REFERENCES

1. Butler WM, Merrick GS. I-125 Rapid Strand™ loading technique. Radiat Oncol Invest 1996; 4:48-49.

2. Edmundson GK, Yan D, Martinez AA. Intra-operative optimization of needle placement and dwell times for conformal prostate brachytherapy. Int J Radiat Oncol Biol Phys 1995; 33:1257-1263.

3. Khan K, Thompson W, Bush S, Stidley C. Transperineal percutaneous iridium-192 interstitial template implant of the prostate: results and complications in 321 patients. Int J Radiat Oncol Biol Phys 1992; 22:935-939.

4. Syed AM, Puthawala A, Austin P, Cherlow J. Temporary iridium-192 implant in the management of carcinoma of the prostate. Cancer 1992; 69:2515-2524.

Chapter 6

Implant design

The dosimetry of prostate brachytherapy is murky, primarily due to target definition uncertainties and to marked dose inhomogeneity. There is no generally accepted method of treatment planning, and substantial variability exists among implant teams. It is not clear that one method is better than the others. The best way to avoid problems when starting a program is to understand why differences exist and the potential pitfalls in transferring techniques from one implant team to another.

PLANNING IMAGES

Implants are planned from images of the prostate, usually taken several days or weeks prior to the procedure. Transverse TRUS images are taken at 5 mm intervals from the prostatic base through the apex. Sagital plane images are helpful in identification of the base and apical boundaries. The patient should be in the lithotomy position, as close as possible to that of the implant procedure itself.

For CT-based implants, the prostate is imaged with 5 mm thick slices, at 5 mm intervals. Scans are taken from approximately 2 cm above the prostate and all the way down to the perineum (see Chapter 9).

THE *'0' PLANE*

The most proximal image is considered the *0 plane*. It is located by visualizing the most proximal image, and usually includes the base of the seminal vesicles (**Figure 6-1**). Cranial-caudal source positions are specified by their distance from the *0 plane*. Other transverse planes are numbered by their distance (in mm) from the *0 plane* (i.e.: the *10 plane* is 10 mm caudal to the *0 plane*).

To help determine the *0 plane* for CT-based implants, dilute dye is placed in the bladder to help differentiate the bladder from the top of the prostate. The *0 plane* is generally taken as the first image distal to the bladder, making some allowance (approximately 4 mm) for the thickness of the bladder wall (**Figure 6-2**).

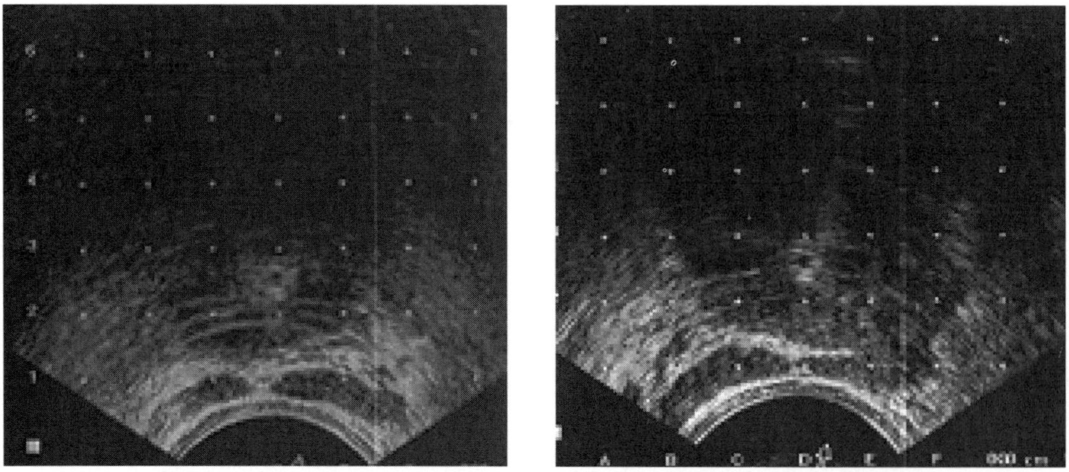

Figure 6-1. Determining the 0 plane on TRUS. On the left is a TRUS image taken at the base of seminal vesicles, and the proximal prostatic capsule. On the right is the next 5 mm image inferior, showing the first image of the prostate. The image on the left is considered the 0 plane.

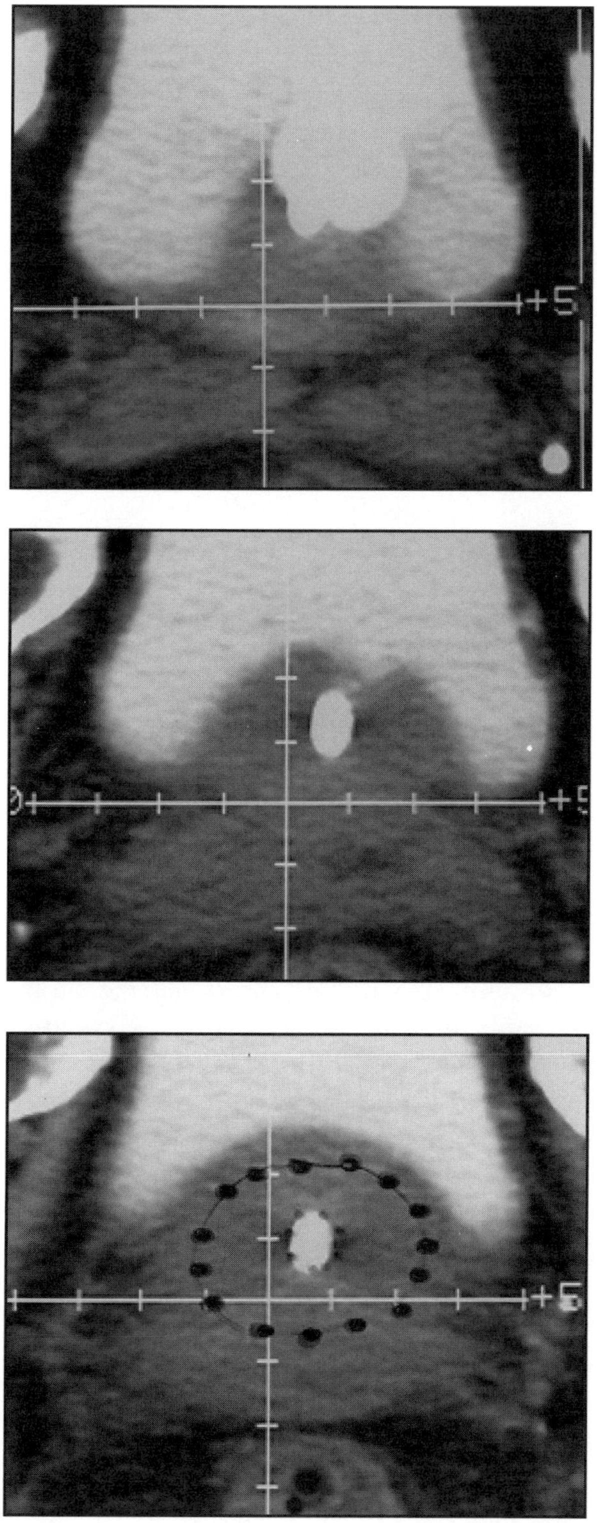

Figure 6-2. Determining the 0 plane by CT. The most proximal slice of the prostate is considered to be four mm distal to the bottom of the catheter balloon, allowing for the bladder wall thickness. Renografin™ (1:50) has been instilled in the bladder to help differentiate the bladder from the prostate. The image at the bottom is taken as the 0 plane.

DRAWING THE TARGET ON THE PLANNING IMAGES

The target is the tissue identified to be treated to a cancericidal dose. All tissue within the target margins should receive the prescription dose or higher. In practice, much of it will receive 1.5 to 2 times the prescription dose, due to high doses near the implanted sources.

The target volume can be derived from TRUS, CT or MR images. Currently, nearly all implants are based on TRUS images (see Chapter 4). Whatever the imaging method, the prostatic margin (target) is drawn on the images and transferred (digitized) into a planning program. The way in which the target is drawn determines the dose to the prostate and to the surrounding tissues. Differences in drawing the prostatic margins on the planning scan are probably the biggest source of variability in prostate brachytherapy.

Regardless of the imaging method, discerning the prostate margins is an "art," because the margins appear fuzzy (see Chapter 4). The target volume can vary substantially depending on who happens to draw the target on the planning images.

Drawing more generous margins will increase the volume irradiated and the total activity required, and should increase the likelihood of tumor eradication. It may also increase the likelihood of complications. Variable image interpretation is one reason that there could be substantial differences in tumor control and complication rates between brachytherapists, despite their using the same prescription dose.

The target is commonly drawn outside of what appears to be the prostatic margins on the TRUS images (**Figures 6-3 & 6-4**). In reality, the margins may still be within the prostate, because the prostate may be larger than the TRUS images indicate (see Chapter 3).

If the target is drawn too large, sources will be placed outside of the prostate, and may migrate in the retroperitoneum or the vasculature. If multiple sources are consistently lost at the time of the procedure or shortly afterwards, either the targets should be drawn tighter, or the dosimetrist should arbitrarily keep sources farther in from the drawn target.

Seminal vesicles

The entire seminal vesicles should not be included in the target volume because reliably placing sources in the seminal vesicles is not feasible. However, a portion of the seminal vesicles adjacent to the prostate is commonly included in the target volume, to create a margin around the prostate.

Base

A moderate margin is drawn at the prostatic base (**Figure 6-5**). In contrast to outlining the apex, generous outlining of the prostatic base leads to source

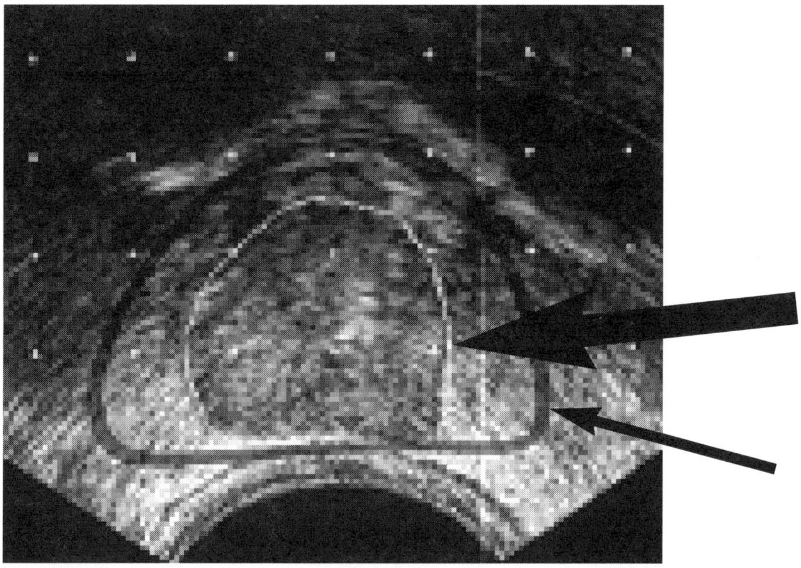

Figure 6-3. There is no generally accepted convention for drawing the target from the planning scan. On this image, the prostatic contour has been traced with a light pen (large arrow). The target, for treatment planning purposes, is drawn with the thick black line (smaller arrow). This discrepancy between the imaged margin and what is drawn as the target can lead to substantial variability in the prostatic, urethral and rectal dose from one brachytherapy team to another, despite the use of a standard prescription dose.

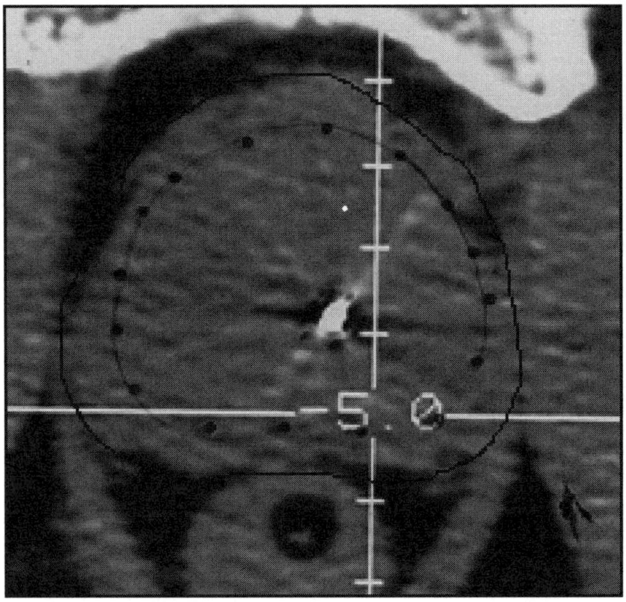

Figure 6-4. This CT image shows the potential for variability in drawing the target on a CT image. The target volumes (dotted line, per K. Wallner) are drawn within the CT-defined prostate margin. Care is taken not to include the puborectalis muscle laterally. Laterally, the muscle must be extrapolated from its posterior course, which is outlined by the perirectal fat medially and ischiorectal space laterally. Anteriorly, the target is drawn tight, to account for the periprostatic venous plexus. Admittedly, this requires a certain amount of imagination. Some brachytherapists might draw the prostate as the solid line, which clearly includes extraprostatic tissues (puborectalis muscle), giving a larger target volume.

placement in loose, periprostatic tissue, resulting in a high probability of source migration.

Mid prostate

The middle portion of the prostate can be drawn generously, laterally and anteriorly. No margin is added posteriorly.

Apex

Surgical resection margins are frequently positive at the prostatic apex, in part because tumor can track outside of the prostate where the neurovascular bundles pierce the capsule posteriorly.[Stamey 1990] Because of the risk of tumor extension through the apical region, the apex should be drawn generously on the planning images. Sources usually stay in the region of the apex even if they are outside of the prostate, because they are imbedded in the pelvic floor musculature.

Generous target definition at the apex does not appear to lead to excessive risk of urinary incontinence or sexual dysfunction. However, in extreme cases over irradiation of the prostatic apex might lead to stricture formation or a higher likelihood of impotence (see Chapter 16).

Urethra

The urethra can be identified, so as to avoid placing sources too near it. Limiting the urethral dose decreases the likelihood of urinary morbidity.[Wallner 1995] A urinary catheter helps to visualize the urethra.

Rectum

Considering the low incidence of rectal complications in most series, no special steps need be taken to avoid the rectum, as long as the prostatic margin is not drawn posterior to what is identified on the planning scan. The common practice of drawing the target several mm anterior to the posterior TRUS prostatic margin is probably not necessary.

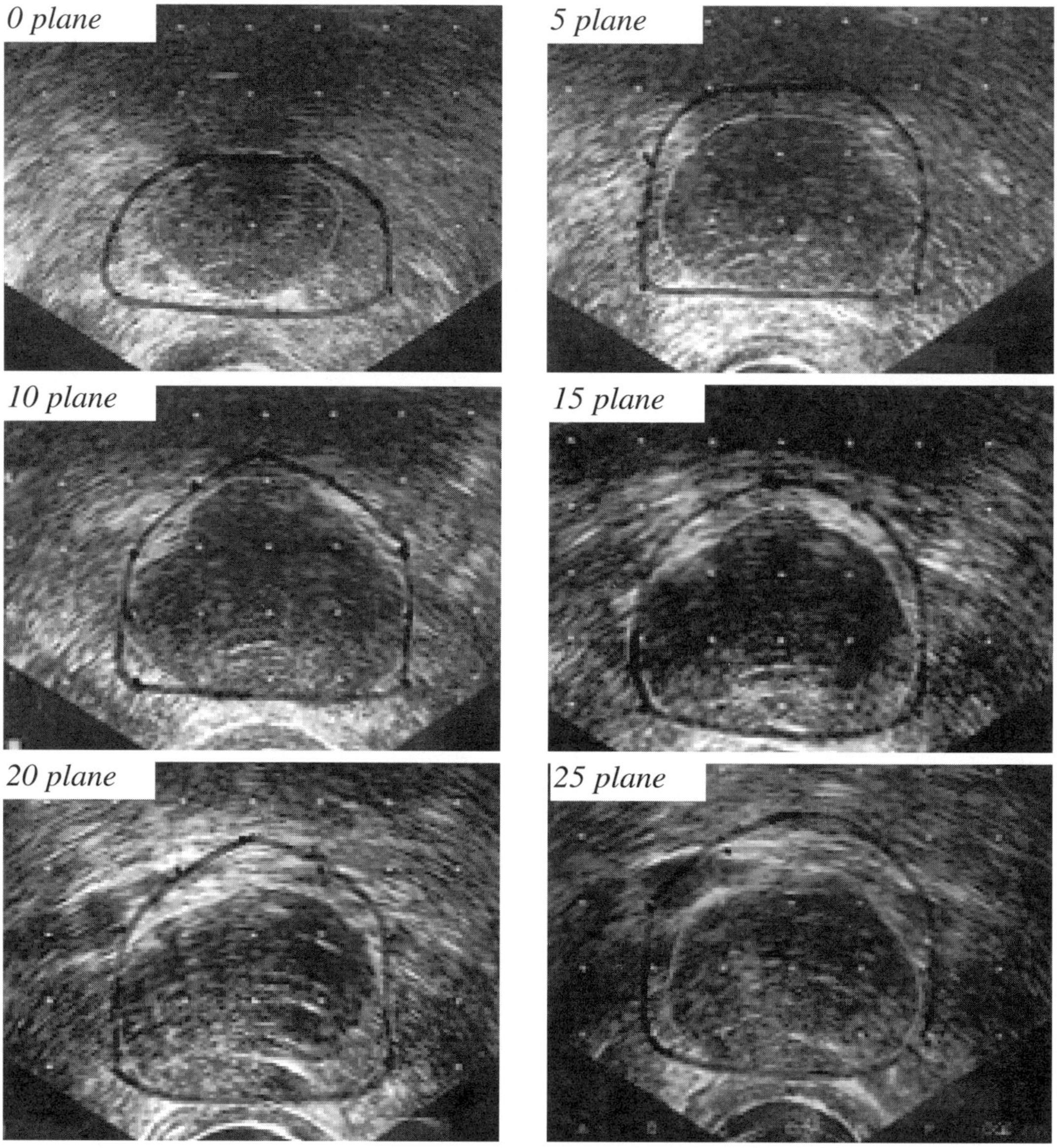
0 plane
5 plane
10 plane
15 plane
20 plane
25 plane

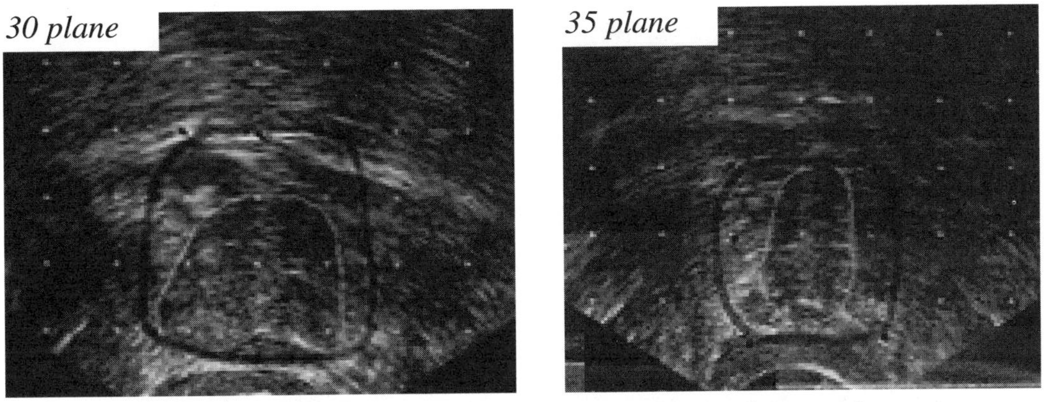

Figure 6-5a. Planning images for I-125 implant, with target drawn by J. Blasko. The apparent prostatic margin is traced in white, using the light pen supplied with the TRUS unit. The target is drawn in thick black ink. Note that the target extends beyond the margin of the prostate anteriorly and laterally. The prostatic apex may be difficult to discern on transverse TRUS images, and is simply drawn generously at the most distal portion of the prostate (30 and 35 plane). Corroborative sagital imaging may help delineate the base and the apex.

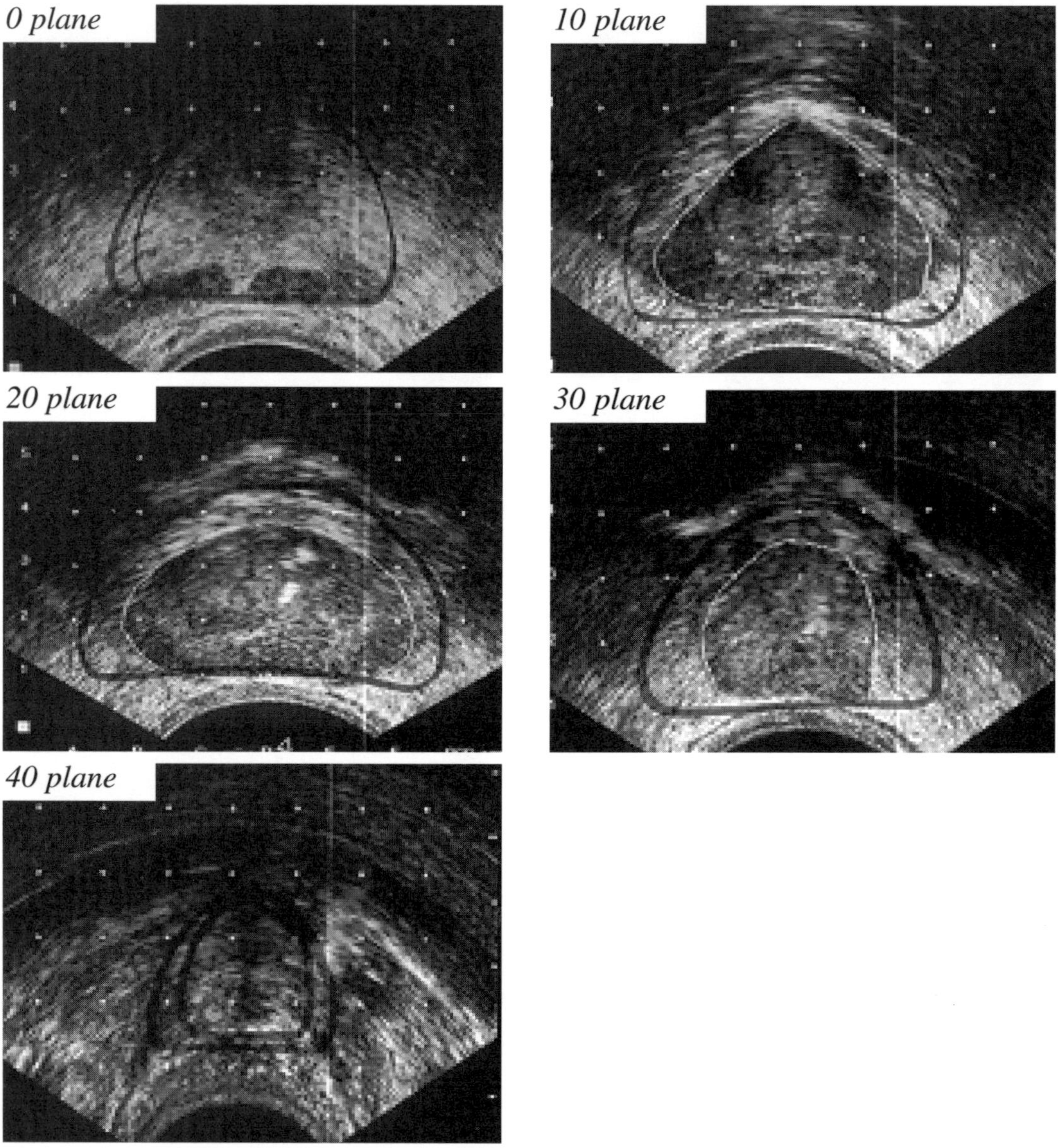

Figure 6-5b. Planning images for 115 Gy Pd-103 implant by M. Dattoli. Note that the target extends considerably beyond the margin of the prostate anteriorly and laterally, even more so than the example of Figure 6-5a. (Only alternate TRUS images are shown here, although every 5 mm image is used for treatment planning. (Fab)

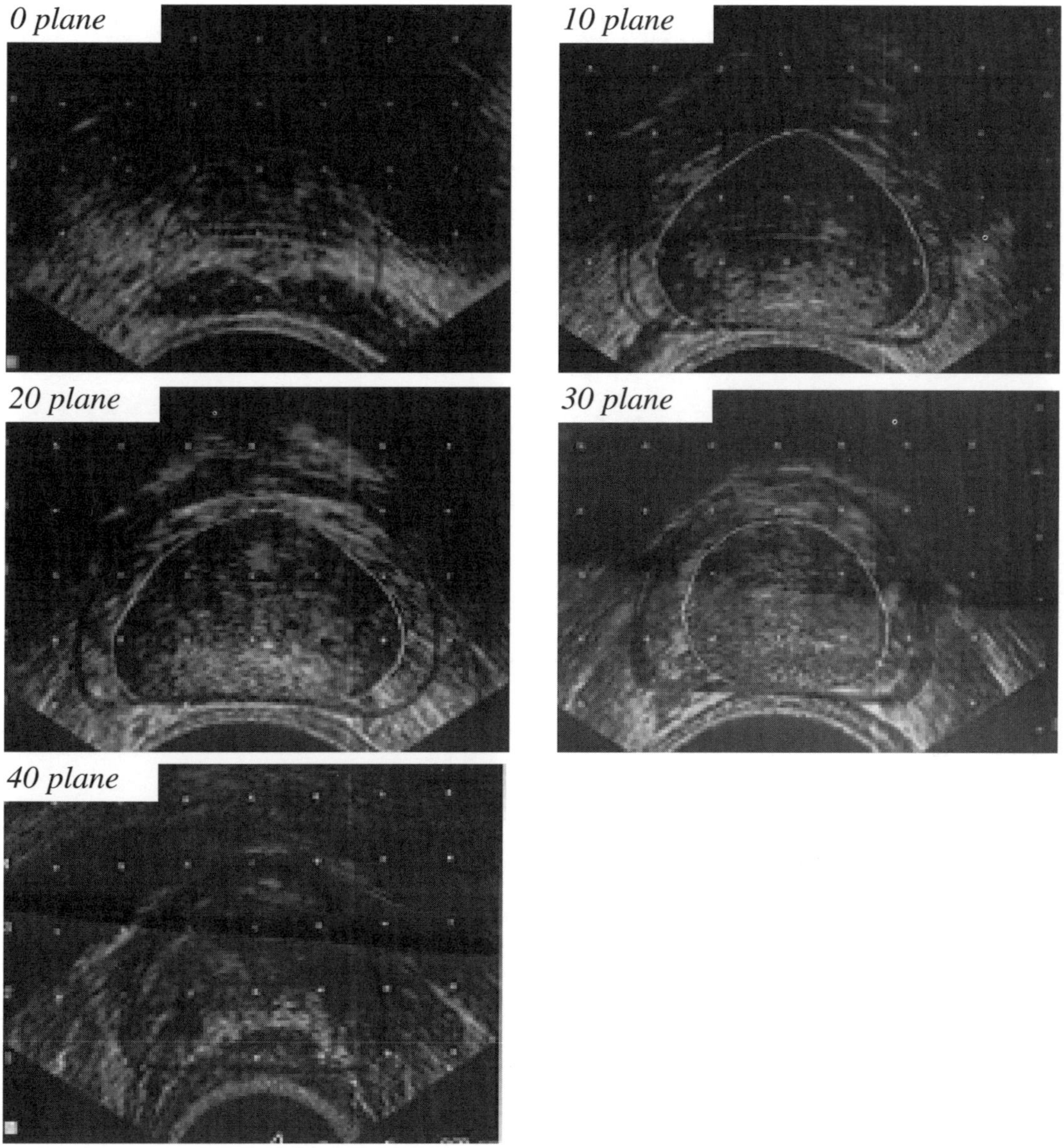

Figure 6-5c. Planning images for 80 Gy Pd-103 implant by M. Dattoli. (Only alternate TRUS images are shown here.) (Har)

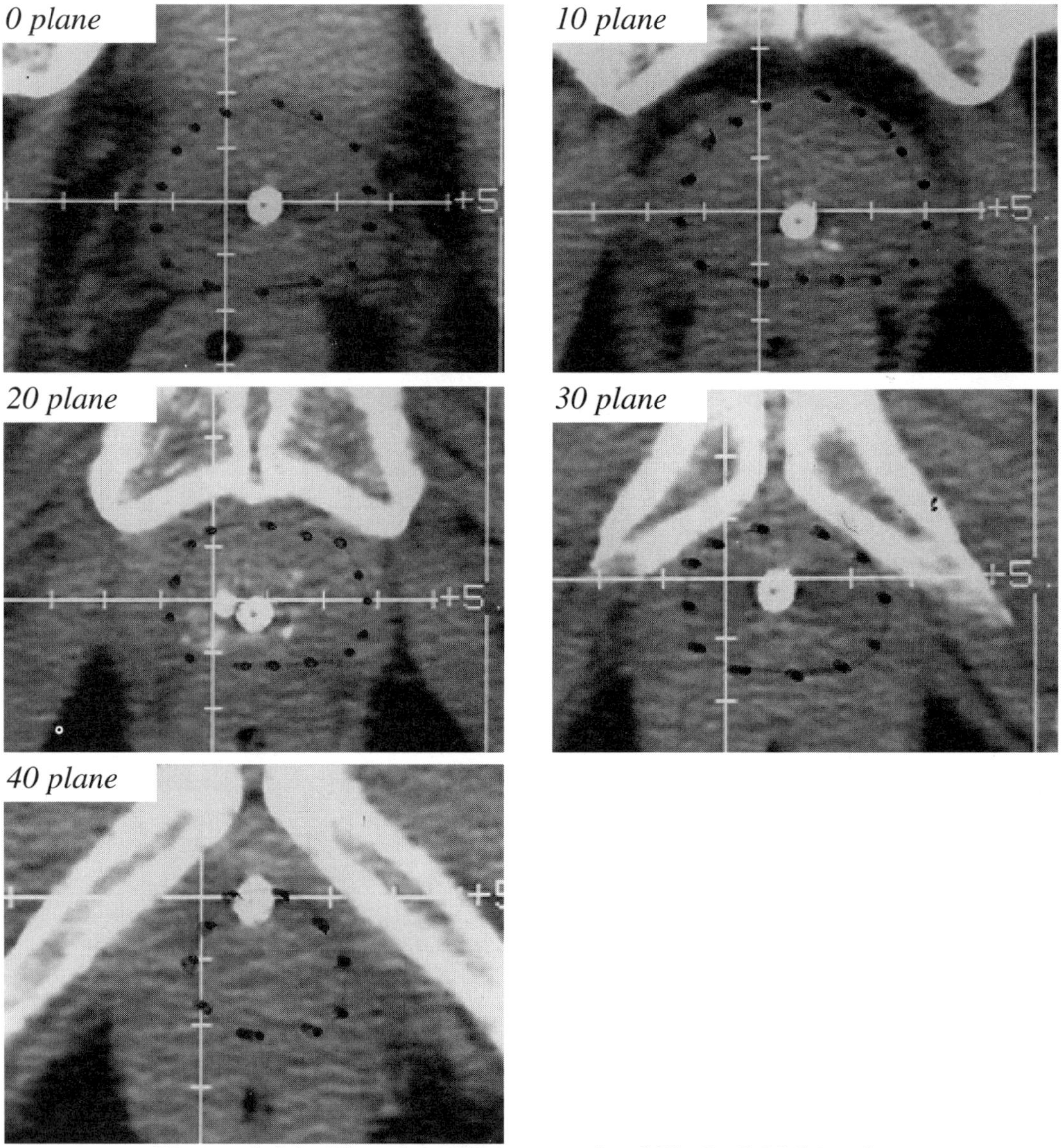

Figure 6-5d. Planning CT images for 150 Gy I-125 implant drawn by K. Wallner. The target (dotted line) is drawn at or slightly within the apparent prostatic margins, except at the apex, where it is probably generous. Only alternate CT images are shown here, although every 5 mm image is used for treatment planning. (JCha)

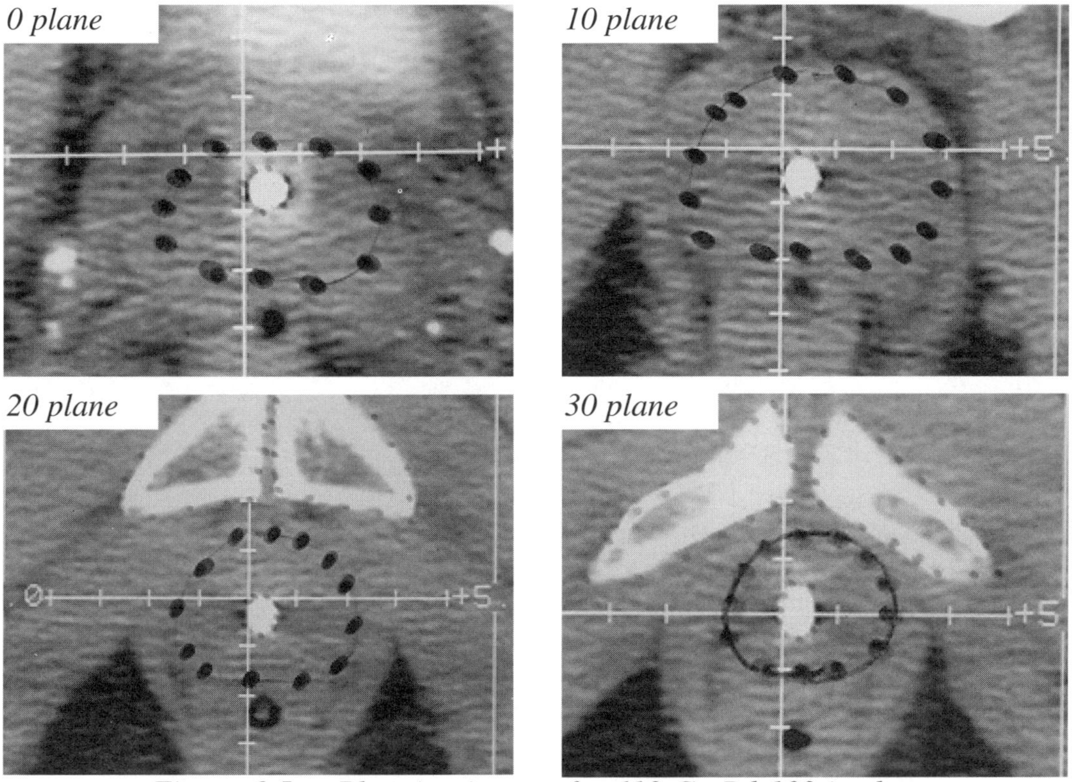

Figure 6-5e. Planning images for 110 Gy Pd-103 implant drawn by K. Wallner. The target is drawn at or slightly within the apparent prostatic margins, except at the apex, where it is probably generous. (MSwa)

TOTAL ACTIVITY

Before the widespread availability of desk-top computers and TRUS-based planning, the total activity needed to treat the prostate was determined from standardized tables, based on past experience and trial calculations. The prostatic volume was estimated using the three orthogonal dimensions and the total activity was dispersed at approximately one cm intervals throughout the prostate.

Dosimetry for permanent implants is now computerized, and can be closely tailored to an individual patient's prostate. No standard tables are needed. Instead, activity is simply placed around the prostate periphery at approximately one cm intervals. After a preliminary source placement on the computer screen, the target coverage is calculated quickly and sources are added or deleted to achieve coverage of the entire target periphery.

Figures 6-6 a-e show the total activity versus the target volume for implants by various teams. The graphs are intended as general guidelines. The actual activity for a given target volume will depend on the shape of a particular prostate, how much effort is made to minimize the rectal and urethral dose, and how closely the prescription dose is tailored to the target margins.

SOURCE STRENGTH

I-125 sources typically vary in strength from 0.2 to 0.9 mCi. Pd-103 sources vary from 0.9-2.0 mCi. By using higher activity sources, fewer total sources are required, the implant requires fewer needles, and it takes less time to perform. However, it has been argued that use of high activity sources could lead to a higher complication rate or less target coverage because the position of each source is more critical. Data regarding the benefit of high versus low activity sources are sparse.

Cumes and colleagues analyzed 14 patients after I-125 implantation and concluded that higher activity sources were more likely to lead to complications.(Cumes 1981) They recommended that individual source strength be limited to less than 0.4 mCi. Their data, however, comes from patients re-implanted at Stanford University Medical Center with the retropubic method following recurrence of cancer after EBRT or prior retropubic implant. Only seven patients had high activity sources.

Contrary to the Stanford experience, a detailed analysis of patients implanted with I-125 at MSKCC showed no relationship between source strength and urinary or rectal morbidity (**Figure 6-7**). The MSKCC experience is more convincing than that of Stanford because it is based on far more patients, who had no previous treatment and were implanted in a uniform fashion. The lack of a relationship between source strength and morbidity should not be surprising. Radiation-related urethral or rectal complications result from the cumulative dose delivered, not the individual source strength.

While it is possible that higher source strength would lead to larger 'hot spots' in the immediate vicinity of the sources and increase the likelihood of complications, there are no good data to support such an argument. At MSKCC, I-125 source strengths of 0.5 to 1.0 mCi have routinely been used since 1988 and the complication rate since 1992 has been low.[Wallner 1996] Rectal complications in the early experience at MSKCC were probably related to suboptimal source placement, rather than to source strength.

Lower source strength = less error?

One argument for using lower strength sources is that there may be less likelihood of underdosing if a few sources are not correctly placed. With a greater number of lower activity sources, the potential for error is spread out over a greater number of sources, so that misplacement of a few is of less consequence. While there is some merit to this argument, significant source misplacement should not occur in experienced hands.

SOURCE SPACING

I-125 or Pd-103 sources are each 4.5 mm long and 0.8 mm wide. There is no evidence that any particular lateral or longitudinal spacing is advantageous. Due to the nature of the templates used, there is at least 5 mm lateral spacing between sources. Sources can be placed end to end if necessary, without intervening space. However, they are usually spaced at 1.0 cm between source centers, along the needle track.

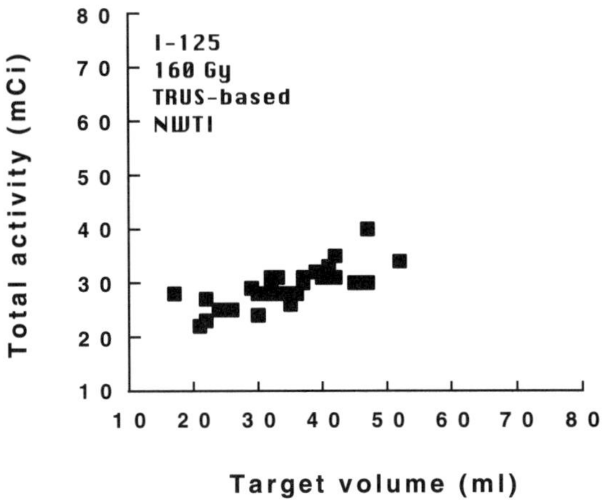

Figure 6-6a. Total activity used for 160 Gy target coverage with I-125 at NWTI.

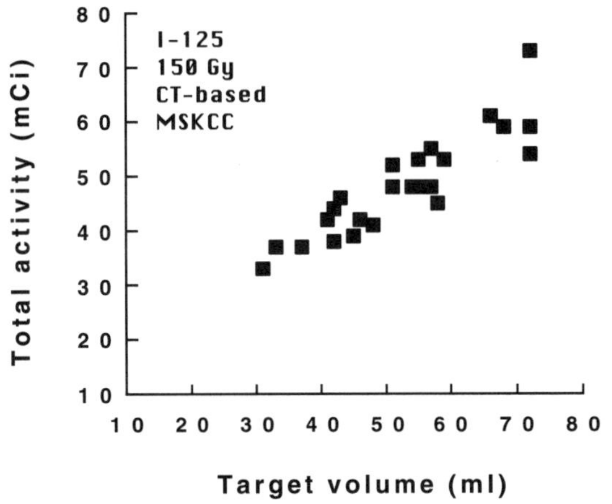

Figure 6-6b. Total activity used for 150 Gy target coverage with I-125 at MSKCC.

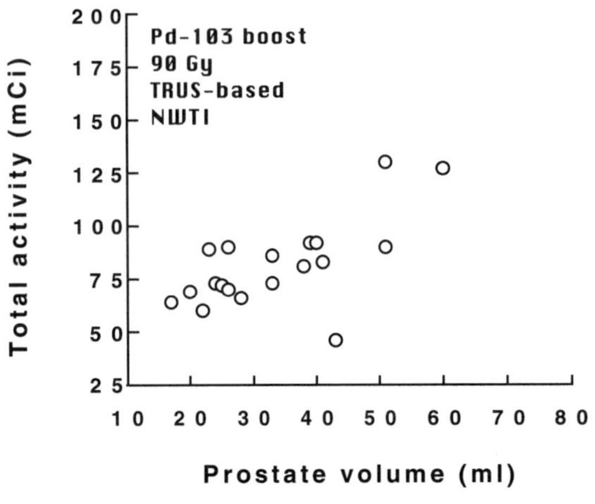

Figure 6-6c. Total activity used for 90 Gy target coverage with Pd-103 at NWTI.

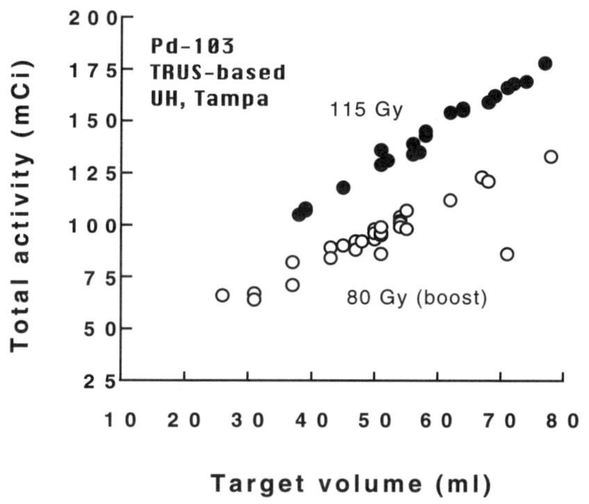

Figure 6-6d. Total activity used for 80 Gy or 115 Gy target coverage with Pd-103 at UCH, Tampa.

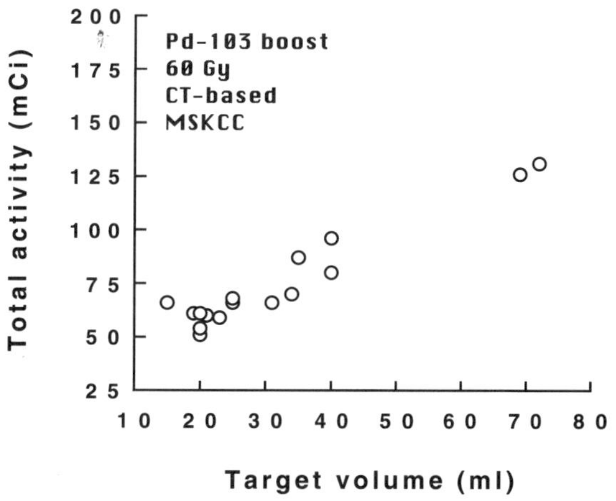

Figure 6-6e. Total activity used for 60 Gy target coverage with Pd-103 at MSKCC.

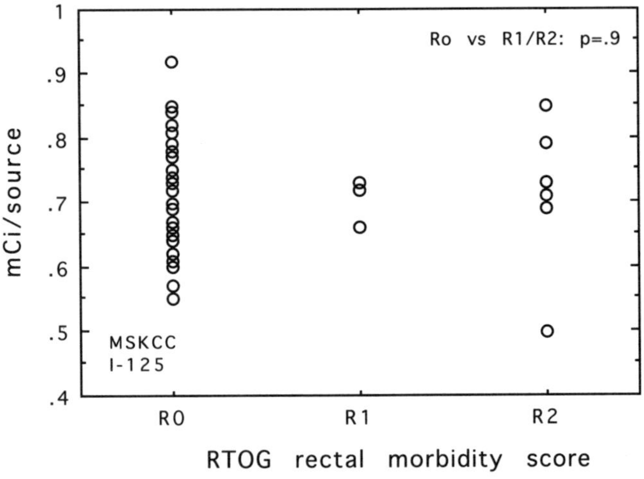

Figure 6-7. Rectal complications versus I-125 source strength following implantation at MSKCC (140-160 Gy). There was no relationship between source strength and the likelihood of rectal morbidity (R1=rectal bleeding, R2=ulceration).

TARGET COVERAGE

Coverage of the entire periphery should be achieved, while keeping the central dose below twice the prescription dose. When the prescription dose cannot be matched precisely to the target margin, it is probably prudent to err on the side of being more generous with target coverage.

Judging from the rarity of rectal complications and the posterior location of most cancers (peripheral zone), the entire target should be covered posteriorly (**Figures 6-8 a-e**).

TARGETING THE TUMOR

Prostatic carcinoma is multifocal in 50 to 80% of cases, so the entire prostate should be treated to at least the prescription dose.[McNeal 1988] It has been suggested that more activity be placed where tumor is known to exist and there is a certain degree of common sense to doing so.

It is not practical to prescribe a higher dose to one portion of the prostate. Instead, the prostatic margin near the tumor-bearing area can be drawn more generously on the planning images. Alternatively, several extra sources could be placed "ad hoc" at the time of the procedure. However, placing more sources than the plan specifies may increase the risk of complications.

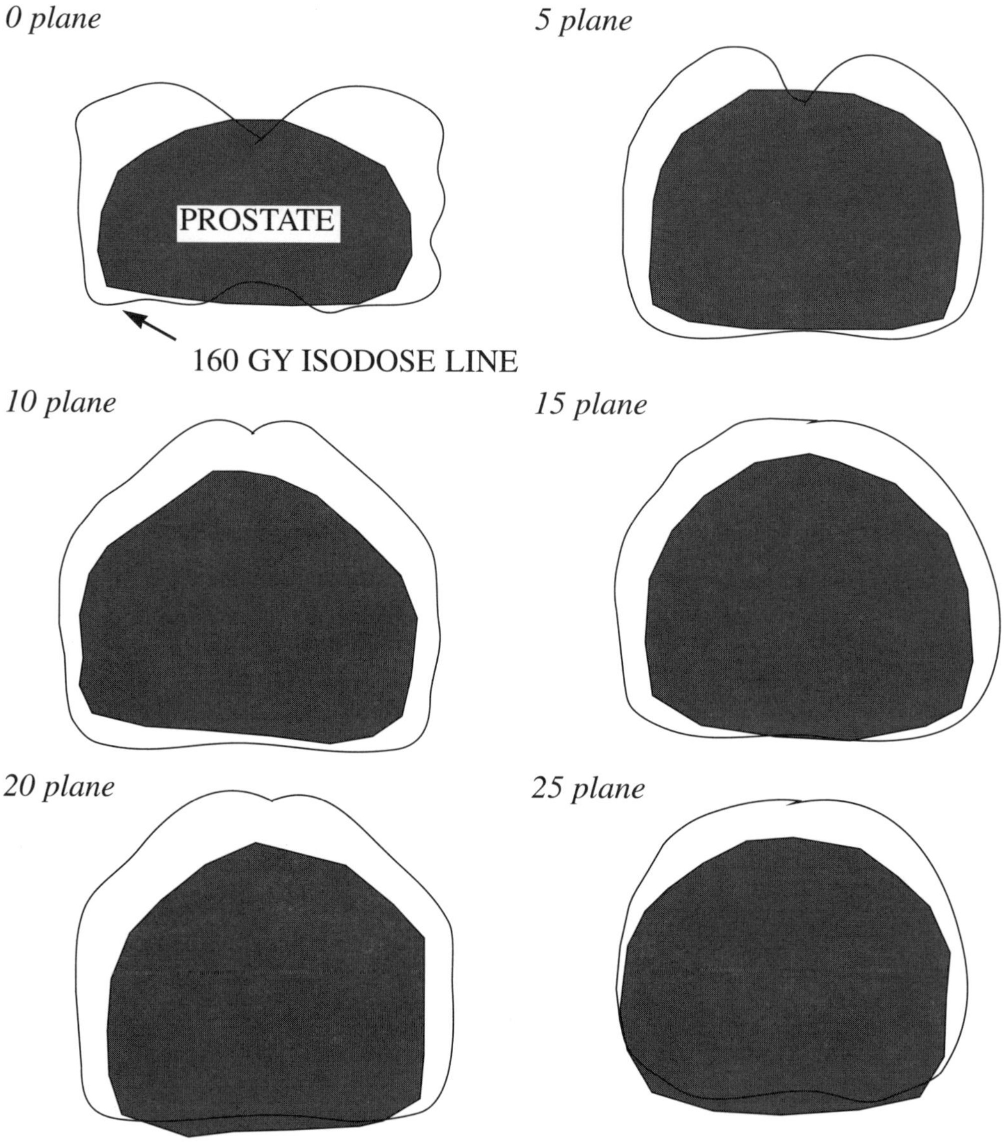
0 plane
5 plane
PROSTATE
160 GY ISODOSE LINE
10 plane
15 plane
20 plane
25 plane

30 plane

35 plane

40 plane

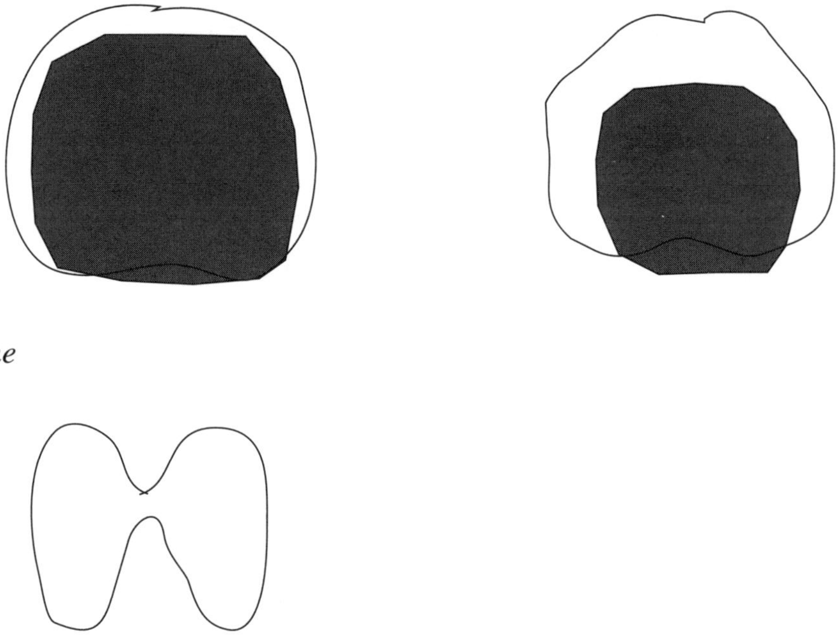

Figure 6-8a. Target coverage by 160 Gy prescription dose with I-125 plan for J. Blasko. This figure corresponds to the TRUS images of Figure 6-5a. The 160 Gy line is slightly generous anteriorly and laterally, and slightly tight posteriorly. Tight posterior coverage is due to reluctance to place sources too close to the anterior rectal wall. Slight over or underdosing of the target is accepted, realizing there is always some degree of uncertainty in target definition and source placement, anyway. Note that the 160 Gy isodose extends to the 40 plane even though no prostate was visible at that level on TRUS, because sources were placed at that plane to assure coverage of the prostatic apex. At the 0 plane, especially, minor crossing of the target volume by the 160 Gy prescription line is accepted because this plane represents a superior margin volume which is primarily bladder neck and proximal seminal vesicle, with only a small amount of prostate centrally.

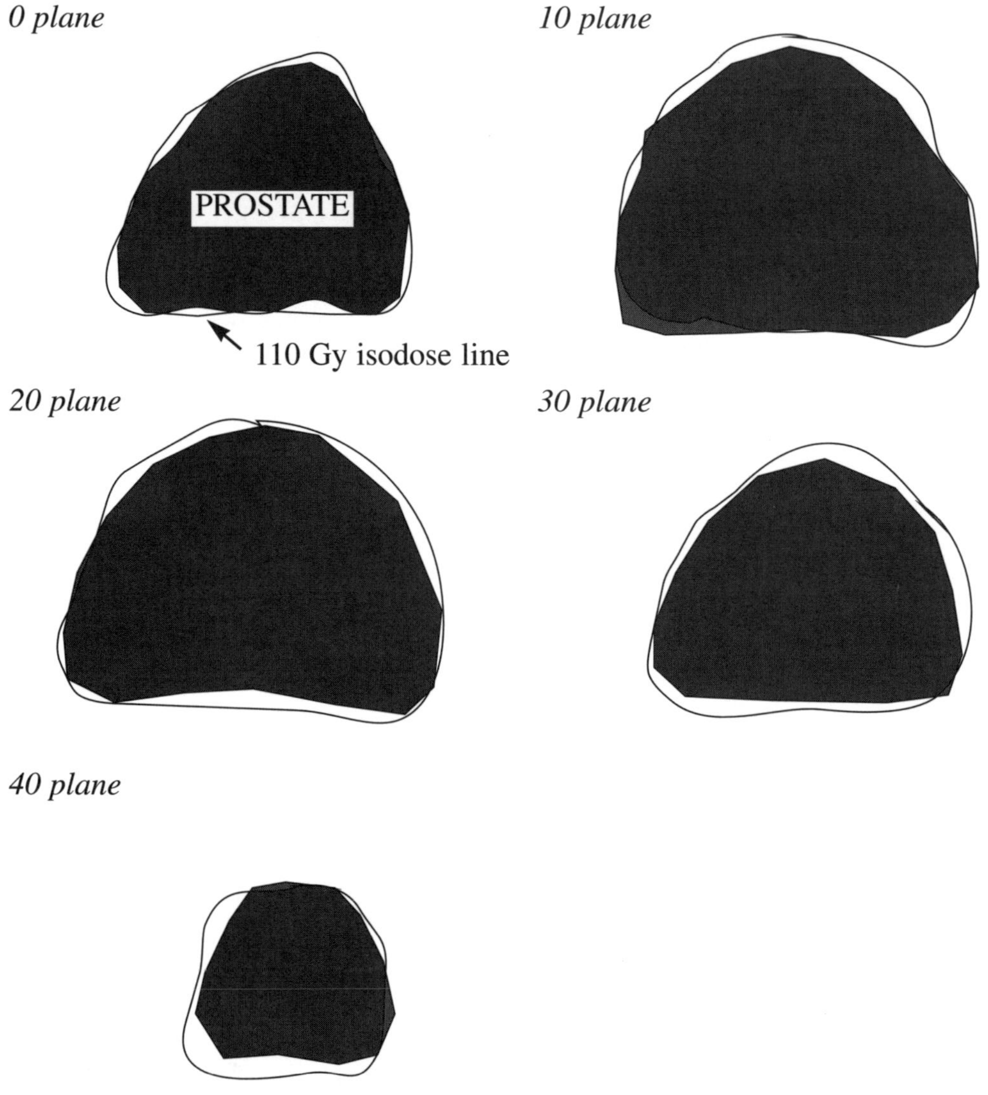

Figure 6-8b. Target coverage for 110 Gy Pd-103 implant by M. Dattoli for patient shown in Figure 6-5b. Isodose plan conforms closely to the target. Slight over or underdosing is acceptable, realizing there is always some degree of uncertainty in target definition and source placement, anyway (Fab).

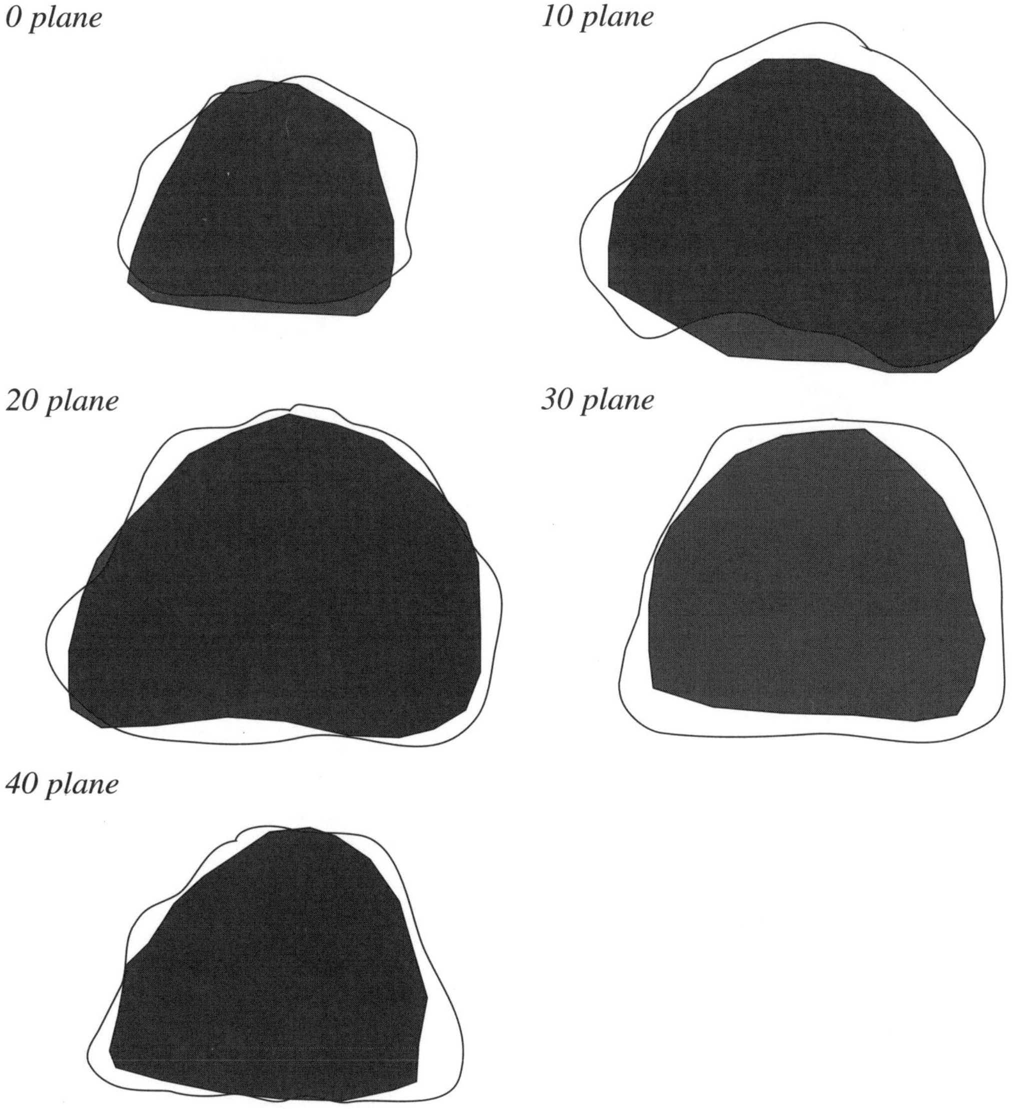

Figure 6-8c. Target coverage for 80 Gy Pd-103 implant by M. Dattoli, for patient shown in Figure 6-5c. Isodose plan conforms closely to the target. Slight over or underdosing is acceptable, realizing there is always some degree of uncertainty in target definition and source placement, anyway. (Har)

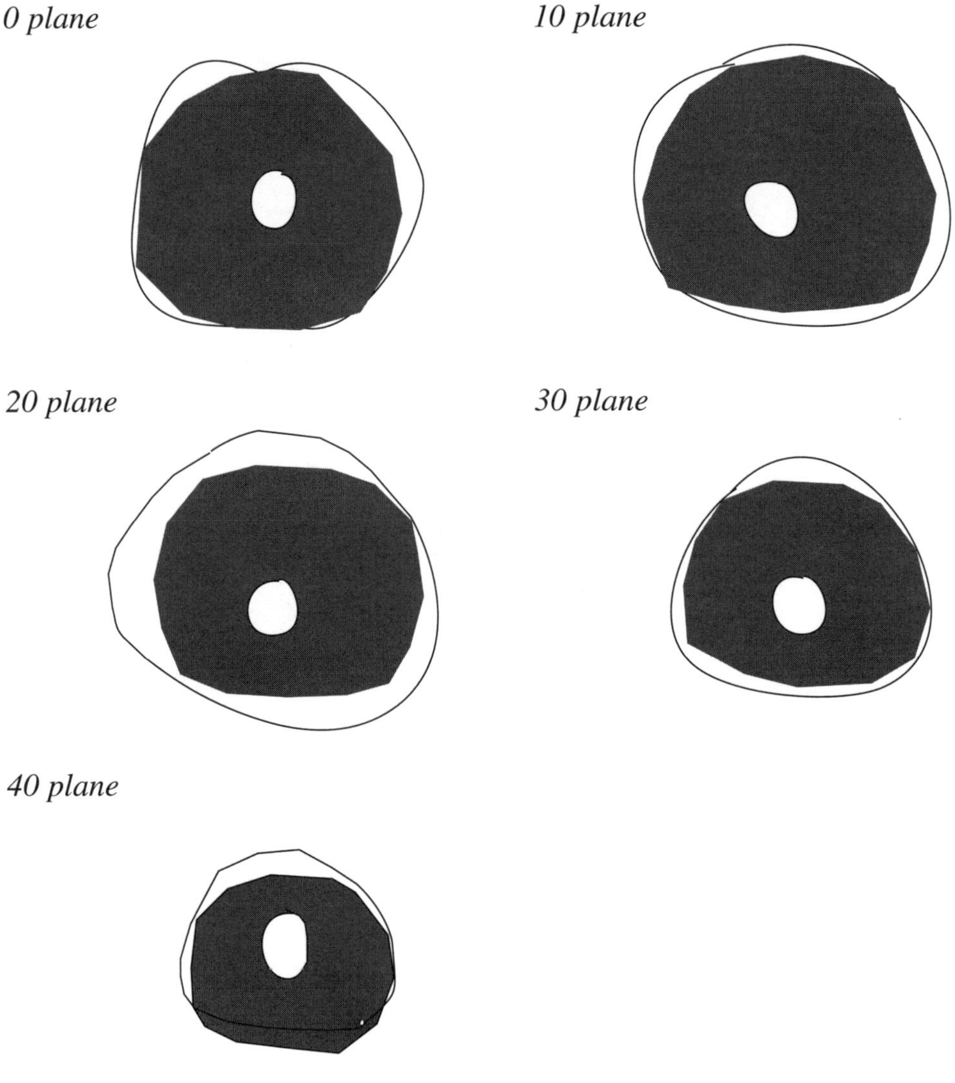

Figure 6-8d. Target coverage by 150 Gy prescription dose for I-125 plan for K. Wallner. This figure corresponds to the CT images of Figure 6-5d. The 150 Gy prescription isodose conforms closely to the target. In this plan, it happens to be slightly tight posteriorly at the apex (40 plane).

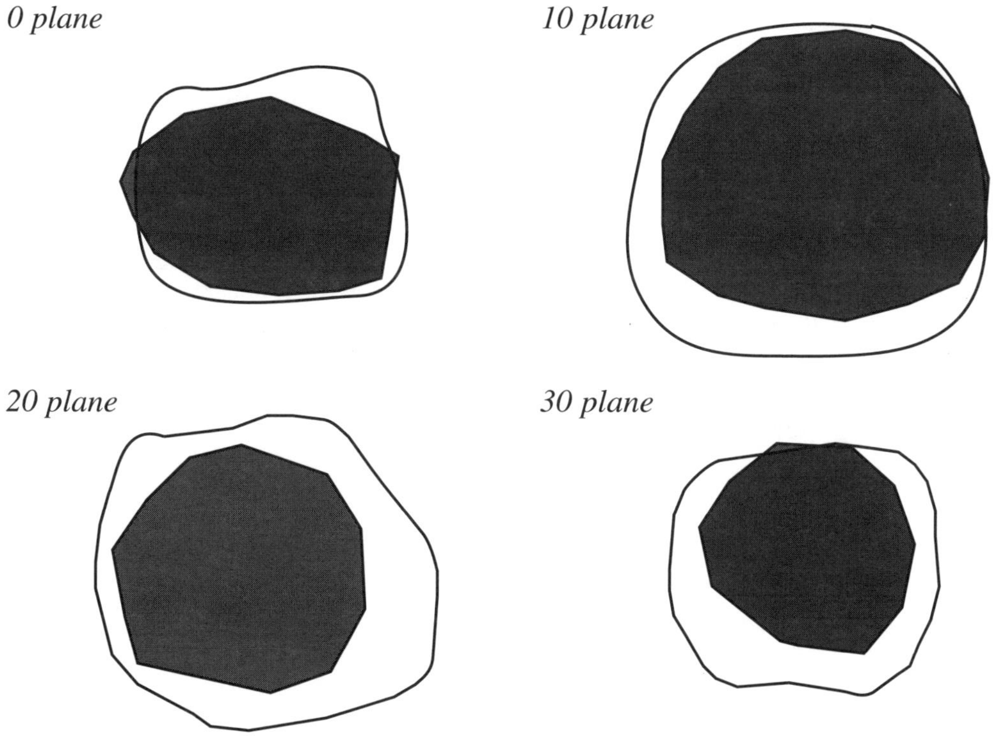

Figure 6-8e. Target coverage by 110 prescription dose for Pd-103 plan for K. Wallner. This figure corresponds to the CT images of Figure 6-5e.

SOURCE PLACEMENT

Homogeneous versus peripheral loading

Sources can be distributed in a regular pattern throughout the prostate or kept toward the periphery. With homogeneous source spacing throughout the prostate, the urethral dose can easily exceed 700 Gy and high urethral doses can lead to urinary morbidity, particularly in patients with a prior TURP.(Wallner 1995)

If sources are preferentially placed at the prostatic periphery, the entire prostate can be treated to the prescription dose without excessive central doses.(Narayana 1996) With a peripheral loading the central dose is usually kept below twice the prescription dose, which should lessen the likelihood of serious urinary morbidity.

In practice, keeping sources at the periphery is often easier said than done. The prostate is a small target, and some sources often have to be placed close to the urethra because there simply is not enough room to achieve coverage of the prostate while maintaining a minimum lateral source distance of 5 mm (**Figure 6-9**). This is especially true for Pd-103, because a large number of sources is required due to the relatively low specific activity.

As a rule of thumb, sources should be kept at least one cm from the urethra. The length of urethra that receives greater than 400 Gy for I-125 alone (without supplemental EBRT) (**Figure 6-10**) or 250 Gy for Pd-103 alone should be kept as low as possible.

SOURCE PLACEMENT MADE EASY

With computer-based planning, source placement can be quickly optimized to keep the central dose low, while achieving the prescription dose at the prostatic periphery. Sources should first be placed around the periphery, at one cm spacing and within 5 to 10 mm of the capsule. Since sources at the periphery alone may not give adequate coverage of the entire volume, additional sources can be placed more centrally and at the capsule's edge. This is usually accomplished by trial and error, moving sources and recalculating the doses until adequate peripheral coverage is achieved.

6.27

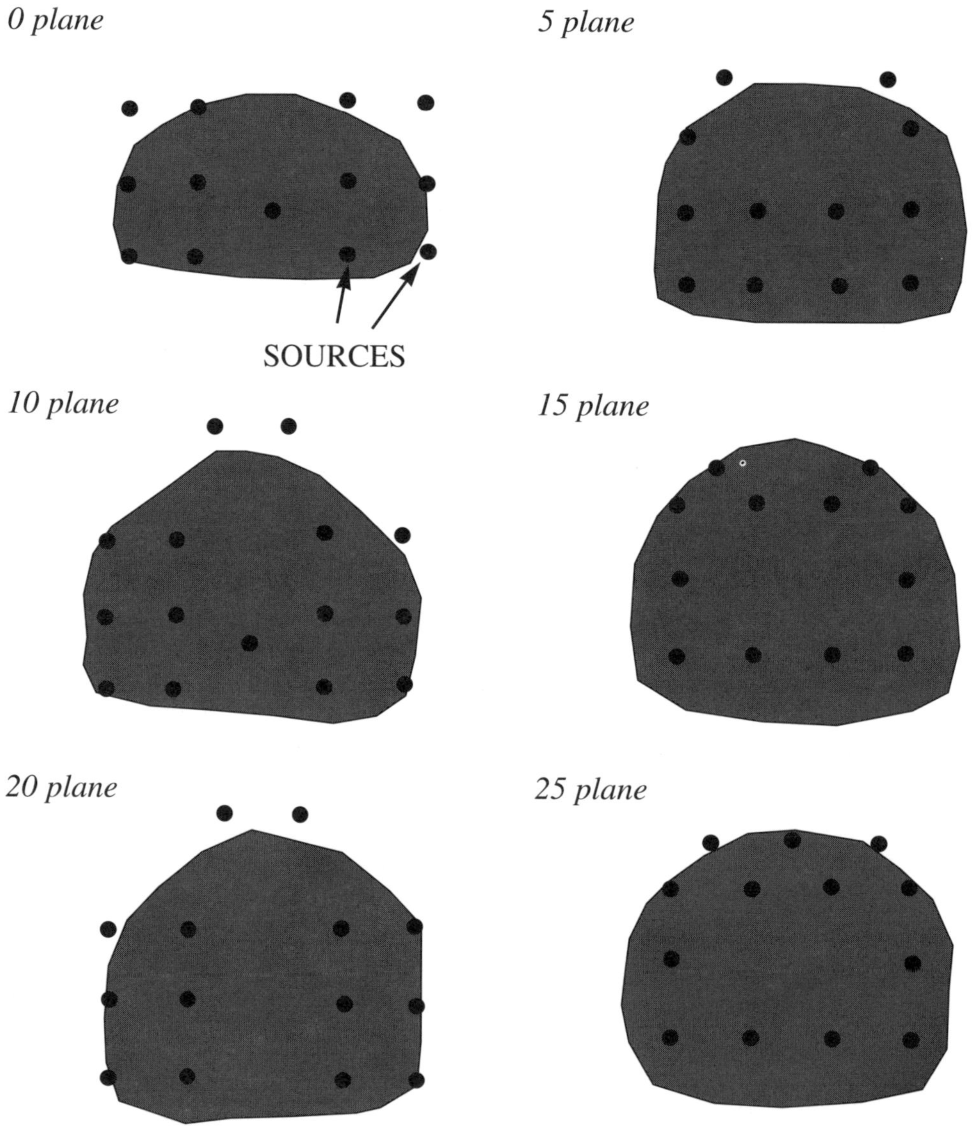
0 plane
SOURCES
5 plane
10 plane
15 plane
20 plane
25 plane

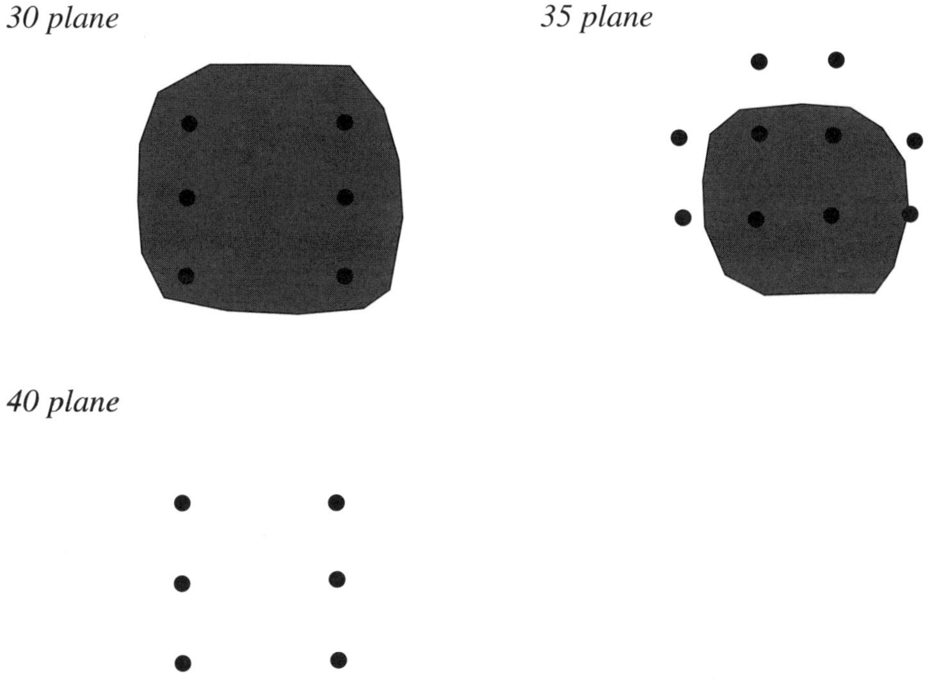

Figure 6-9a. I-125 source (.34 mCi/source) placement plan for J. Blasko. This figure corresponds to the TRUS images of Figure 6-5a. Sources are placed toward the prostatic periphery to limit the urethral dose to approximately 220 Gy. A few sources are placed outside the prostate on image planes 0 through 35. Most will not migrate, if placed just outside of the prostate. Note that sources are placed at the 40 plane, even though no prostate is visible at that level on TRUS. Placing sources at plane 40 helps guarantee coverage of the prostatic apex. The sources will not usually migrate at the inferior planes, because they are imbedded in the pelvic floor musculature. A urinary catheter is not placed for the planning scan, so the precise position of the urethra is not known.

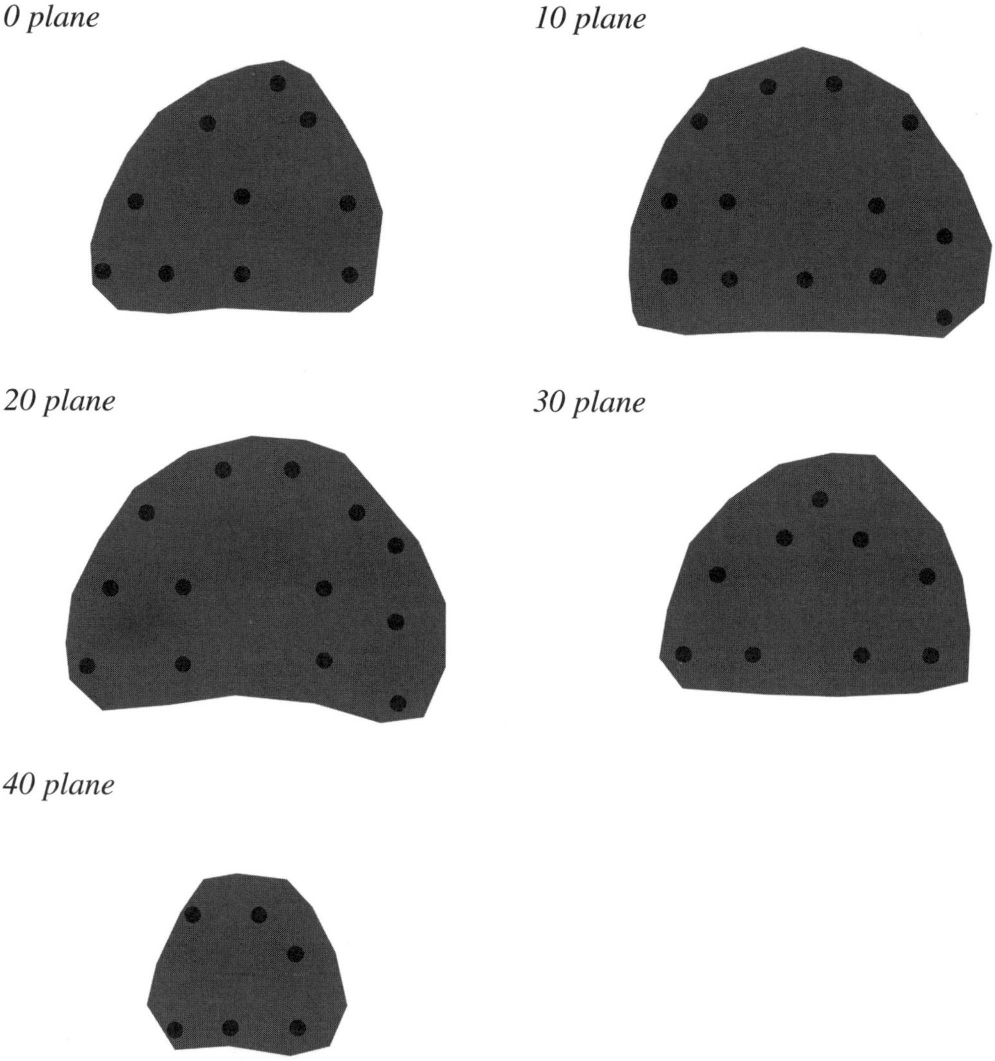

Figure 6-9b. Source placement plan for 115 Gy Pd-103 implant by M. Dattoli. This plan corresponds to the TRUS scan in Figure 6-5b. Sources are placed toward the prostatic periphery, but for a 115 Gy Pd-103 implant, some sources must be placed centrally simply to accommodate the total number needed. (Fab) Only alternate TRUS images are shown here, although every 5 mm image is used for treatment planning.

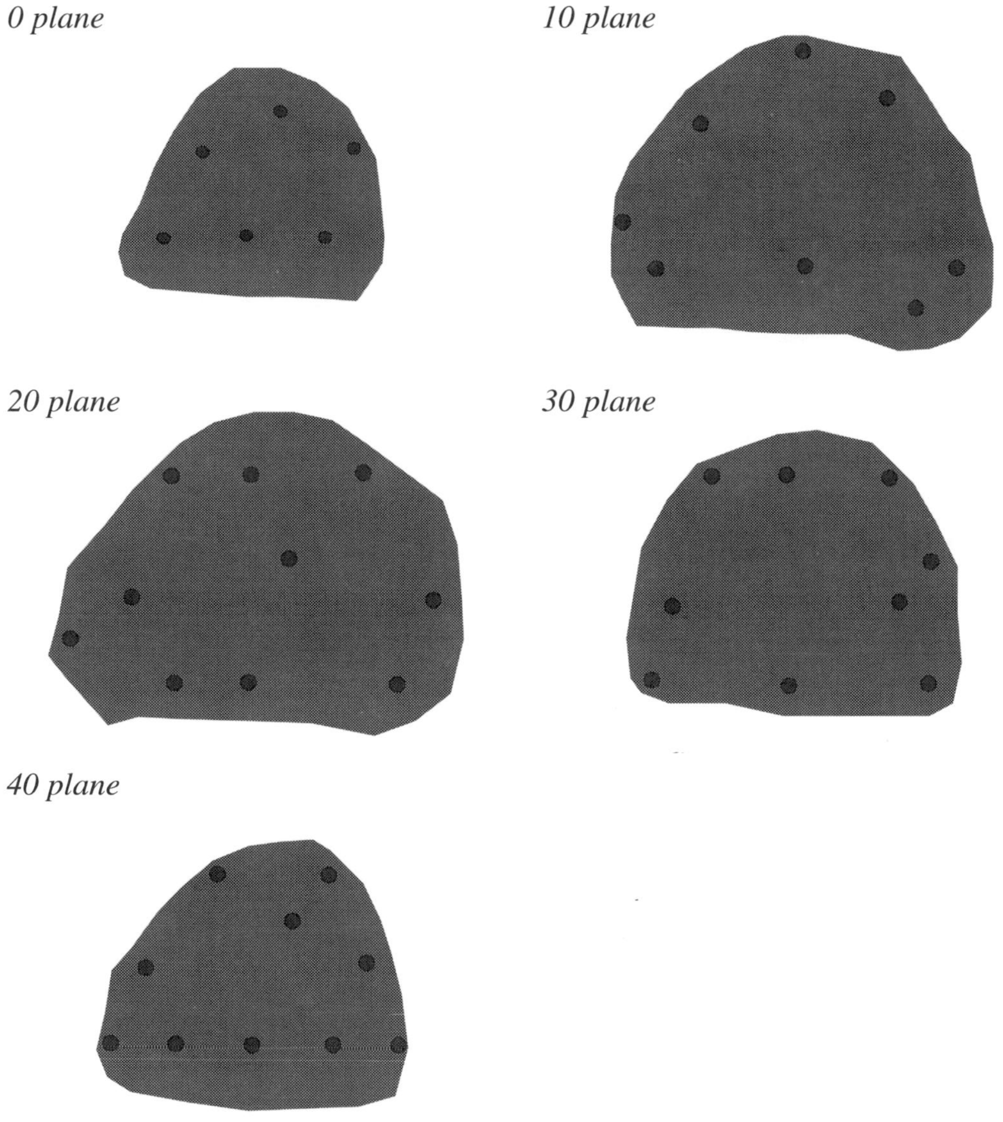

Figure 6-9c. Source placement plan for 80 Gy Pd-103 (1.4 mCi/source) implant by M. Dattoli. This plan corresponds to the TRUS scan in Figure 6-5c. Because the total activity required for an 80 implant is less than for a 115 implant, fewer sources need to be placed in the central portion of the gland, compared to Figure 6-9b. (Har)

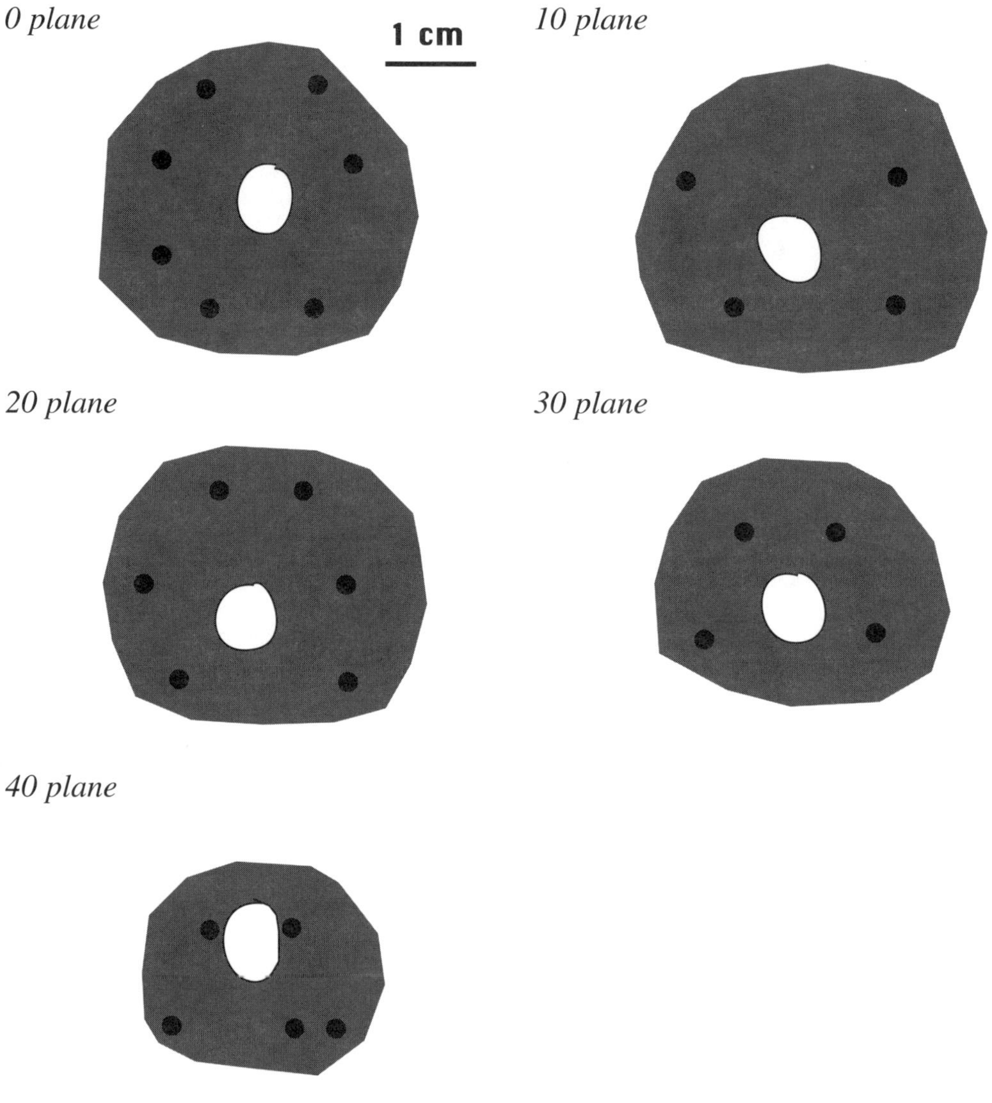

Figure 6-9d. Typical source placement plan for 150 Gy I-125 implant by K. Wallner. Sources are placed toward prostatic periphery, but limited prostate size allows only so much distance from the urethra (JCha). Note the relatively small number of sources, compared to the 160 Gy implant by J. Blasko in Figure 6-9a, due to the higher source activity (.69 mCi) in this patient. (Only alternate CT images are shown here, although every 5 mm image is used for treatment planning.)

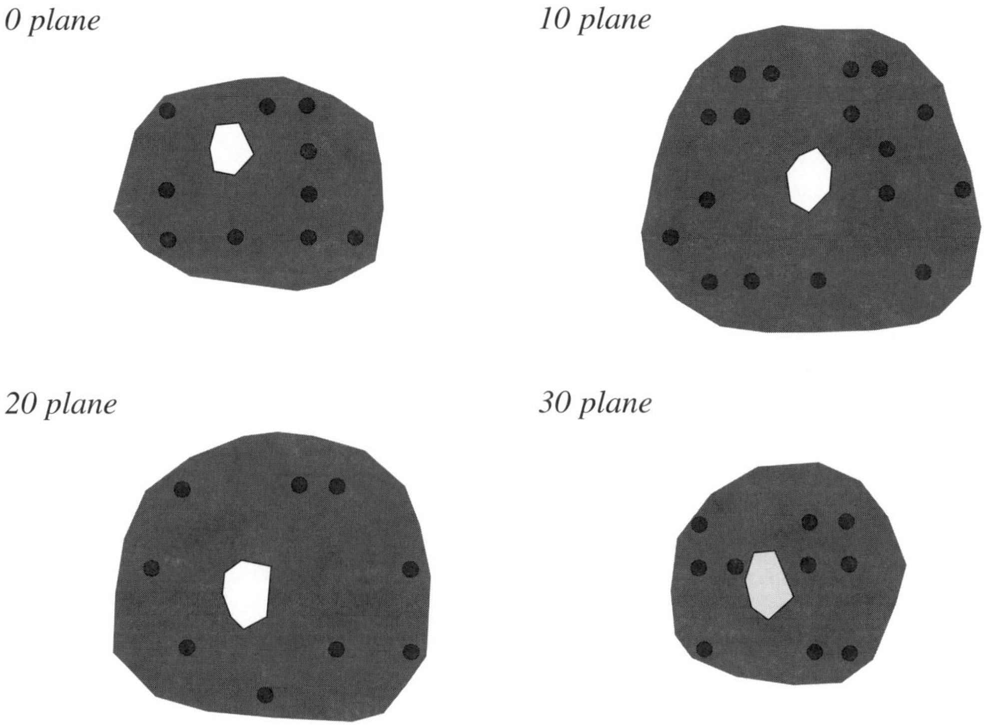

Figure 6-9e. Source placement plan for 110 Gy Pd-103 plan for K. Wallner (1.4 mCi/source). Sources are placed toward the prostatic periphery, but some sources must be placed centrally simply to accommodate the total number needed (MSwa).

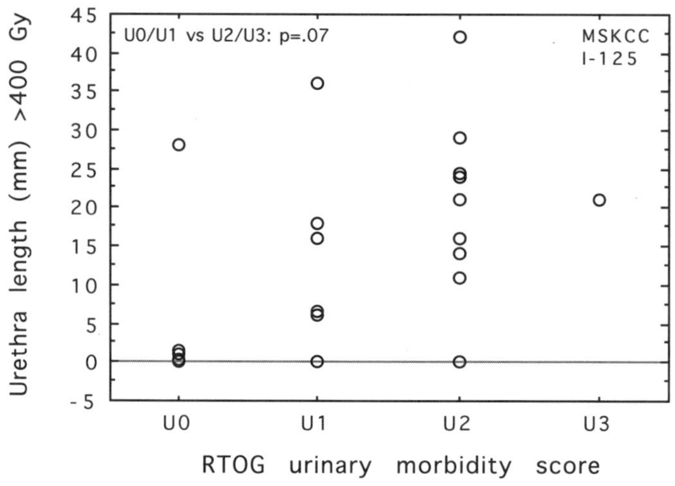

Figure 6-10. RTOG (Radiation Therapy Oncology Group) urinary morbidity versus the length of the urethra that receives less than 400 Gy.

ADDING SOURCES AD HOC

It is common practice to add extra sources at the time of implant, beyond what is called for in the computer-generated plan. Extra sources are commonly added to areas where biopsies are known to be positive, or to regions where source placement appears to be suboptimal. Adding sources ad hoc is a somewhat risky practice, and could lead to overdosing the urethra or rectum. If one chooses to add sources, it is prudent to place them laterally to minimize additional radiation to the tissue between the urethra and the rectum.

K. Wallner's practice is to arbitrarily add six extra sources after completing the computer-generated plan. Extra sources are generally placed at the proximal and distal portions of the prostate (**Figure 6-11a**). If one region of the implant does not look optimal on fluoroscopy, another one or two sources are placed there.

M. Dattoli typically adds eight to twelve additional sources after completing the planned source placement. Extra sources are generally placed in areas that appear more devoid of sources on fluoroscopy and/or TRUS.

J. Blasko typically adds six additional sources after completing the planned source placement. Extra sources are generally placed in regions that are biopsy-positive for cancer, or that appear more devoid of sources on fluoroscopy and/or TRUS. Extra sources are kept far from the urethra and the anterior rectal wall (**Figure 6-11b**).

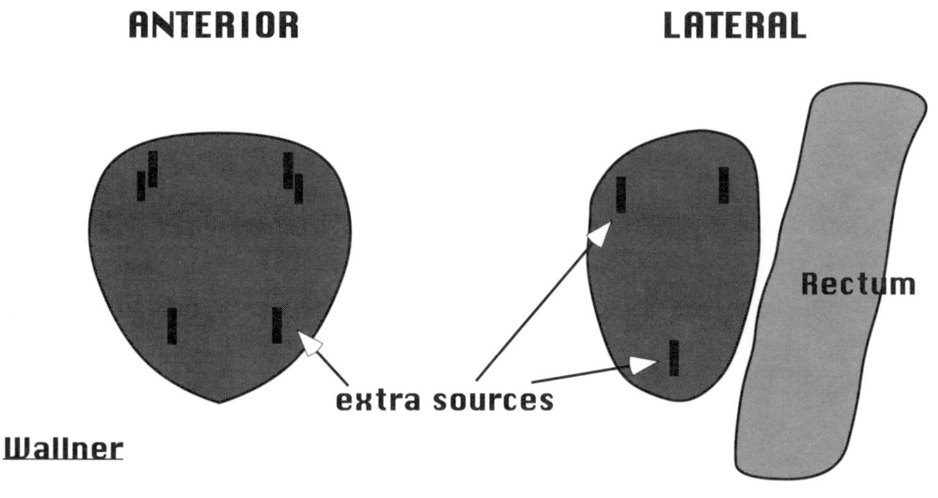

Figure 6-11a. Typical placement of six extra sources by K. Wallner. This is commonly modified, depending on the actual source placement during the implant.

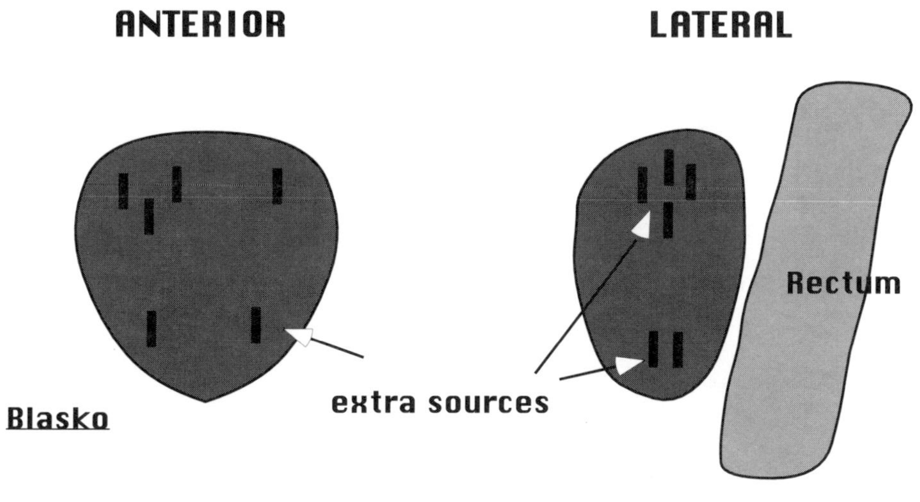

Figure 6-11b. Typical placement of six extra sources by J. Blasko. This is commonly modified, depending on the tumor site and the actual source placement during the implant.

DOSIMETRY AND HORMONAL DEPRIVATION

Androgen deprivation reduces the prostate size by approximately 40% to 50%.(Shearer 1992) When pre-treatment androgen deprivation is used, dosimetry should be based on the reduced prostate volume (**Figure 6-12**). Most of the shrinkage occurs in the first two to three months of androgen deprivation, and sufficient time should be given to allow near maximal shrinkage before obtaining the planning images. Very prolonged hormonal deprivation may lead to excessive shrinkage, making an implant more difficult due to very small target size.

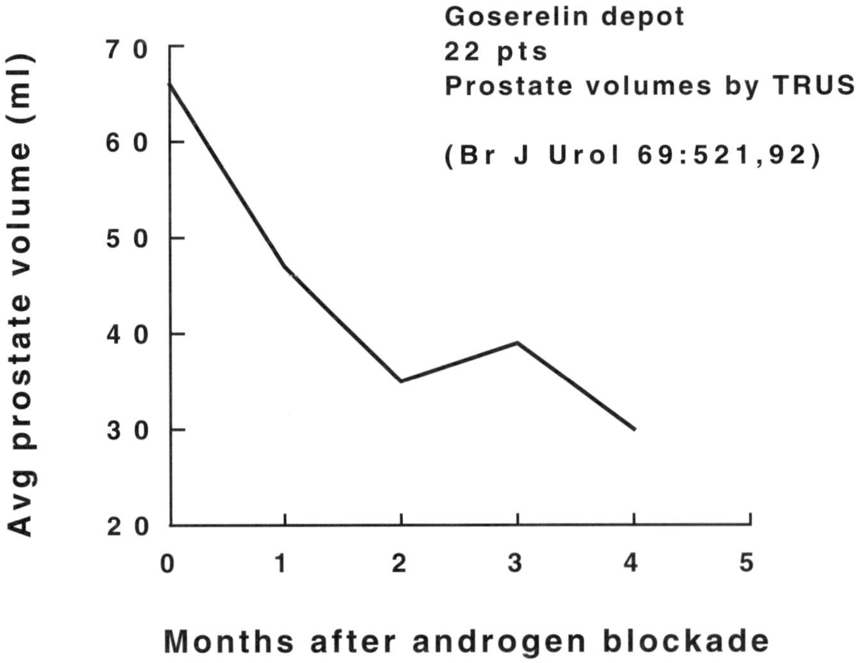

Figure 6-12. Prostate volume reduction after initiating androgen blockade. The volume reduction slows at two months, although there is some variability from patient to patient.

SUPPLEMENTAL EBRT

Combining an implant with supplemental EBRT (external beam radiation) has become a widely used treatment for patients at higher risk of extraprostatic disease extension. There are many possible combinations of brachytherapy and supplemental EBRT. The sequencing, radionuclides and doses can all be varied. While there is no lack of opinions as to how modalities should best be combined, little data exists to support one scheme versus another.

Sequencing

The most common practice is to give supplemental EBRT first, followed by brachytherapy. The rationale is that EBRT may shrink the prostate and facilitate coverage by the implant. This reasoning is probably flawed as it is unlikely that the prostate shrinks substantially during several weeks of EBRT. No systematic study of prostate volume changes during EBRT has been done.

There is concern that doing the implant first could lead to a higher incidence of rectal complications, because of an excessive total daily dose of radiation from the implant and simultaneous EBRT. In one report from Europe, patients who received their implant first had a very high incidence of rectal complications.(Iversen 1989) However, in addition to doing the implant first, the investigators gave large fractions of EBRT (2.37 Gy/day to the whole pelvis) and a full dose I-125 implant. Other investigators are currently treating patients with implant prior to EBRT. Longer follow-up will show whether or not it is safe.(Stone/Stock)

Time between modalities

The time between implant and EBRT varies from two to eight weeks (**Table 6-1**). There are currently no data regarding treatment results versus the time interval. Studies regarding the effect of overall treatment time with EBRT alone for prostate cancer have been mixed.(Amdur 1990)(Lai 1991) However, a short-

Table 6-1. Implant boost treatment schemes used by various groups.

Investigator	1st modality	EBRT dose	Isotope	Imp dose	Time between
Blasko	EBRT	45 Gy	Pd-103	90 Gy	2-4 wks
Wallner	EBRT	50 Gy	Pd-103	60 Gy	2-4 wks
Dattoli	EBRT	41 Gy	Pd-103	80 Gy	2-6 wks
Blasko	EBRT	45 Gy	I-125	120 Gy	2-4 wks
Stone/Stock	Implant	60 Gy	Pd-103	80-90 Gy	8 wks

er time between EBRT and brachytherapy for the treatment of cervical carcinoma may result in better tumor control rates, strengthening the argument for a shorter interval between brachytherapy and supplemental EBRT in the treatment of prostatic cancer. Considering the very low likelihood of rectal complications with any of the time intervals used, it would seem reasonable to use an interval closer to two weeks.

EBRT fields

The EBRT field sizes commonly used range from just large enough to cover the prostate and seminal vesicles to those that cover the pelvic lymph nodes (**Figures 6-13a-b**). Given the negative RTOG study regarding radiation of pelvic lymph nodes, most would argue that the fields should cover only the periprostatic tissue.(Asbell 1988)

Brachytherapy dose

The implant dose is generally 50-80% of that which would be delivered without supplemental EBRT. The brachytherapy doses commonly used range from 90 to 120 Gy with I-125 and 60 to 90 Gy with Pd-103 (**Table 5-3**). Caution should be used when extrapolating combined brachytherapy and EBRT doses between institutions, due to potential differences in how target volumes are drawn.

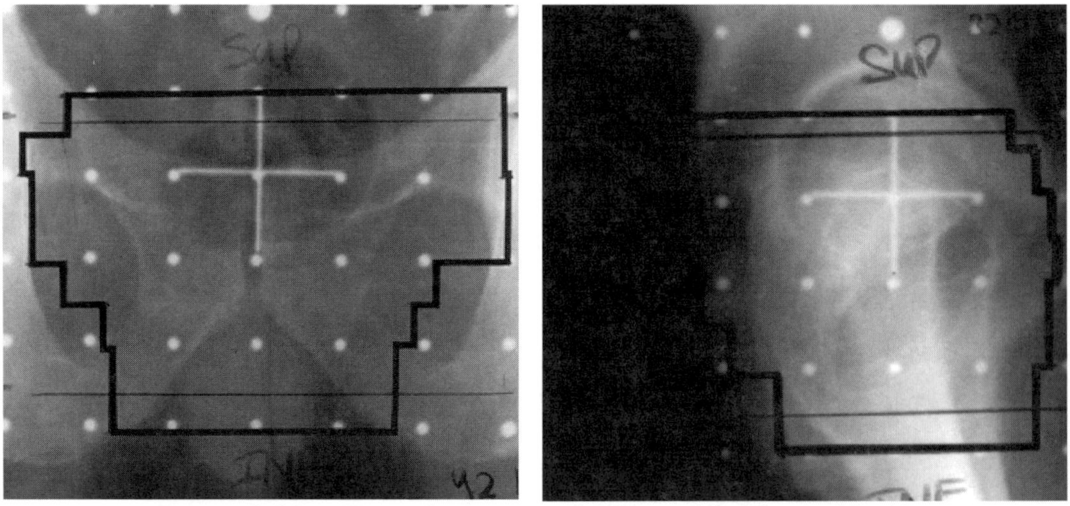

Figure 6-13a. Typical anterior and lateral fields used by K. Wallner.

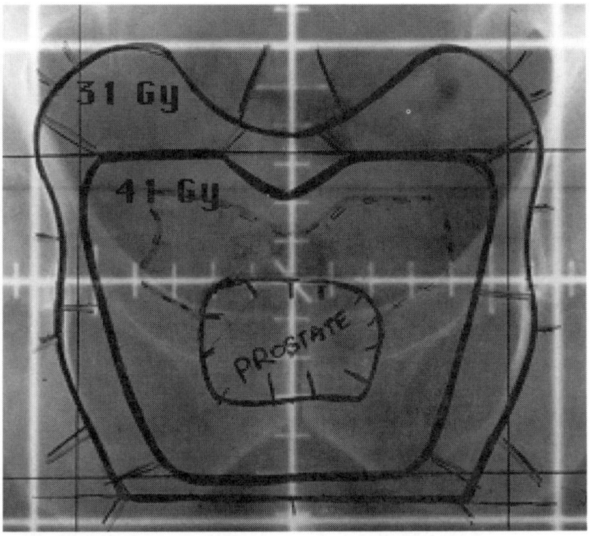

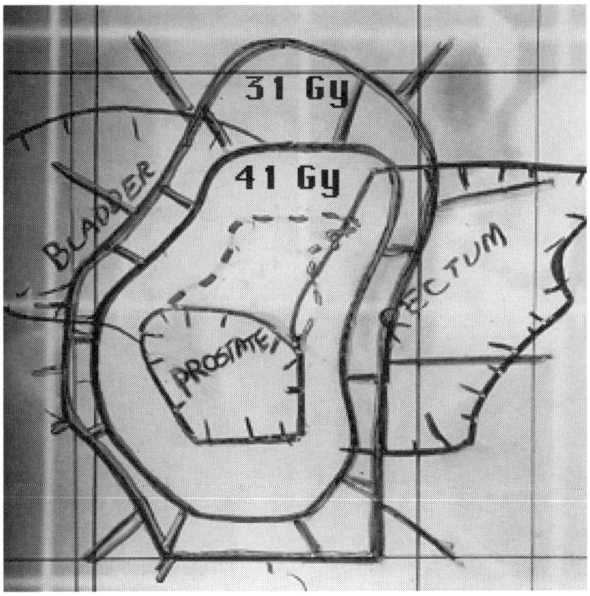

Figure 6-13b. Typical anterior and lateral fields used by M. Dattoli.

EBRT dose

Supplemental EBRT is given to allow more generous coverage of potential microscopic extraprostatic tumor extension (see Chapter 12). Doses of 40 to 60 Gy are used, extrapolating from combined radiation modality treatment of cancer of the cervix, head & neck, and sarcomas. Doses for all sites have been arrived at empirically.

RADIONUCLIDES

The choice of sources is based on personal preference rather than data (see Chapter 3). Encouraging results with both I-125 and Pd-103 have been reported.

TG-43

All of the clinical data presented in this text for I-125 implants are based on single-seed dosimetry in use prior to the publication of Task Group 43 recommendations (Med Phys 22:209, 1995). Re-evaluation of these data using the new dosimetry would result in lower I-125 doses. The precise dose effect has not been agreed upon at the time of this writing.

THE ART OF PROSTATE BRACHYTHERAPY

This chapter, more than any other, points out the differences among brachytherapists in how they perform prostate implants. "Art" is a euphemism for the striking variability in how implants are designed. Much of the variability is due to personal bias rather than legitimate data. But there are probably many ways to obtain an effective implant. Just because the methodology is not standardized does not mean that prostate brachytherapy does not work. It is important to understand the nuances of implant design, in order to achieve adequate target coverage and to avoid complications. Despite the multitude of uncertainties in brachytherapy treatment planning and the widely varying treatment schemes, the clinical results appear almost uniformly favorable.

REFERENCES

1. Amdur RJ, Parsons JT, Fitzgerald LT, Million RR. The effect of overall treatment time on local control in patients with adenocarcinoma of the prostate treated with radiation therapy. Int J Radiat Oncol Biol Phys 1990; 19:1377-1382.

2. Amdur RJ, Parsons JT, Fitzgerald LT, Million RR. Adenocarcinoma of the Prostate Treated with External Beam Radiation Therapy. Radiother Oncol 1990; 18:235-246.

3. Blasko JC, Ragde H, Grimm PD. Transperineal Ultrasound-Guided Implantation of the Prostate: Morbidity and Complications. Scand J Urol Nephrol Suppl 1991; 137:113-118.

5. Cumes DM, Goffinet DR, Martinez A, Stamey TA. Complications of 125-Iodine implantation and pelvic lymphadenectomy for prostatic cancer with special reference to patients who had failed external beam therapy as their initial mode of therapy. J Urol 1981; 126:620-622.

6. Dattoli M, Wallner K, Sorace R. Pd-103 brachytherapy and external beam irradiation for clinically localized, high-risk prostatic carcinoma. Int J Radiat Oncol Biol Phys 1996; 35:875-879.

7. Iversen P, Nielsen L, Bak M, et al. Ultrasonically Guided 125Iodine Seed Implantation with External Radiation in Management of Localized Prostatic Carcinoma. Urol 1989; 34:181-186.

8. Lai PP, Pilipich MV, Krall JM, Asbell SO. The effect of overall treatment time on the outcome of definitive radiotherapy for localized prostate carcinoma: the Radiation Therapy Oncology Group 75-06 and 77-06 experience. Int J Radiat Oncol Biol Phys 1991; 21:925-933.

9. McNeal JE, Price HM, Redwine EA, Freiha FS, Stamey TA. Stage A Versus Stage B Adenocarcinoma of the Prostate: Morphological Comparison and Biological Significance. J Urol 1988; 139:61-65.

10. Narayana V, Roberson PL, Winfield RJ, Kessler ML. Optimal placement of radioisotopes for permanent prostate implants. Radiol 1996; 199:457-460.

11. Shearer RJ, Davies JH, Gelister JSK, Dearnaley DP. Hormonal cytoreduction and radiotherapy for carcinoma of the prostate. Br J Urol 1992; 69:521-524.

12. Stamey TA, Villers AA, McNeal JE, Link PC, Freiha FS. Positive surgical margins at radical prostatectomy: importance of the apical dissection. J Urol 1990; 143:1166-1173.

13. Wallner KE, Roy J, Harrison L. Dosimetry guidelines to minimize urethral and rectal morbidity following transperineal I-125 prostate brachytherapy. Int J Radiat Oncol Biol Phys 1995; 32:465-471.

14. Wallner KE, Roy J, Harrison L. Tumor control and morbidity following transperineal I-125 implantation for Stage T1/T2 prostatic carcinoma. J Clin Oncol 1996; 14:449-453.

Chapter 7

Patient preparation

Proper patient preparation should facilitate the implant procedure, and decrease the risk of post-operative morbidity. There is a wide variety of preparatory practices, with minimal or no objective information to support one over another.

BOWEL PREPARATION

The rectum should be cleared of feces to facilitate proper TRUS imaging. Lower gastrointestinal clearing may also decrease the risk of infection should the rectum inadvertently be pierced with a needle. There is a variety of combinations of enemas, diets and laxatives that can be used, all with a 80 to 90% likelihood of success.(Shapiro 1990) Some regimens are more onerous than others (**Table 7-1**). It would seem wise to use the least expensive and most convenient regimen.

INFECTION CONTROL

In the late 1800s the general, post-operative infection rate fell from nearly 100% to less than 5%, primarily due to adoption of hand-washing and clothing changes. Since that time, a large number of high technology and expensive antiseptic (tissue) and disinfectant (inanimate objects) maneuvers have been introduced, without any clearly documented further reduction in the likelihood of infection.

SKIN SHAVING

It is common practice to shave the perineal skin prior to transperineal implantation, the value of which is highly questionable. Several investigators have reported a higher likelihood of infection after general surgery if the skin is shaved.(Seropian 1971)(Bird 1984) An increased risk of infection with shaving could result from microscopic skin breakage.

Considering that no case of perineal skin or subcutaneous infection after transperineal prostate brachytherapy has been reported, and that shaving may actually increase the likelihood of infection, it is a practice that should probably be avoided.

SKIN CLEANSING

Whether or not the skin is shaved, it should be cleansed with an antiseptic. There is no substantial difference between commonly used skin cleansers regarding their anti-microbial effect.(Ritter 1980) Alcohol (70%) is as effective as any other cleanser, but carries a risk of causing skin irritation. Free iodine (tincture) is

Table 7-1. Lower GI clearing protocols.

	Diet	Enema	Laxative
Blasko	low fiber (24 hr) NPO after midnight	night before & AM of implant	none
Dattoli	NPO after midnight	night before & AM of imp	none
Wallner	clear liquids (24 hours)	none	magnesium citrate (10 oz) (evening prior)

no longer used, due to its risk of skin irritation. Iodine complexed with povodine (10% povodine-iodine solution, Betadine™) is less likely to irritate the skin than is free iodine. It works as well as tincture of iodine, and reactions to it are rare.

ANTIBIOTICS

In general, prophylactic antibiotics (ATBs) are prescribed far more frequently than is supported by the medical literature. Data to support their use for transperineal implantation are scarce.

Two randomized trials have shown that prophylactic ATBs can decrease the incidence of bacteriuria or bacteremia following trans*rectal* biopsy.(Ruebush 1979)(Crawford 1982) However, no significant decrease in clinically recognized sepsis or urinary infection was shown. Patients with bacteriuria or bacteremia nearly always clear the bacteria with natural defenses.

Amazingly, the negative data regarding prophylactic antibiotics for transrectal biopsy have been ignored and antibiotics are routinely given with transperineal brachytherapy. Ignoring negative transrectal biopsy data and using prophylactic ATBs for transperineal implantation is especially questionable because transrectal biopsies are done through a contaminated rectal mucosa, whereas transperineal procedures are generally sterile.

No randomized trials have tested the benefit of routine ATBs for transperineal biopsy or implantation (**Table 7-2**). In a non-randomized retrospective trial, Packer and colleagues found no benefit to ATB use in patients with a documented negative urine culture prior to transperineal biopsy.(Packer 1984)

MSKCC experience without antibiotics

At MSKCC prophylactic ATBs were not used routinely for transperineal prostate brachytherapy.(Wallner 1996) The primary reason was the lack of support-

Table 7-2. Clinical data supporting the use of prophylactic antibiotics with transperineal prostate brachytherapy.

Table 7-3. Febrile episodes following transperineal implantation at MSKCC, with or without prophylactic antibiotics.

	No. of patients	Febrile episodes
No ATBs	114	2 (2%)
no catheter	95	2 (2%)
catheter	19	0 (0%)
ATBs	17	0
no catheter	16	0
catheter	1	0

ive data. Additional reasons included efforts to minimize exposure of patients to unneeded therapy at unnecessary cost and to minimize the emergence of drug-resistant bacterial strains.

From 1987 through 1995, 131 patients underwent I-125 implants at MSKCC. None of the 17 patients who received prophylactic ATBs had a postoperative febrile episode. One hundred fourteen patients did not receive prophylactic antibiotics, 17 of whom required Foley catheter drainage one day or longer for post implant urinary retention. Two patients (2%) who did not receive ATBs developed a post-implant febrile episode within two weeks of surgery (**Table 7-3**). One patient was treated empirically as an outpatient with trimethoprim/sulfamethoxazole (TMP/SMX) and defervesced. The second patient had a 10-year history of chronic lymphocytic leukemia (CLL) and was probably immunocompromized from chlorambucil therapy. He developed E. Coli sepsis 24 hours after the procedure, and required inpatient antibiotic therapy.

Cost

Stopping the routine use of prophylactic ATBs would save money (**Table 7-4**). The actual charge to the patient could be two to three fold higher than the wholesale costs listed in Table 7-4.

One reason for the routine use of prophylactic antibiotics is the fear of a lawsuit from a patient who is not given ATBs and develops a serious post-operative infection. Such legal fears should be dismissed, considering the lack of supportive data and the published data regarding brachytherapy without ATB use. Dropping the routine use of prophylactic antibiotics would be a service to patients and would help control medical costs.

Table 7-4. Common ATB regimens used.

Brachytherapist	*Antibiotic(s)*	*Dose*	*Timing*	*Cost ($US)*
Blasko	Cipro™@	400 mg IV	intra-op	$20
	Cipro™	250 mg PO	b.i.d. x 5 days	$40
Dattoli	Unasyn™*	1.5 gm IV	after procedure	$42
	Cipro™	500 mg	bid x 7 days	$55
Wallner	none			$0

*ampicillin/subactam
@ciprofloxacin

When use of antibiotics is more justifiable

There are some more compelling circumstances for the routine use of antibiotic prophylaxis, including rheumatic heart disease, prosthetic devices or immune compromise.(Dajani 1997)

The significance of a previous history of prostatitis is unclear. Such patients have generally not been given prophylactic antibiotics at MSKCC, with no apparent increase in complications, but their post-implant course has not been specifically studied.

If prophylactic antibiotics are used, they should be given immediately (within one hour) pre-operatively, so they are present at the time of the procedure. They should be effective against the most likely contaminants - presumably *E. Coli* and *Enterococcus faecalis*.

PRE-OPERATIVE URINE CULTURE

Patients can have routine, pre-procedure urine culture. The likelihood of asymptomatic urinary infection is so low, however, that it is difficult to justify routine cultures in all patients. It would probably be wise to do so only in patients with a past history of infection, or in those with some suggestive symptoms.

PRE-OPERATIVE BLOOD WORK

Patients typically get a complete blood count (CBC) and a check of blood clotting function (PT/PTT) before implantation. Routine electrolyte or liver function tests, in otherwise healthy patients without specific indications are probably not necessary.

ANTICOAGULANTS

Non-steroidal anti-inflammatory agents (NSAID) should be stopped two weeks prior to the implant procedure. Coumadin should be stopped three days prior. With these policies, post-operative bleeding problems are rare. (These policies are probably overly cautious considering the rarity of bleeding problems with transperineal implantation.)

DVT PROPHYLAXIS

A high incidence of venous thrombosis has been demonstrated in patients undergoing orthopedic procedures. For implantation, patients are in the lithotomy position for approximately one to two hours. The incidence of deep venous thrombosis (DVT) or symptomatic thromboembolism with prostate brachytherapy has never been reported. Presumably they are very low, and prophylactic measures are not routinely used. However, prophylactic heparin (6,000 units immediately prior to the procedure) may be warranted in patients with a past history of thrombosis or some other predisposing condition. Venous compression could also be used.

OBESE PATIENTS

Obese patients are more likely to experience adverse post-operative events, including thromboembolism and heart failure. No excess risk of complications has been reported specifically for transperineal implantation of morbidly obese patients, but prophylaxis against DVT may be warranted.

STERILE BARRIERS

Like prophylactic antibiotics, sterile barriers are used far more than is supported by objective data. It seems sensible that liberal use of sterile gowns or drapes would decrease the likelihood of infectious complications, but this has never been shown. The current liberal use of disposable sterile barriers is probably unnecessary and wasteful (**Table 7-5**).

Table 7-5. Approximate hospital cost for sterile barriers.

Gown	$3
Leg drapes	$6
Mask	$.5

Sterile gowns

The use of sterile gowns for any type of operative procedure has not been studied. Considering that transperineal implantation is a minimally invasive procedure, and that the skin is cleansed immediately pre-operatively, the use of sterile gowns is probably not necessary. Sterile gowns are not used by J. Blasko or K. Wallner.

Sterile drapes

Use of sterile leg and pelvic drapes is another common anti-infection practice without supporting data. The use of drapes may actually increase the likelihood of infection, because they may trap and promote propagation of bacteria on the warm, moist surface under the barrier. The routine use of sterile drapes might be justified as a way to define and preserve a sterile field, but it should not be necessary in experienced hands.

Masks

Understandably, it is assumed that masks will prevent infectious contamination of the operative site. However, even the use of face masks has never been shown to decrease the risk of infection. In a large, randomized trial from Sweden, the use of masks did not decrease the infectious rate for open operations.(Tunevall 1991)

ANESTHESIA

Anesthesia for prostate implantation can be either spinal (epidural) or general. There is a perception that spinal anesthesia is safer. On the contrary, for 262 orthopedic patients randomized to general or spinal anesthesia at Cornell University Medical College, there was no safety advantage, from either a cardiac or cognitive standpoint.(Williams-Russo 1995)

The primary advantage of general anesthesia is that induction is quick. Patients may also recover bladder function more quickly with general than with spinal anesthesia.

No matter what the implant team's experience, considerable maneuvering is required to get the needle and source placement correct. Some patients find it upsetting to hear any uncertainty from medical personnel during the procedure, which is another argument in favor of general anesthesia.

Many brachytherapy teams prefer spinal anesthesia. In addition to providing anesthesia for the procedure, it helps prevent perineal discomfort in the immediate post-operative period.

PROPHYLACTIC CORTICOSTEROIDS

Approximately 10% of patients develop post-implant urinary retention, requiring temporary catheter drainage. Older patients with large prostate glands are at higher risk (see Chapter 16). Prophylactic corticosteroids might decrease the likelihood of post-operative urinary retention, the rationale being that they will

Table 7-6. Dexamethasone schedule used by M. Dattoli.
•10 mg IV intra-operative
•4 mg IV at 8 PM
•4 mg IV at 6 AM
•discharge with 1-2 week taper schedule

prevent post-implant tissue swelling. Corticosteroids are routinely given by M. Dattoli (**Table 7-6**).

Although the concept is appealing, there is no statistical evidence that corticosteroids decrease the likelihood of post-operative urinary obstruction. They are not currently prescribed by K. Wallner or J. Blasko. A controlled trial would be helpful to ascertain their usefulness.

HOSPITALIZATION

The vast majority of implants are performed on an outpatient basis. Post-operative complications have been low in all known series. Without data to the contrary, it is hard to justify routine overnight hospitalization.

Patients occasionally request to be hospitalized in case they develop a post-operative problem. Such hospitalization, in the absence of extenuating circumstances, should be discouraged. It is expensive, and has not been shown to decrease the likelihood of post-operative problems. Additionally, hospitalization might increase the likelihood of hospital-derived infection from drug-resistant organisms. Overnight hospitalization might be used for patients with other serious health conditions that might warrant closer observation.

An alternative to overnight hospitalization that constrains costs yet still provides the patient some feeling of security is "23 hour hospitalization," whereby the patient is observed overnight but spared the full charge of an overnight hospitalization. M. Dattoli uses 23 hour hospitalization routinely. The urinary catheter is removed at 4 AM to allow a voiding trial before discharge.

WHAT TO TELL PATIENTS BEFOREHAND

What and how much to tell patients beforehand is largely a matter of personal practice. However, we have learned a few things the hard way. Patients commonly get the impression from the news media or overly zealous brachytherapists that side effects with brachytherapy are minimal. When considered in comparison to radical prostatectomy, this is true. But there is still a fairly high risk of acute urinary retention, and a very high risk of longer-term radiation-related prostatitis. It is probably in the patient's and the physician's interest to make sure that patients are warned in some detail about these probabilities.

Urinary symptoms

Patients should be warned that they have a 10% likelihood of requiring a catheter to relieve urinary retention in the first few days following their procedure. A small percent of patients require a catheter (or self-catheterization) for much longer. They should be told to expect burning with urination, frequent daytime urination, and perhaps a very slow stream, especially during the night. The use of alpha blockers to alleviate radiation-related urinary symptoms should be mentioned beforehand. It is especially important to tell patients that they can expect to have some radiation-related urinary symptoms for 6 months to a year, and sometimes longer.

Rectal symptoms

Patients should be told that they are likely to experience frequent bowel movements, loose stools, and some rectal urgency for several months after implantation. Rectal symptoms usually resolve within six to twelve months of the procedure, usually earlier than urinary symptoms.

Return to activities

Nearly all patients experience some dysuria for several days after the procedure, but the general physical discomfort is surprisingly mild. Patients should be advised to limit strenuous physical exertion for 1-2 days. Mild exertion, including brisk walking, may be helpful regarding their post-implant urinary obstructive symptoms (mechanism unknown). Many patients return to work the following day, and no serious problems have been reported. Driving a car should be postponed until the following day,because of possible residual anesthetic effects.

Sexual function

Considering that many patients choose brachytherapy because of their desire to have a better chance of maintaining potency, it is especially important to warn sexually active patients that they are likely to experience pain with orgasm for several months, and that they are likely to have less ejaculate volume. They should also be warned that a small percent of patients are impotent immediately after the procedure, with some chance that they will improve over time.

Physicians commonly instruct implant patients to refrain from sexual activity for some time after the implant, but there is no evidence that abstinence is necessary. It would seem prudent for patients to use a condom for 2 months following Pd-103 implantation and six months after I-125, until the risk of passing a radioactive source was minimized.

Late Complications

Patients should be told that there is a small risk of permanent urinary incontinence, and a very small risk of rectal bleeding or ulceration, requiring colostomy.

General warning

Patients should be reminded to call their physician if they experience any symptoms in excess or different from what they have been told to expect. As well, the possibilities of post-operative fever and bleeding should be mentioned.

REFERENCES

1. Bird BJ, Chrisp DB, Scrimgeour G. Extensive pre-operative shaving: a costly exercise. N Z Med J 1984; 97:727-729.

2. Crawford ED, Haynes AL, Story MW, Borden TA. Prevention of urinary tract infection and sepsis following transrectal prostatic biopsy. J Urol 1982; 127:449-451.

3. Dajani AS, Taubert KA, Wilson W, Bolger AF. Prevention of bacterial endocarditis: Recommendations by the American Heart Association. JAMA 1997; 277:1794-1801.

4. Packer MG, Russo P, Fair WR. Prophylactic antibiotics and foley catheter use in transperineal needle biopsy of the prostate. J Urol 1984; 131:687-689.

5. Pound DC. Flexible sigmoidoscopy: Techniques and utilization. Baltimore: Williams & Wilkins, 1990:83.

6. Ruebush TK, McConville JH, Calia FM. A double-blind study of trimethoprim-sulfamethoxazole prophylaxis in patients having transrectal needle biopsy of the prostate. J Urol 1979; 122:492-494.

7. Seropian R, Reynolds BM. Wound infections after preoperative depilatory versus razor preparation. AM J Surg 1997; 121:251-254.

8. Wallner KE, Roy J, Harrison L. Low risk of perioperative infection without prophylactic antibiotics for transperineal prostate brachytherapy. Int J Radiat Oncol Biol Phys 1996; 36:681-683.

9. Williams-Russo P, Sharrock NE, Mattis S, Szatrowski TP. Cognitive effects after epidural vs general anesthesia in older adults. JAMA 1995; 274:44-50.

Chapter 8

TRUS implants: The procedure

The phenomenal renewed popularity of prostate brachytherapy is primarily due to the introduction of real-time transrectal ultrasound (TRUS) in the early 1980s. Although TRUS has drawbacks (see Chapter 3), it is a simple, direct way to verify proper needle placement within the prostate during transperineal brachytherapy.

SET-UP

Patient positioning

After induction of anesthesia, the patient is placed in the lithotomy position (**Figure 8-1 a and b**). It is best to reproduce the relationship between the TRUS probe and the prostate that was used at the time of the planning scan. However, the position of the prostate in relation to the pelvis is not fixed, and some deviation is unavoidable. The legs should be symmetrically rotated and extended at the hips and knees to avoid rotating the pelvis.

The extended lithotomy position will help reduce pubic arch interference when placing needles in the anterior portion of the prostate (**Figure 8-2**). The extended position requires bringing the knees toward the chest, thus tilting the pelvis back, which moves the pubic bones away from the anterior portion of the prostate. This position can be achieved by adjusting the leg stirrups (**Figure 8-1**). A wedge pillow under the buttocks may also help tilt the pelvis back.

CATHETER

A urinary catheter can be inserted to help visualize the urethra and bladder neck (**Figure 8-3**). If fluoroscopy is used during the procedure, the catheter balloon helps to locate the prostate base. During the set-up, moderate traction should be placed on the catheter, to ensure that the balloon is pulled against the prostate.

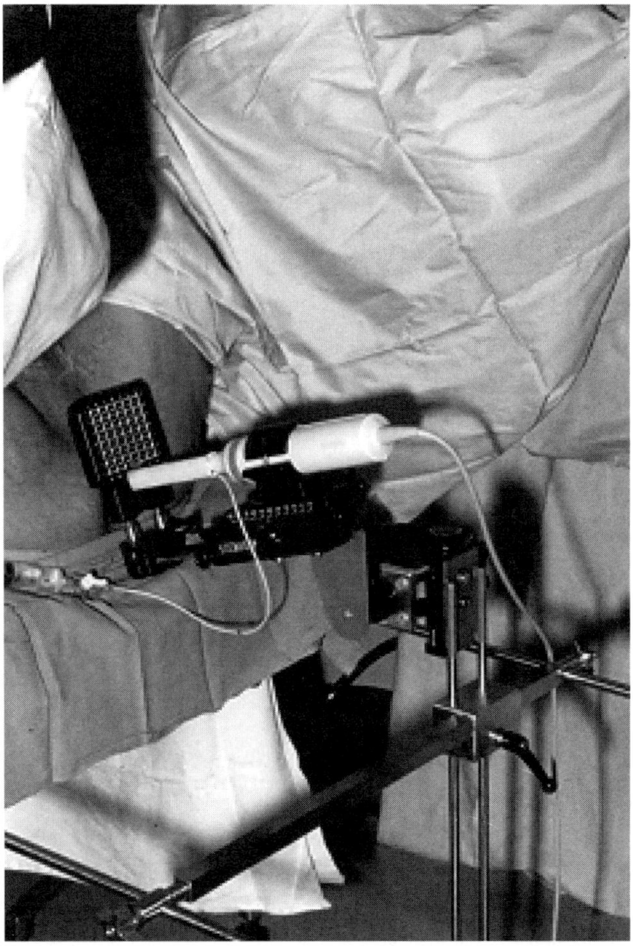

Figure 8-1a. Typical patient positioning at the University of Washington (J. Blasko).

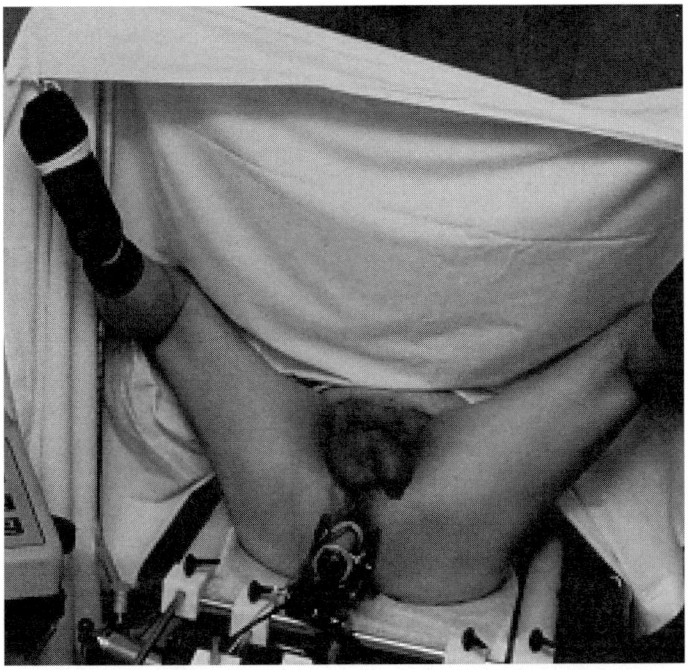

Figures 8-1b and c. Patient set-up by M. Dattoli. The hips are highly flexed in the extended lithotomy position, to avoid striking the pubic bones with the anterior needles. The patient above is having a TRUS planning scan in the office. The patient below is being prepped for the actual implant procedure.

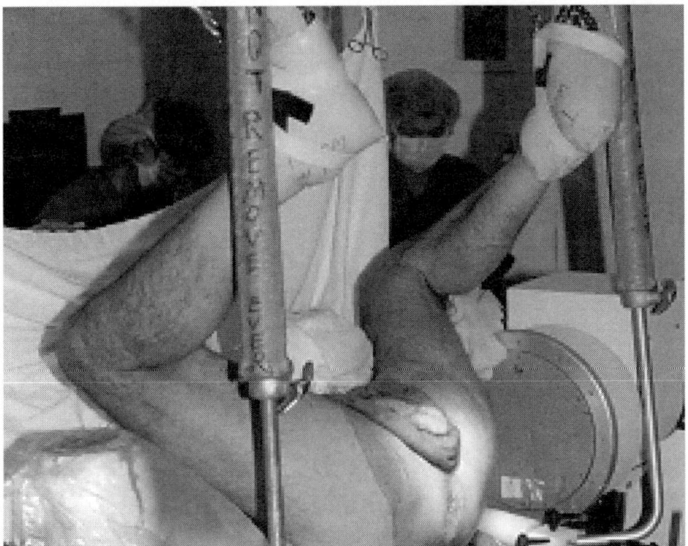

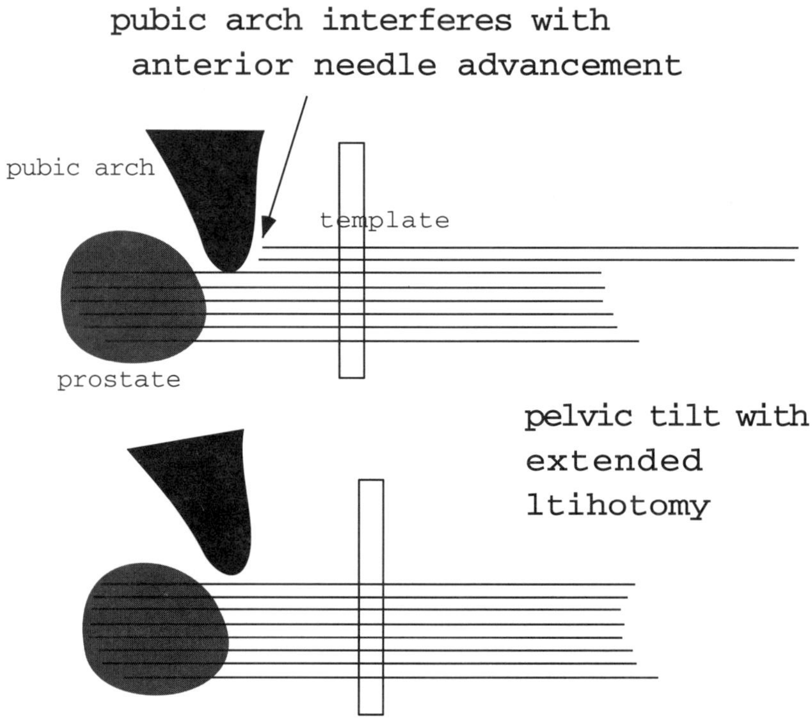

Figure 8-2. Effect of the extended lithotomy position on the pubic arch relationship with the anterior prostate. By tilting the pelvis back, there is more room to get past the pubic bones anteriorly.

If a urinary catheter is not used during the procedure, one can be placed temporarily prior to inserting needles, in order to inject 50 cc of water or dye into the bladder to help distinguish the prostate from the bladder base, both by ultrasound and fluoroscopy.

As an alternative to keeping a catheter in during the procedure, M. Dattoli places a catheter prior to starting the case and places 50 cc of 100% Renografin™ into the bladder, and takes a lateral fluoroscopic view. This reference image is held on the second fluoroscopy screen throughout the procedure itself, to show where the urethra is. After the reference image is taken, the catheter is removed for the implant procedure itself (**Figure 8-4**). The dye is left in the bladder during the procedure to help visualize the interface between bladder and the prostate on lateral or anterior fluoroscopy.

J. Blasko does not use a catheter during the procedure. Instead, 30 cc of Renografin™ is injected into the bladder, followed by 15 ml of aerated gel, held

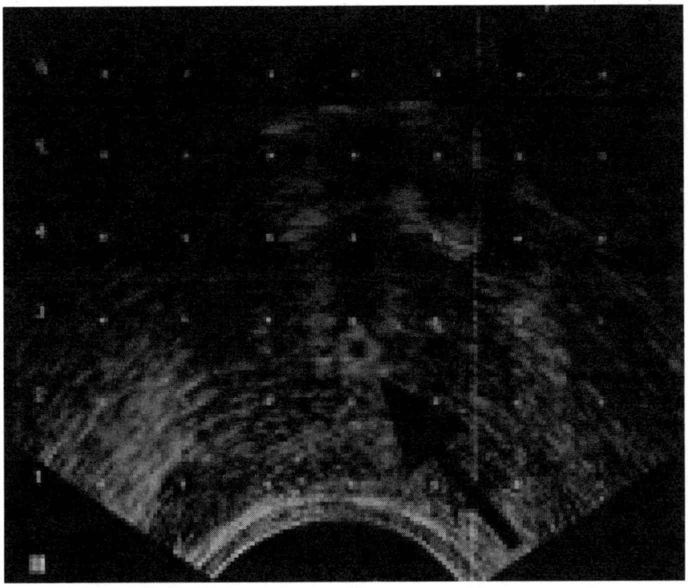

Figure 8-3. Axial TRUS image with urinary catheter in place (arrow). Identifying the urethra can help to avoid piercing it with needles.

inside the urethra by a penile clamp. The aerated gel provides accurate identification of the urethra by ultrasound during the procedure, without introducing artifact or prostate distortion from a catheter.

SCROTUM

The scrotum should be kept away from the perineum. It can be held up to the abdominal wall with tape or with a clear plastic tape sheet. A rolled up, wet reusable towel can be used (**Figure 8-1c**). Towel clips can be used to clip the scrotum against the abdominal wall, but add unnecessary trauma to the procedure.

TRUS PROBE

Both uniplane and biplane probes are available. The biplane probe allows the greatest flexibility, especially for looking at needle depth (**Figure 8-5**). Frequencies of 5, 6 or 7.5 megahertz are commonly used. The optimum choice of frequency depends on the prostate size, presence of calcium deposits, and other factors.

The probe should be covered generously with lubricant. An outer condom can be used, but may interfere with image quality. If an outer condom is used, it should be coated generously with lubricant.

The ultrasound probe is inserted into the rectum and attached to the stepping unit. Approximately 5 to 10 ml of fluid should be inserted into the balloon, and adjusted to minimize air artifact from the rectum. Excessive water should be avoided, as it may distort the image. The probe should be angled so that the nee-

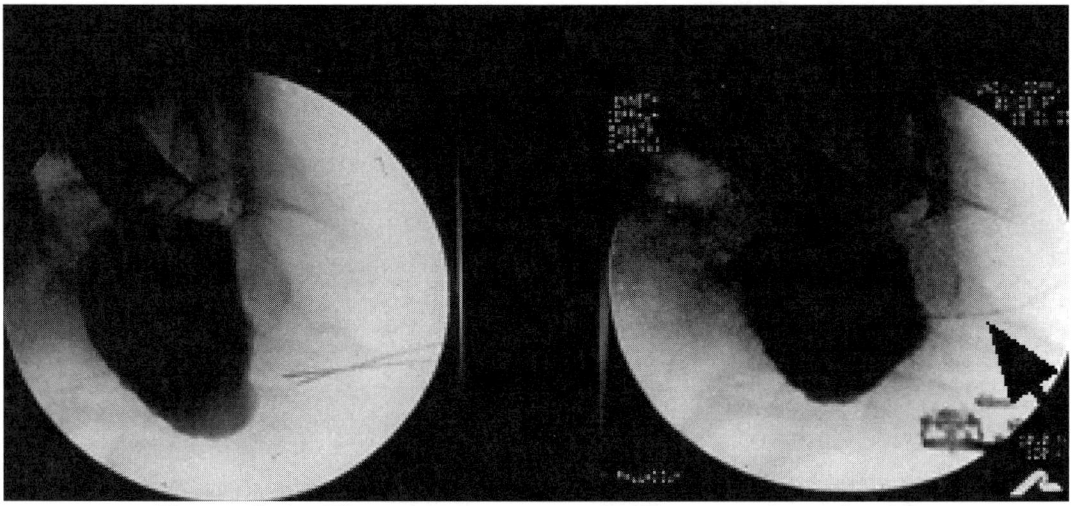

Figure 8-4. Fluoroscopy screen during procedure, for M. Dattoli. On the right is a pre-procedure view with a urinary catheter in place (arrow), and 50 ml Renografin™ in the bladder. The right-sided image is kept during the procedure, to help identify the urethra. The left screen is used during the procedure to help monitor needle and source placement. (Note posterior crossing stabilization needles on the left screen)

dle pathway will be as parallel to the rectal wall as possible so as to avoid needles passing through the rectal wall at the apical portion of the prostate.

The probe is held in place with a stepping unit connected to a mounting apparatus, that allows the probe to be moved caudad or cephalad at 0.5 cm intervals. A variety of stepping units are available. The unit must be capable of holding the probe steady, without obstructing access to the perineum (**Figure 8-5**). Ask for advice from an experienced colleague before choosing a system.

RECREATE THE PREPLANNING TRUS CROSS SECTIONS

Cross-sectional imaging of the prostate is affected by the angle of the probe. Ideally, the imaging planes during the implant procedure should match those for the planning images. The images often not do not match well. Lack of reproducibility may be due to day-to-day changes in the prostate shape and volume, or to technical factors.

To get identical views, one needs to slightly tilt the probe in various directions. It is easiest to do so at mid-prostate. The correlation with pre-planning images should be checked at other levels, once the mid-level section matches well with that of the planning scan.

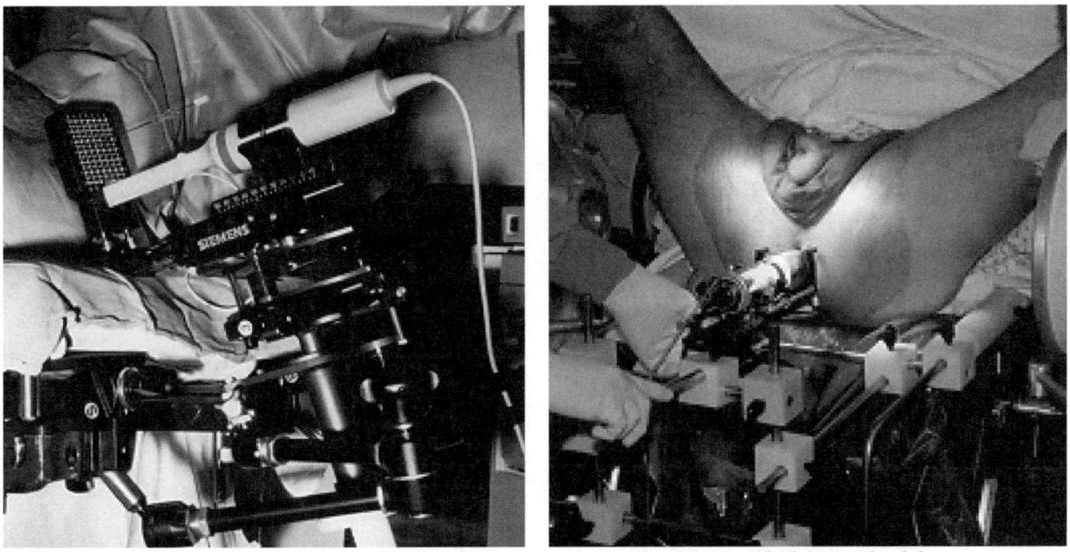

Figure 8-5. A variety of stepping units are available to hold the probe steady in relation to the patient without obstructing access to the probe and perineum.. A commercial system is used by J. Blasko at the University of Washington (left). A custom built device is used by M. Dattoli at University Community Hospital, Tampa.

NEEDLE-GUIDE TEMPLATE

A needle-guide template is positioned on the ultrasound probe, against the perineum. There should be 1 to 3 cm of space between the skin surface and the template, to allow for manual adjustment of the needles if necessary (**Figure 8-6**).

NEEDLE INSERTION

Once the TRUS probe positioning is adequate, needles are inserted through the template holes and the perineal skin. Piercing the skin can be difficult because of thick skin, or because of tangential orientation of the needles to the skin. If the skin is caught tangentially, the needle should be retracted and the skin held taught while the needle is re-inserted. To pierce thick skin, the needle should be pressed firmly against the skin surface and then advanced with a sudden, controlled thrust.

NEEDLE DEFLECTION

During insertion, needles are often deflected by the skin, the tissue planes, or anteriorly by the pubic bones. Deflection will cause the needle to appear in some other spot on the TRUS image than that predicted by the template coordinate at which it was inserted. Needle deflection is obvious on fluoroscopy. When

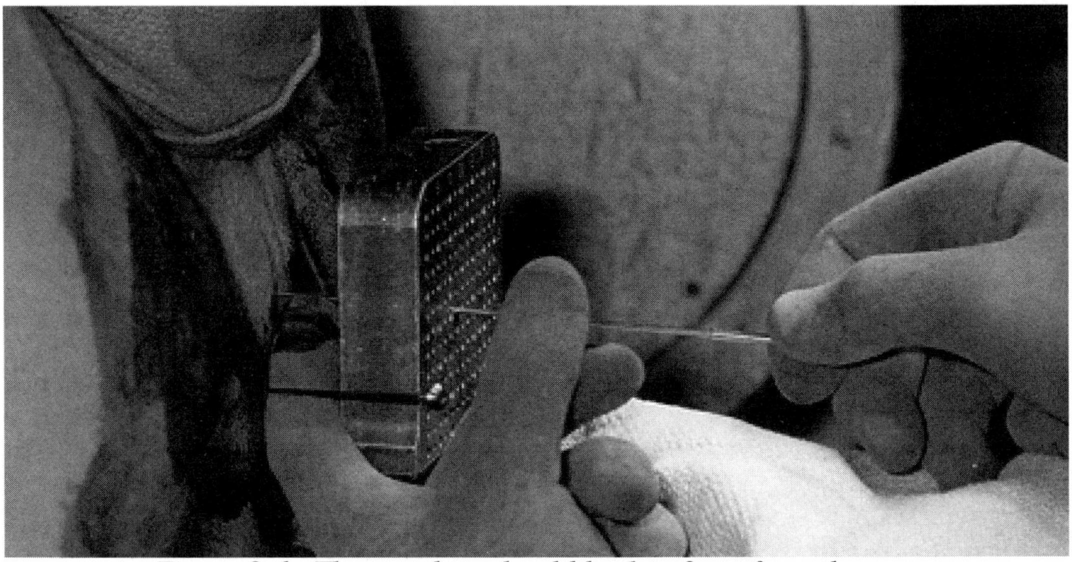

Figure 8-6. The template should be 1 to 3 cm from the perineal skin surface, to allow for digital manipulation of the needle.

deflection occurs, the needle should be withdrawn several centimeters, and re-inserted. Try twisting the needle during insertion may help get it through the offending tissue plane with less deflection. The needle path can be altered by pulling on the needle on the patient side of the template, as the needle is advanced (**Figure 8-6**). If the deflection still occurs, withdraw the needle and check that it is straight.

Hitting the pubic bones

The most anterior needles may strike the pubic bones. If they hit the bone squarely, they simply will not advance. If a needle glances the bone, it will deflect medially and/or posteriorly.

If the pubic bones are obstructing the needle path, the TRUS probe can be depressed posteriorly to give more room to clear the bones. However, doing so will alter the angle at which the prostate is imaged, which in turn will make some alteration in the shape and size of the prostate. Alternatively (additionally) the patient's legs can be positioned in a more extended lithotomy position, if feasible.

VISUALIZING NEEDLES

Once several needles are inserted, discerning others can be difficult, due to image degradation from ultrasound reflections (**Figure 8-7**). Burnished tip needles are easier to see on ultrasound, and provide more certainty as to where the

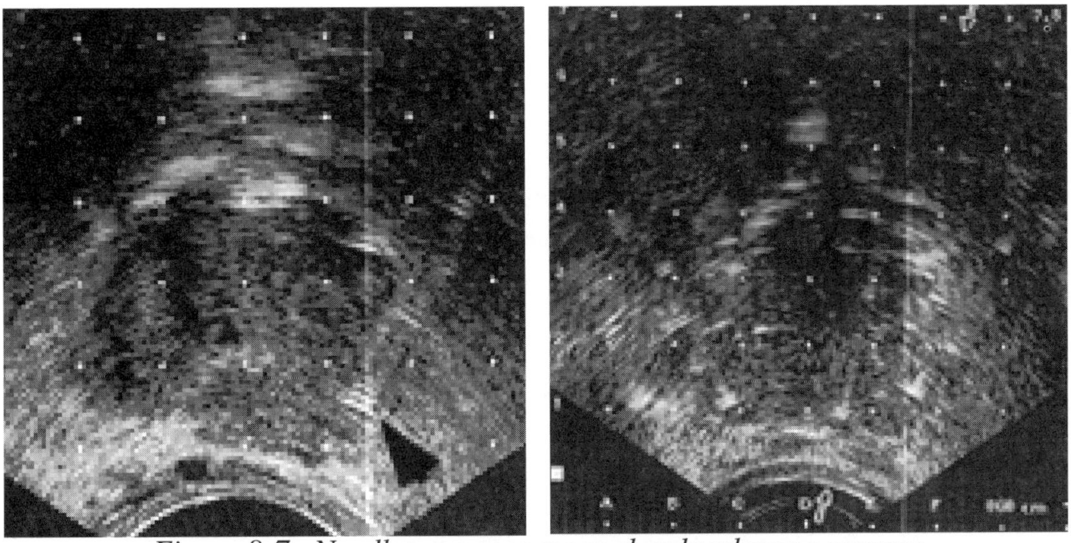

Figure 8-7. Needles are seen more clearly when no sources have been placed (left). Once a number of sources have been dropped, the position of other sources and needles is considerably obscured, and it is difficult to be certain of their proper position within the prostate (right). In this situation, fluoroscopy can be helpful as a check on proper placement.

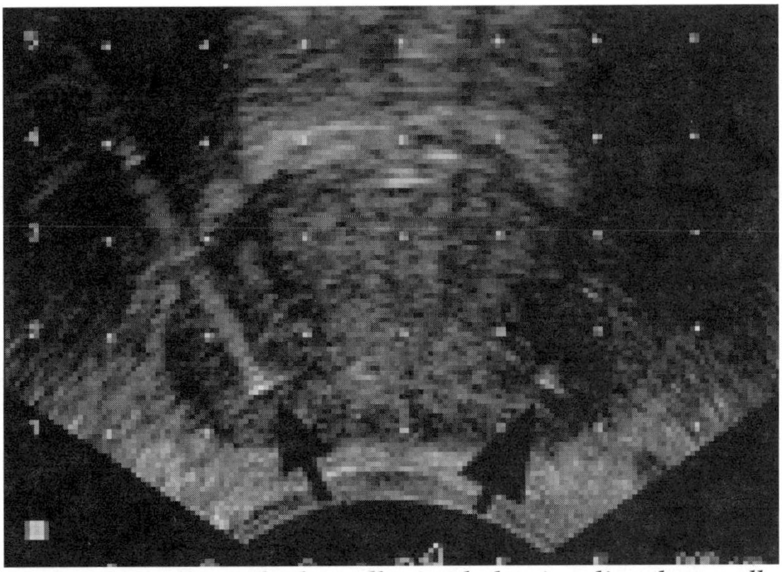

Figure 8-8. Burnished needle tips help visualize the needle on TRUS. The needle on the right of the page (larger arrow) has an unburnished tip. That on the left has a burnished tip, which enhances ultrasound reflection.

needle tip is (**Figure 8-8**). Image degradation can be minimized by inserting and loading the more anterior needles first, and then proceeding to the more posterior needles. This prevents the posterior needles from obscuring those more anterior.

NEEDLE DEPTH

Determining needle placement depth is as important to proper source placement as is correct positioning to the cross-sectional images. There are several ways to determine needle depth, and these methods can be combined to give extra confidence.

From the *0 plane*

Once the probe is positioned so the images match those of the pre-plan ones, the depth at which loading is to start should be determined. The deepest plane is at the bladder/prostate interface, the most reliable landmark for which is the junction of the seminal vesicles and bladder with the prostate (referred to as the *0 plane*) (**Figure 6-3**). This should match the deepest plane of the planning images.

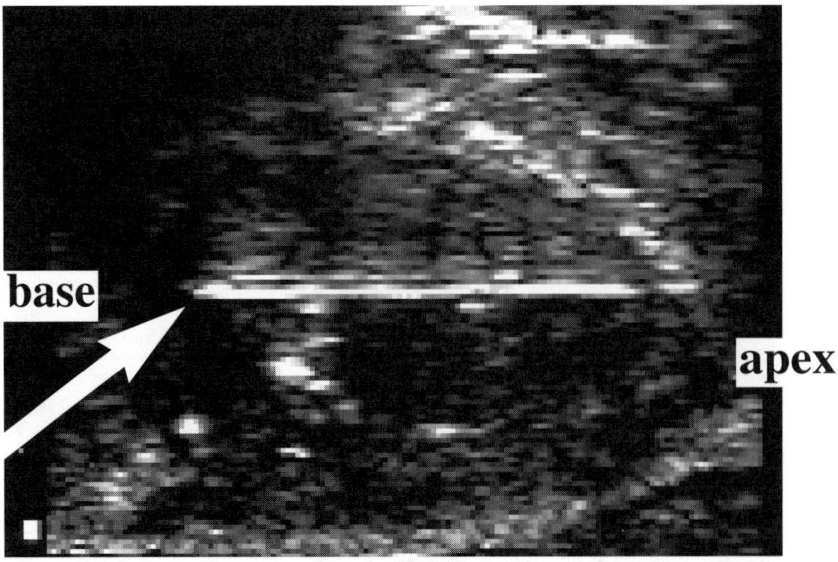

Figure 8-9. Longitudinal TRUS image, showing entire course of needle through the prostate. The tip (arrow) can be identified with more confidence when the length of the needles is visible (Courtesy of Richard Stock).

Longitudinal TRUS imaging

Visualizing a needle tip on cross-sectional images is often difficult, especially if multiple needles or sources are already in place. It may be easier to check the needle depth with longitudinal TRUS imaging because then the entire needle length can be imaged at once (**Figure 8-9**).

Fluoroscopy

Fluoroscopy can be used to check needle depth relative to the Foley balloon. The bottom of the balloon should be resting on the base of the prostate, which should be checked by tugging gently on the catheter. If the needle tip is at the prostate base, the tip of the needle should be within 2 to 4 mm of the inferior edge of the balloon.

In some patients the balloon is not a reliable indicator of the prostatic base location because of enlargement of the median lobe. Median lobe enlargement may be better appreciated with TRUS, and should be considered when interpreting fluoroscopic views.

PIERCING THE URETHRA

The urethra is probably pierced commonly during an implant procedure. To help visualize the urethra and to minimize the likelihood of piercing it, a catheter or aerated gel can be left in during the procedure (**Figures 8-3 and 8-4**).

It is unknown whether piercing increase the acute or chronic urethral morbidity, but it seems prudent to minimize doing so. It could be that urethral piercing increases the likelihood of acute urinary retention, although it has not been our impression that an inordinate number of needle insertions, as occurs in more difficult cases, leads to a higher likelihood of post-implant urinary retention.

PROTECTING THE RECTUM

If the prescription dose conforms closely to the posterior prostatic margin, and the plan is implemented correctly, there should be a minimal risk of rectal complications, which have been very infrequent in most implant series.

Nonetheless, one practical method commonly used to further ensure that rectal doses are not excessive is simply to make sure, using axial and/or lateral TRUS views, that no needle is closer than 0.5 cm to the anterior rectal wall.

PROSTATE MOTION

The prostate is highly mobile, as has been documented in the EBRT literature.[Crook 1995] The primary motion, in the absence of needle insertion, is in the anterior/posterior direction. During needle insertion, fluoroscopy commonly shows lateral and cephalad motion of one cm or more. Anterior displacement occurs when posteriorly placed needles strike the posterior surface tangentially.

Presumably, the prostate can also twist around its longitudinal axis, though the degree of twisting has not been documented. These motions can easily be viewed fluoroscopically, by looking at the change in the positions of the catheter balloon and of any sources already implanted.

Prostate mobility varies substantially from patient to patient, possibly due to differences in periprostatic fat, periprostatic veins, looseness of pelvic tissues, or changes in the organ's general muscle tone.

Several methods have been proposed to anchor the prostate, minimizing its motion. None is foolproof, though motion can be substantially decreased.

Tissue-gripping needles

One way to decrease prostate motion is to insert tissue-gripping needles that can hold the tissue and prevent motion along the needle tracks. Prostate fixation needles are commercially available (**Figure 8-10**). They are inserted on each side of the prostate, and have retractable hooks to grip the tissue once they are inserted. They diminish the degree of prostate mobility but some motion still occurs, partly because portions of the prostate can still move, independent of portions that contain stabilizing needles.

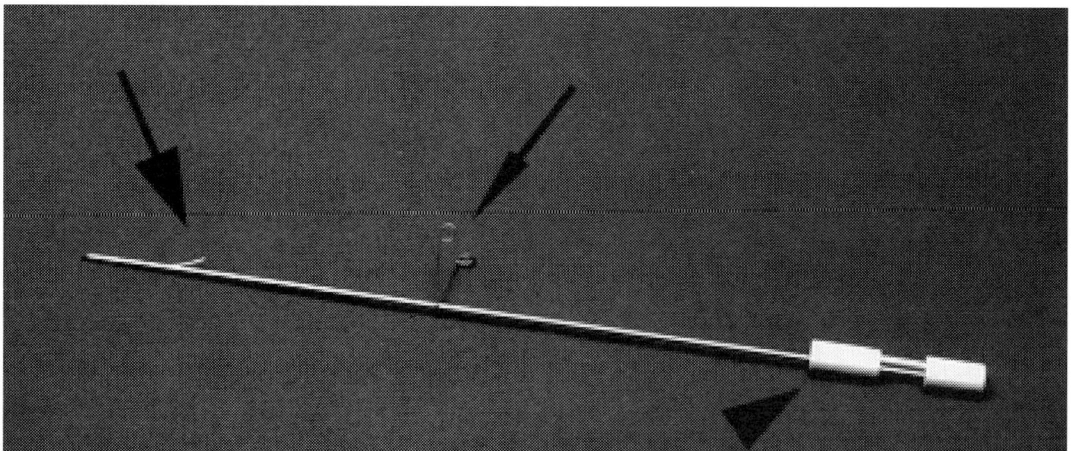

Figure 8-10. At least two types of stabilizing needles are commercially available. One is a Morganstern needle™, which has a single retractable tissue hook. The more proximal clip (arrow head) is snugged against the template, to prevent the needle from sliding in or out of the template once the needle is fixed in the tissue.

Crossing needles

Another method to decrease prostate motion is the insertion of two crossing needles through the prostate (**Figure 8-11**).(Dattoli 1997) Crossing needles limit prostate motion, presumably by piercing the pelvic floor musculature at an angle, thus limiting the likelihood that the prostate can slide cephalad along their length. This method works quite well, and does not require specialized needles. As with Morganstern needles™, some motion still occurs, making it important still to monitor the prostate position with TRUS and/or fluoroscopy.

SOURCE PLACEMENT

Placement of sources can be done with a variety of tools and techniques (See Chapter 5). Regardless of technique, a variety of errors can occur, requiring some adjustment in source placement during the procedure. Concentration and attention to detail can make the difference between a good and bad implant, regardless of one's experience.

The most likely problems during source placement are sliding of free sources along the needle track as the needle is withdrawn. This is apparently a vacuum phenomenon and can be largely avoided by moving needles slowly. Watching the sources under fluoroscopy during insertion is one way to guard against source misplacement. Often, source displacement can be corrected with judicious re-insertion or retraction of the needles, while watching the sources under fluoroscopy or ultrasound.

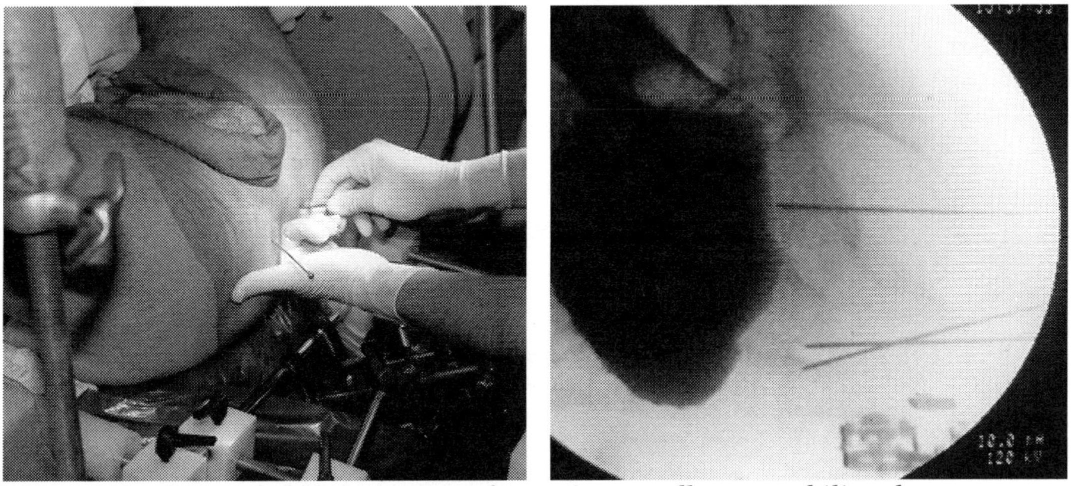

Figure 8-11. Insertion of crossing needles to stabilize the prostate, as done by M. Dattoli. On the right is a fluoroscopic view of the two crossing needles (arrow).

IMPLANTING THE ANTERIOR PROSTATE IN DIFFICULT CASES

The pubic arch often obstructs anterior needle placement, because the needles strike the inferior border of the pubic arch. This is more likely to occur in patients with larger prostate glands and in those with a narrow pelvis. While there are guidelines as to the largest prostate volume that should be implanted, such guidelines are not based on firm data. Patients with larger prostate glands can be adequately implanted if their pubic arches are wide enough. Several maneuvers can facilitate anterior needle placement.

Freehand

It is possible to remove the TRUS template, and place the sources by hand, using TRUS or anterior and lateral fluoroscopy to check for proper positioning in relation to the other sources or to the Foley catheter.

More extended lithotomy

By placing the patient in the extended lithotomy position, the pubic bones can be moved superiorly which allows more room under the pubic arch. To rotate the pelvis significantly, the hips must be flexed almost to where the thighs touch the abdomen. Less motion will not move the pubic bones enough, because there is considerable play at the hip joint. In using the extended lithotomy position, it should be kept in mind that the prostate orientation relative to the TRUS probe may change, leading to differences from the images used to plan the implant.

Angling the probe

Angling the probe posteriorly can help get under the pubic bones. One potential problem with probe angulation is that it changes the relationship of the probe to the prostate, which could lead to some shifting of the source location from what was intended.

FLUOROSCOPY

Most brachytherapists have fluoroscopy available during the implant procedure, as a supplemental imaging modality. Fluoroscopy helps give a general overview of how the procedure is proceeding, and is especially helpful after multiple sources have been placed, because artifact may make it difficult to see individual needles and sources with TRUS (**Figure 8-12**). Such artifact may arise from sources, calcium deposits, or hematoma formation in the course of the implant procedure.

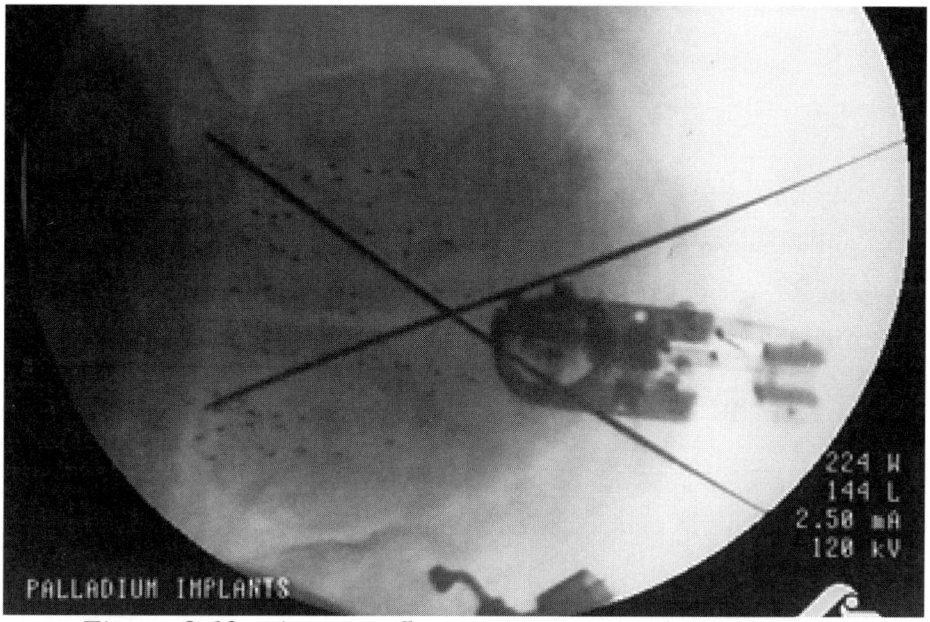

Figure 8-12. Anterior fluoroscopic view of TRUS procedure, upon completion of source placement. Fluoroscopy helps give a general overview of how the procedure is proceeding, and is especially helpful after multiple sources have been placed, because artifact makes it difficult to see individual sources by TRUS (see Figure 8-7).

POST-PROCEDURE CYSTOSCOPY

Cystoscopy is commonly performed immediately after the implant procedure to remove stray sources from the bladder and perhaps to remove sources that protrude into the urethral lumen. Bleeding points in the bladder could be cauterized and any clots removed lest they cause post-implant urinary obstruction. While all of these reasons for doing post-implant cystoscopy seem obvious, it should be pointed out that many brachytherapists do not routinely perform post-implant cystoscopy, with no known untoward effects from omitting it (see Chapter 16).

DO AWAY WITH PRE-PLANNING (?)

Stone, Stock and Dywngaart have reported extensively on TRUS-based implants, done without the use of pre-planning images. The prostate size is estimated from pre-implant TRUS, and the approximate number of sources needed is determined from a nomogram. At the time of the procedure, two thirds of the activity is placed at the prostatic periphery, and the remainder in the interior of the

Table 8-1. Pros and cons of pre-planning.

Pros	Cons
Better tailored to prostate contour	Prostate contour may change
Can anticipate difficult implants	More time-consuming (for physicist)
Helpful for less experienced teams	

gland. Satisfactory dosimetry is achievable with their method.(Stock 1995) There are pros and cons to pre-planning (**Table 8-1**).

THIS IS JUST A START

There are many ways to do transperineal implants. The methods described here are a general summary of the salient features of the authors' current techniques. Other brachytherapists use modifications of methods described here, some of which may be better than those described. Probably all brachytherapy teams change and improve their techniques over time. Good results are more dependent on the skill and experience of the brachytherapy team than on the particular methods used.

REFERENCES

1. Crook JM, Raymond Y, Salhani D, Yang H. Prostate motion during standard radiotherapy as assessed by fiducial markers. Radiother Oncol 1995; 37:35-42.

2. Dattoli M, Wallner K. A simple method to stabilize the prostate during transperineal prostate brachytherapy. Int J Radiat Oncol Biol Phys 1997; 38:341-342.

3. Stock RG, Stone NN, Wesson MF, DeWyngaert JK. A modified technique allowing interactive ultrasound-guided three-dimensional transperineal prostate implantation. Int J Radiat Oncol Biol Phys 1995; 32:219-225.

Chapter 9

CT-based implants

Nearly all prostate brachytherapy teams use TRUS to plan and implement their implants. It is generally assumed that TRUS is the reason that better quality implants became possible. Only partly true. Prostate brachytherapy improved with newer transperineal techniques which allowed assessment of the size and shape of the prostate, and verification of proper needle and source placement. While TRUS is the most commonly used method to make these determinations, CT scanning can accomplish the same end.

There is some skepticism among TRUS enthusiasts as to the legitimacy of CT-based implants. Keep an open mind. Each modality has advantages and disadvantages (see Chapter 3). CT-based implants have been performed at MSKCC since 1987, with biochemical-based tumor control rates comparable to those reported with TRUS-based methods.

The CT-based techniques described here sound complicated. However, they are not. Admittedly, they are not as intuitive as TRUS-based methods. In practice, though, they are quite simple and accurate. CT-based techniques continue to evolve, and those described here are somewhat different than previously reported.(Wallner 1991)(Wallner 1994)

BRIEF OVERVIEW

The urethra is the primary landmark for planning and verifying proper needle placement for CT-based implants. A urinary catheter is placed for the planning CT scan, to visualize the urethra on CT images. The prostate cross sections are then digitized, and a three-dimensional source placement plan is devised, as described in Chapter 5. The urethral position is marked on the planning images. The needle position relative to the urethra determines how the needles should appear on anterior and lateral fluoroscopic views at the time of the procedure.

At the time of the implant, a urethral catheter with a wire inside with lead markers at one cm intervals is inserted. The markers are readily visible on anterior and lateral fluoroscopy, and allow translation from a three-dimensional cross-sectional plan from the computer, to orthogonal fluoroscopic views taken in the operating room.

PLANNING SCAN

The planning CT scan is obtained several days prior to the procedure to allow sufficient time for dosimetric preparation and to order sources. The patient follows a standard lower GI preparation, and is scanned in the supine position. The patient is not in the lithotomy position during the scan. Moving the legs from supine to the standard lithotomy position does not substantially alter the position of the prostate in relation to the pubic arch (unpublished observation by K. Wallner).

A urinary catheter is placed for the CT scan. A coude catheter is used because it shows up well on CT images, and is usually easier to insert. No dye is placed in the catheter balloon, as it is easily visible on CT images. Fifty ml of 2:50 dye (diatrizoate meglumine/Renografen-60™) is placed in the bladder, to help distinguish the bladder wall from the prostate on the CT images (see **Figure 6-2**).

The prostate is scanned with 5 mm thick images, taken at 5 mm intervals from the top of the catheter balloon to the perineum, so that the entire needle path (prostate to perineum) is visualized. Only the cross-sectional images are printed. Scout views are not needed. Soft tissue CT window setting is used.

PREPARING THE PLAN

The prostatic margins, pubic arch, and urethra are digitized. A standard template pattern (0.5 cm spacing) is overlaid on the digitized images and preliminary source placement is entered to cover the periphery with the prescribed dose (**Figure 9-1**). The process of choosing source locations relative to the target, urethra and rectum is identical to that for TRUS-based implants, as described in Chapter 6.

Avoiding the pubic bones

A major advantage of CT-based treatment planning is that the pubic bones are well visualized, so that pubic arch interference can be anticipated and necessary adjustments in template position can be planned. To do so, the needle orientation is superimposed on the digitized planning images, and only those needles that avoid the pubic bones are used for source placement. If the anterior prostate cannot be covered adequately, the template can be shifted posteriorly and angled anteriorly to allow the more anterior needles to get under the pubic arch (**Figures 9-1 and 9-2**).

PATIENT POSITIONING

For the implant procedure, the patient is placed in the lithotomy position. The extended lithotomy position isn't necessary, because the template position will be adjusted, based on the CT-derived plan, to avoid the pubic bones (**Figure 9-3**).

A Foley catheter with radio-opaque markers at every one cm inside is placed. The markers are standard dummy sources (pre-loaded cable dummy ribbon, Best Medical International). Eight cc of diatrizoate meglumine (50% in water) is placed in the Foley balloon to allow easy visualization on fluoroscopy. No dye is placed inside the bladder.

TEMPLATE STAND

A template stand is used to hold the template steady, while allowing spatial adjustments. Various stands have been devised.[Wallner 1991] A commercial version is available from Mick Nuclear (**Figure 9-4**).

NEEDLE PLACEMENT

Anterior needles

The needle guide template is mounted against the perineum and three needles are inserted (**Figure 9-3**). The first two needles are chosen by studying the cross-sectional planning images. They should be just posterior to midplane, on each side of the urethra. Ideally, they should bracket the urethra evenly, to make it easier to judge their proper positioning. In patients with asymmetry of the

0 plane

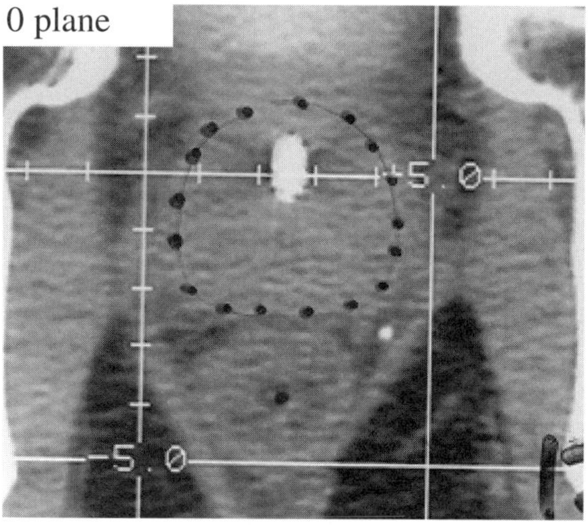

0 plane

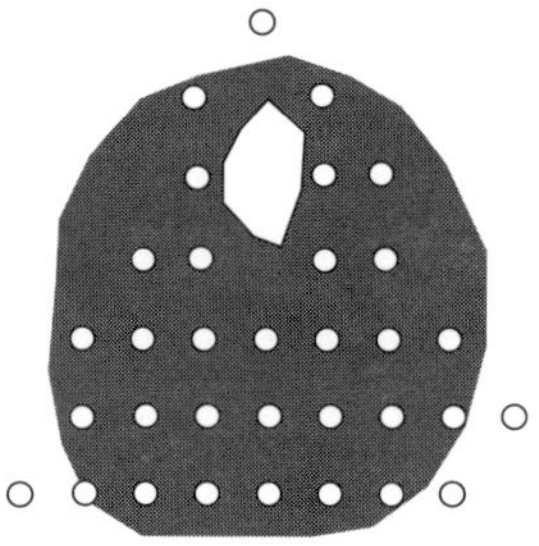

10 plane

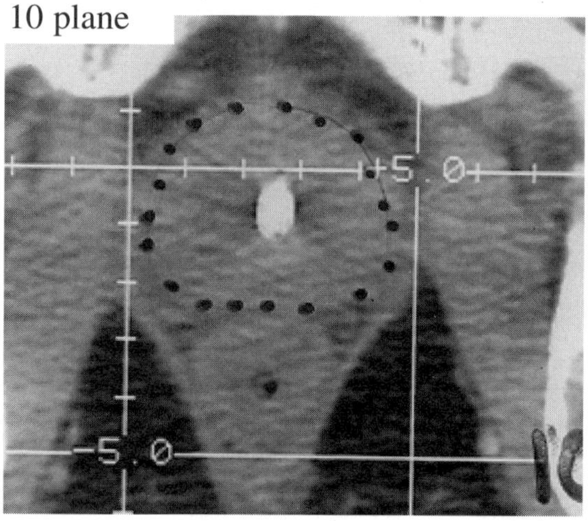

10 plane

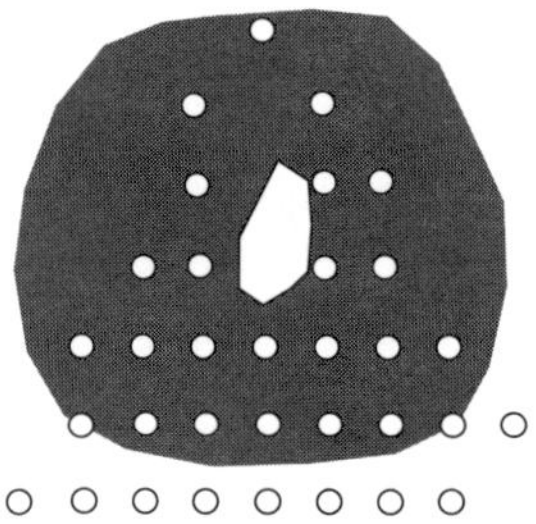

20 plane

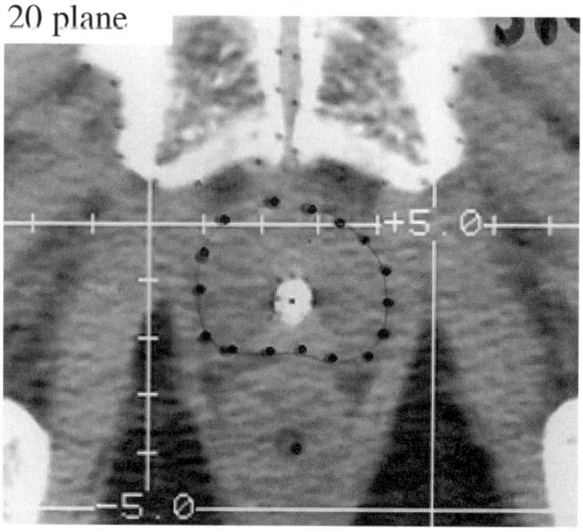

20 plane

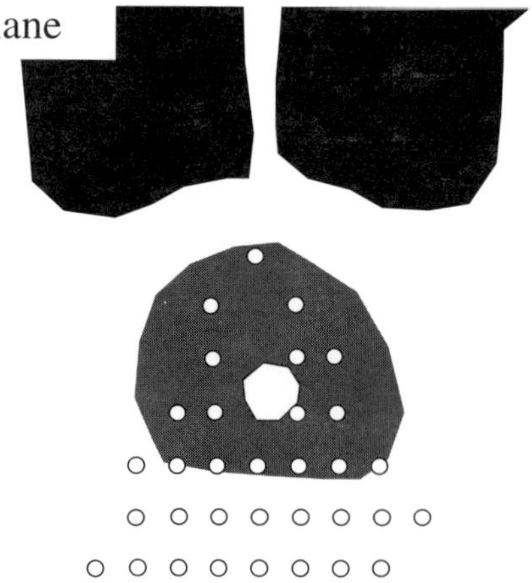

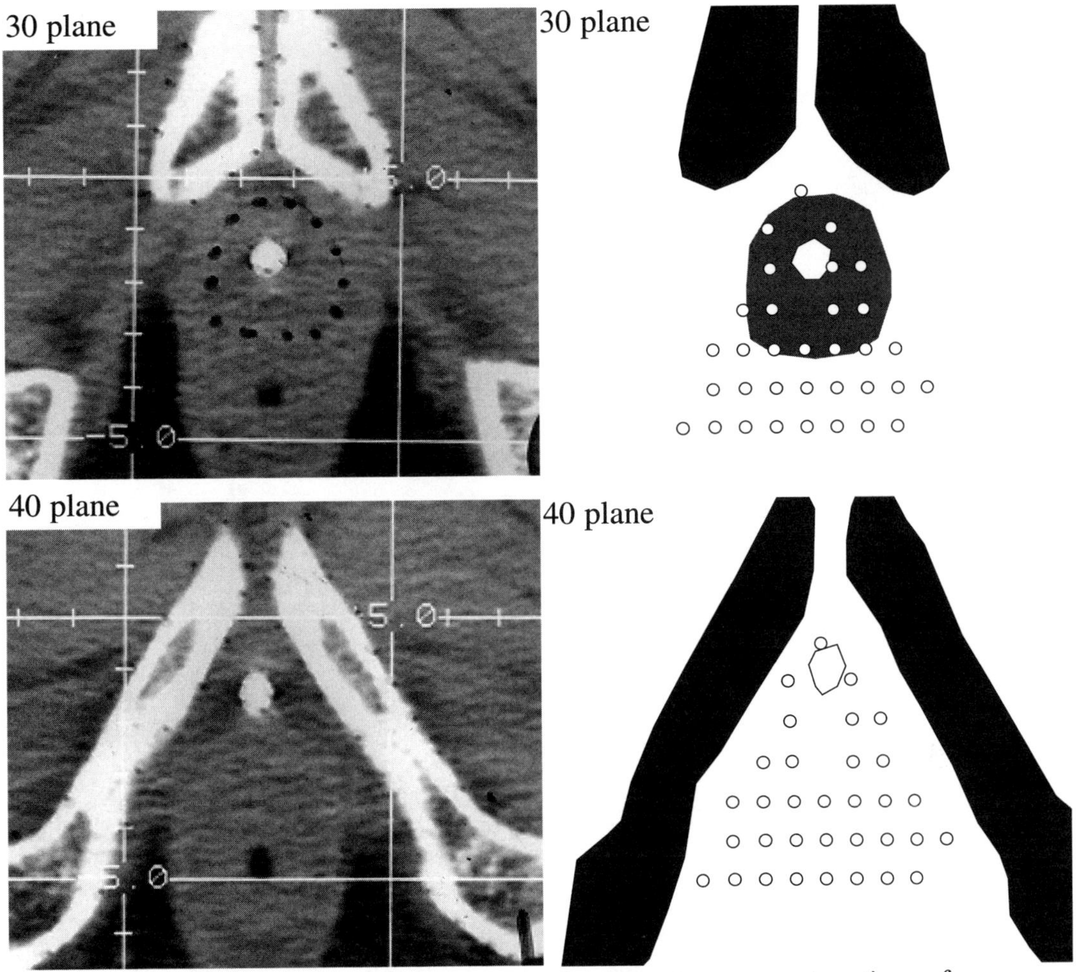

Figure 9-1. CT images and computer reconstruction of actual case. Only those needles which do not strike the pubic bones are used for source planning. This assures that the implant is planned with only those needles whose placement is possible. If not enough anterior needle positions are available to cover the anterior prostate, the template can be moved posteriorly and/or angled more anteriorly (Figure 9-2). (This figure shows an extreme case, in which the pubic arch is narrower than usual.)

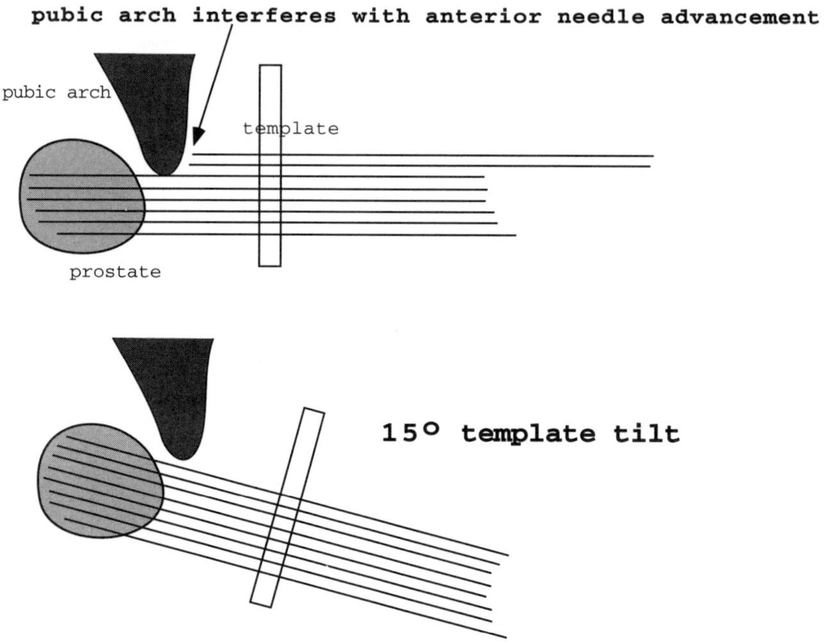

Figure 9-2. CT-based implants allow visualization of the pubic bones, which are digitized for planning. By doing so, pubic arch interference is anticipated, and the template can be tilted and/or moved posteriorly to avoid striking the pubic bones with the needles.

prostate gland, the urethra may deviate, and no needles will bracket the urethra perfectly (**Figure 9-5**). The actual choice of needles does not make much difference, as long as their position on anterior and lateral fluoroscopy matches that of the CT-based plan.

The first two needles are inserted simultaneously, to minimize lateral movement of the prostate. The position of the needles is checked on anterior and lateral fluoroscopy. If their relationship to the urethra does not match that on the plan, they are withdrawn, the template is moved right or left, and they are re-inserted. This process is repeated until the needles bracket the urethra as they do on the pre-implant CT scan images (**Figures 9-5a and 9-5b**).

Of course, things often don't happen in real life the way textbooks tell us they will. For example, often the urethra is not perfectly midline, and the needles do not bracket it in a nice parallel fashion. No matter. The technique still works; it's just not as pretty. **Figures 9-6a and b** show an actual case, with the initial two needles seen on anterior and lateral fluoroscopy.

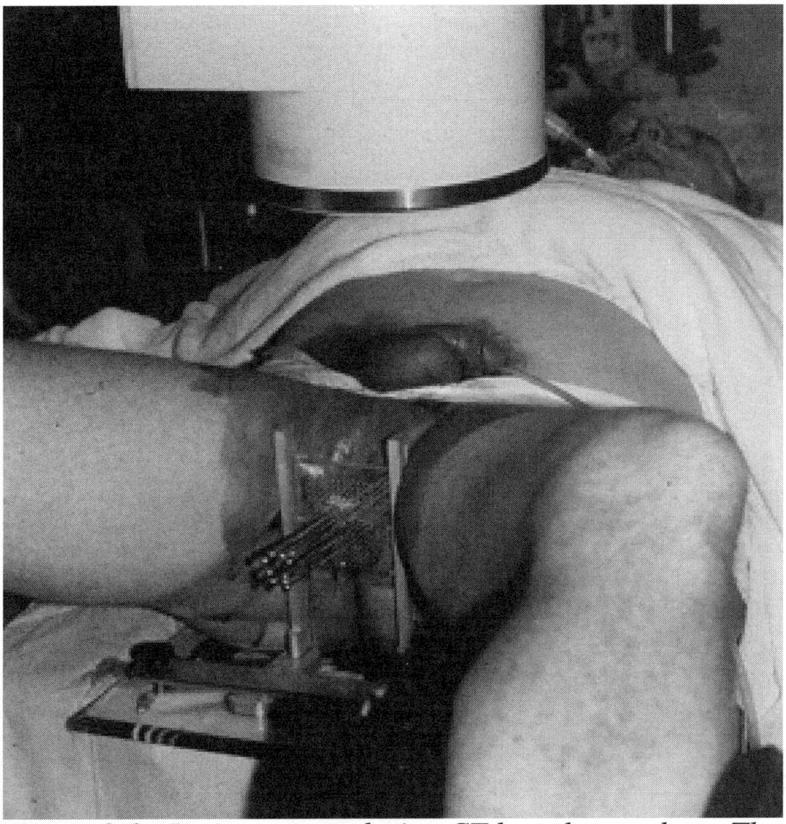

Figure 9-3. Patient set-up during CT-based procedure. The template stand is not sterile, but the template is. The template is re-positioned with the left hand (non-sterile), while needles are placed with the right hand (sterile).

Template positioning is the most time-consuming part of the procedure, because several repositionings may be required before satisfactory placement is achieved. It is done most efficiently by moving the template with the left hand, while keeping the right hand glove sterile to remove and insert the needles. By doing so, correct positioning can usually be achieved in several minutes.

Once the initial needles are properly positioned, to place the sources additional needles are inserted and withdrawn in groups.

NEEDLE ORDER

The prostate is remarkably mobile in all directions. To help minimize the effect of prostate mobility, it is advisable to insert all the anterior needles first. The anterior sources are then placed, leaving only 2-4 needles at midplane (**Figures 9-7, 9-8**). Then the posterior needles are inserted. These are inserted separately because of their tendency to displace the prostate anteriorly, even when several anterior needles are already in place.

The posterior needles also tend to deflect posteriorly as they strike the posterior capsule, potentially placing sources too close to the rectum. In practice, to compensate for posterior deflection, the template usually must be tilted superiorly (anteriorly on the patient) when placing the posterior needles. The more anterior needles still in place should not be re-inserted once the template tilt has been changed. Their position would change if they were withdrawn and replaced after the template tilt had been changed.

JUDGING DISTANCES ON FLUOROSCOPY

The 1 cm urethra markers are used to judge distances on the fluoroscopic images. With magnification of the fluoroscopic images, one can judge distances accurately to within 1 to 2 mm. That's close enough.

SOURCE PLACEMENT

Sources can be inserted with a Mick applicator™, pre-loaded needles, or RAPIDStrand™. K. Wallner uses a Mick applicator™, because it provides for the adjustment of source placement slightly, depending on the degree of source misplacement that may have occurred during the procedure.

NEEDLE DEPTH

The needle depth is determined from the lower edge of the Foley balloon, as visualized fluoroscopically. The deepest (most caudal) plane is usually just inferior to the lower edge of the balloon. However, in patients with a prominent median lobe, the most cephalad slice may actually be more proximal than the inferior balloon edge.

When using the Mick applicator™, the needle is pulled back, from the *0 plane* to appropriate CT planes, at 5 mm intervals. With experience, the distances are estimated by looking at the position of the needle tip in relation to the 1 cm markers in the urethra; this way is faster and allows adjustment in needle withdrawal to accommodate motion of the prostate as the needle is being withdrawn.

One way to verify that the needle tip is at the base of the prostate is to gently advance the needle several mm past that point, while watching fluoroscopically. If the needle tip is against the prostatic base, further advancement moves the entire prostate, visible by watching the catheter balloon and/or the sources already implanted (**Figure 9-9**).

WATCH WHAT'S HAPPENING

As each needle is withdrawn, the actual source placement should be viewed fluoroscopically and compared with the planned separation between

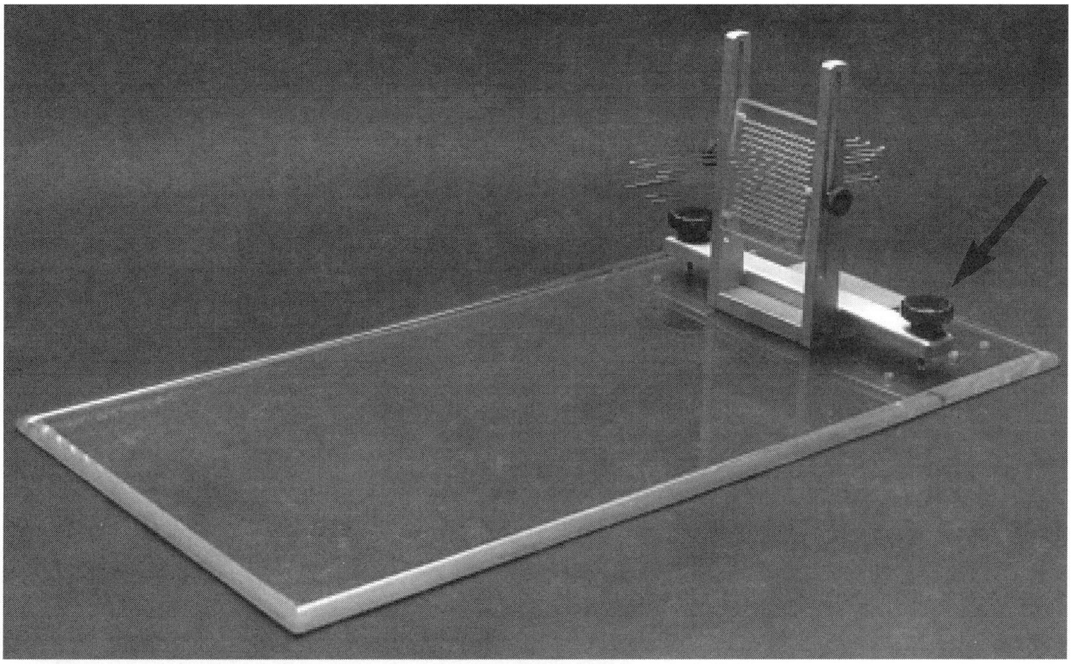

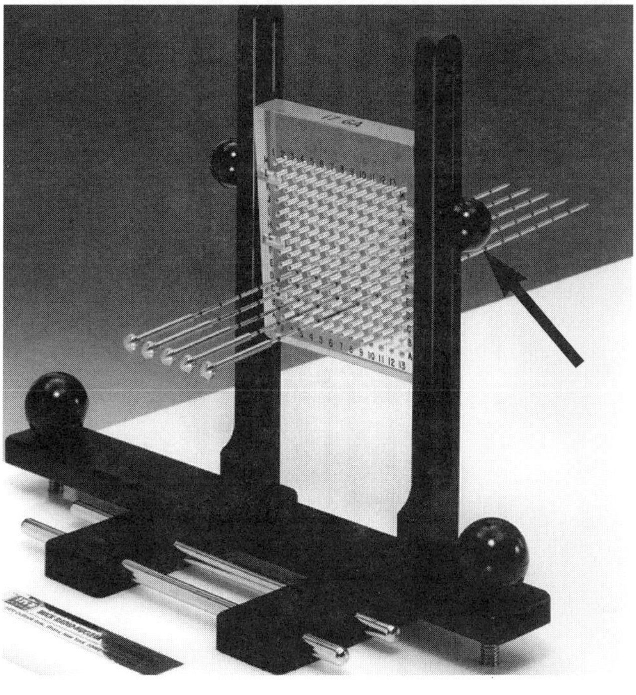

Figure 9-4. A variety of template stands have been used. Above is a recent version used by K. Wallner. It was custom designed and built. The template can be adjusted in all directions, by loosening the base plate screws or the screws holding the template to the stand (arrow). To the left is a template stand manufactured by Mick Nuclear. The template is tilted, raised and lowered by loosening the side mount screws (arrow). The template can be angled to the left or right by first loosening the base plate screws.

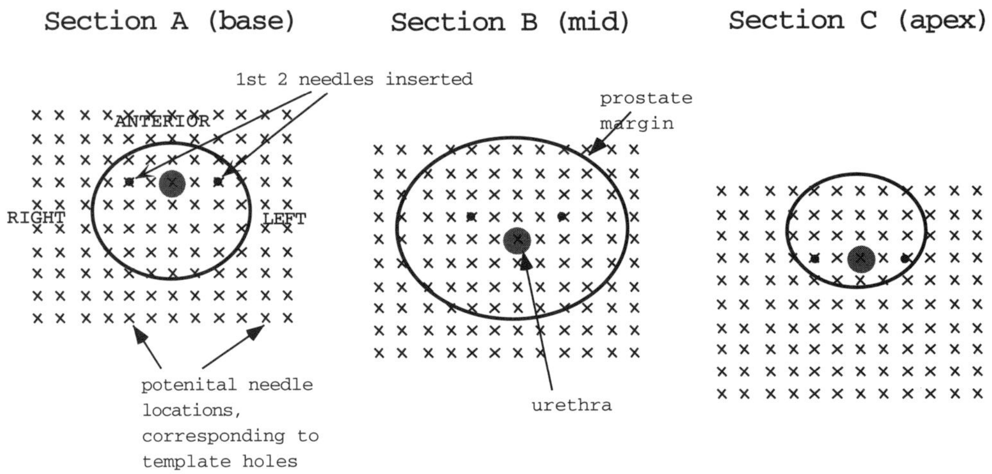

Figure 9-5a. Cross sections through the prostate, digitized from the planning CT scan. Potential needle paths, corresponding to the 0.5 cm spacing of the template, are marked by Xs. The urethra is identified on each CT slice, and its location is used to determine proper needle placement fluoroscopically during the implant procedure.

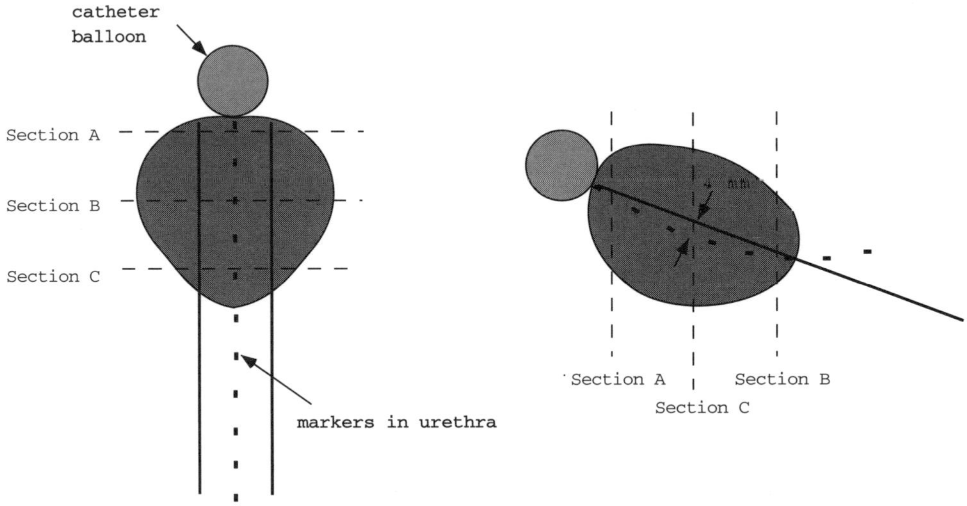

*Figure 9-5b. Schematic, fluoroscopic view of needle paths in the anterior and lateral projection, with two needles shown on planning images above (***Figure 9-5a***). The needles are symmetric to the urethra on the anterior projection, as in the CT scan images. On the lateral projection, the needles are level with the urethra at the prostate base and apex, and 4 mm anterior to the urethra at the mid prostate.*

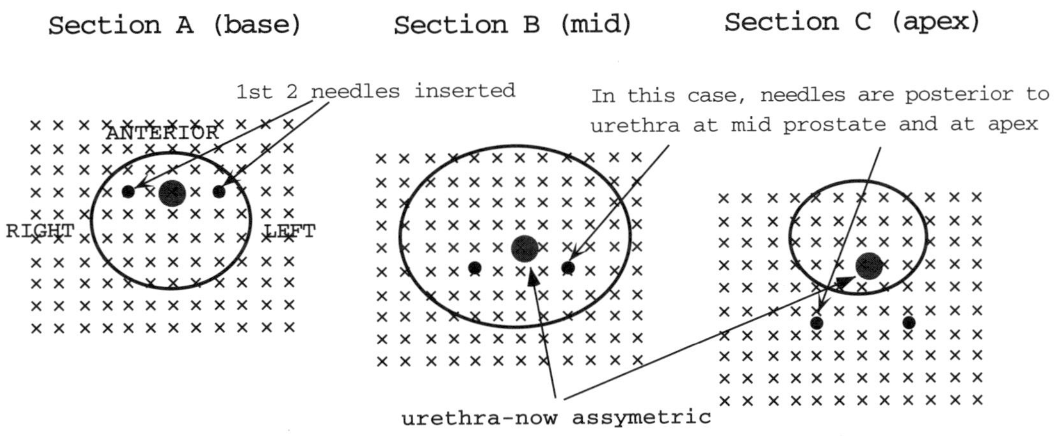

Figure 9-6a. Cross sections through prostate, digitized from the planning CT scan from an actual patient, whose urethra deviates from right to left, moving caudad.

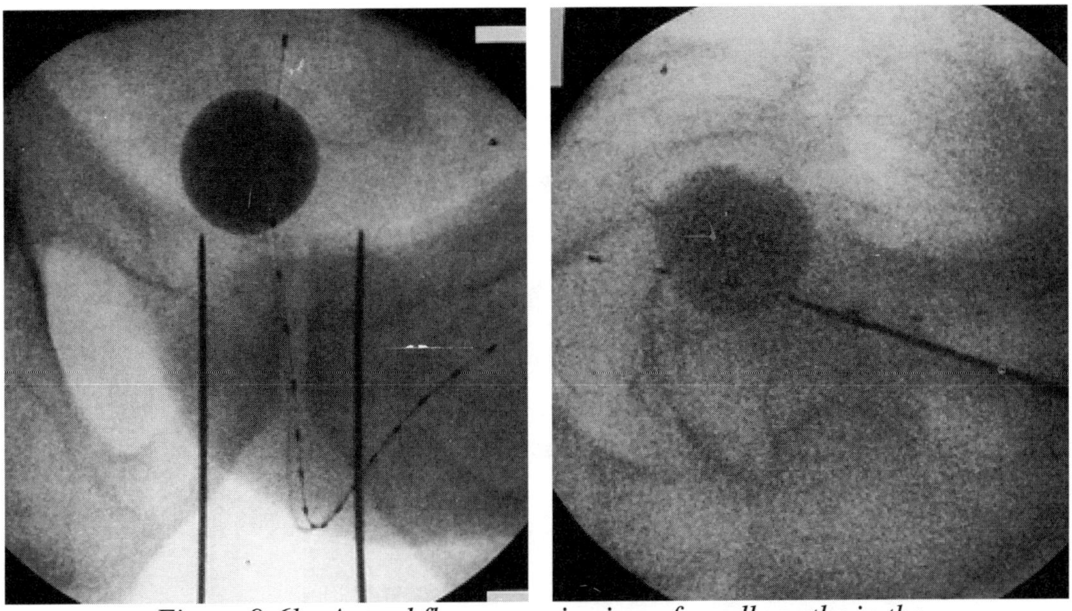

Figure 9-6b. Actual fluoroscopic view of needle paths in the anterior and lateral projection for the patient in 9-6a. Unlike the ideal case in Figure 9-5, the needles are asymmetric around the urethra on the anterior projection, as predicted from the CT scan images. On the lateral projection, the needles are level with the urethra at the prostate base, and 4 mm posterior to the urethra, 2 cm distal to the base.

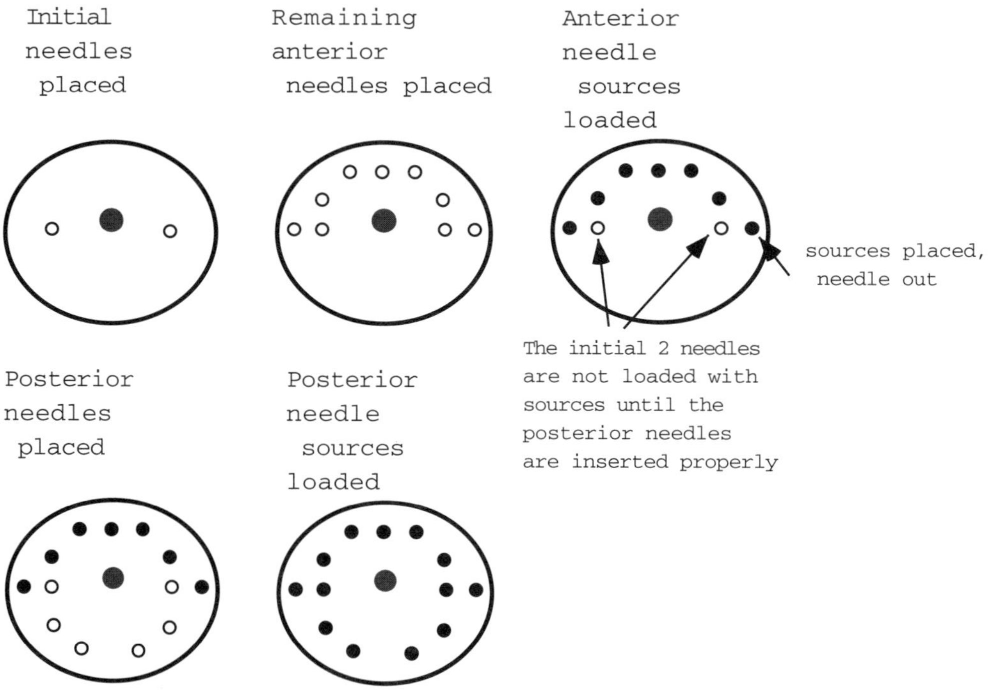

Figure 9-7. Schematic of the order in which anterior and then posterior needles are positioned and then loaded.

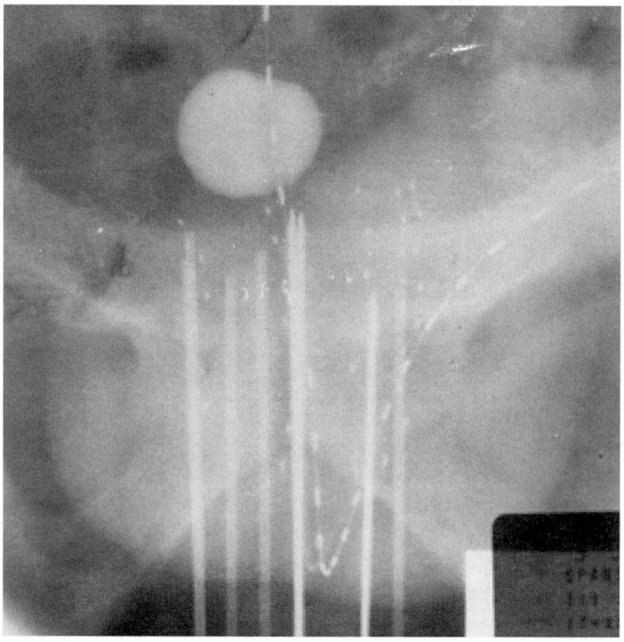

Figure 9-8. Fluoroscopic view during procedure, after the anterior sources and several posterior needles have been placed.

sources. To accommodate imperfect source placement along needle tracks, adjustments in subsequent source placement are made during the procedure.

FLUOROSCOPY TIME

With the CT-based implant method described here, fluoroscopy is the primary tool used to confirm proper needle and source placement. In experienced hands, the total fluoroscopic time is approximately five minutes, comparable to a cardiac catheterization procedure (**Figure 9-10**).

RECTAL MARKER

The use of a rigid rectal marker has been described in earlier publications regarding CT-based implantation techniques.(Nori 1990)(Wallner 1991) For performing the technique as described above, a rectal marker is not necessary and potentially misleading. The location of a rectal marker can vary, due to distensibility of the rectum. If the needle and source positionings are done properly, using the urethra as the landmark, the sources will be the proper distance from the rectal wall.

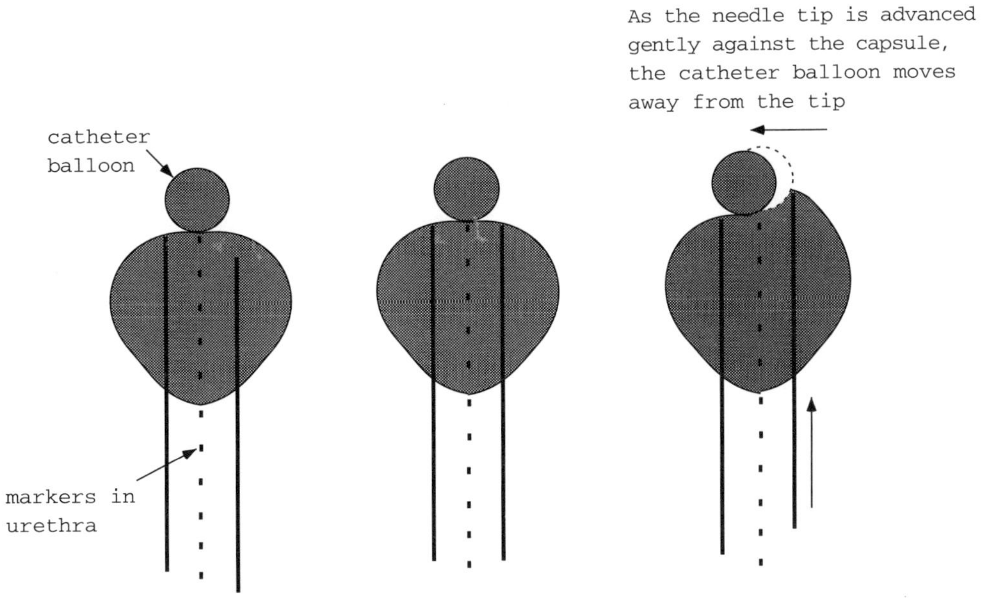

Figure 9-9. Use of fluoroscopy to help verify that a needle tip is against the prostatic capsule. When the needle tip is pushed against the capsule, the catheter balloon moves to the left, as the prostate is deformed.

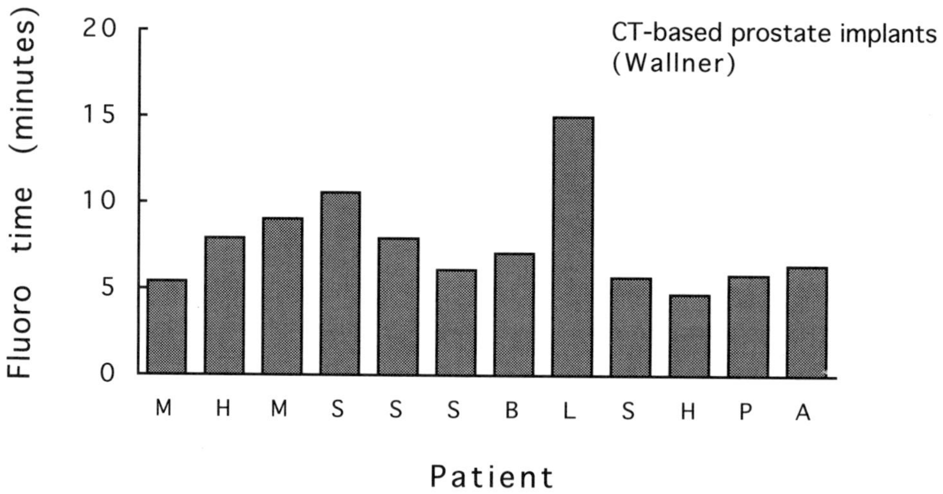

Figure 9-10. Fluoroscopy time for 10 patients implanted by K. Wallner in 1996. The times can be far greater if a resident trainee helps.

THIS COULD BE DONE WITH MR

The method described here could just as easily be done with magnetic resonance images (MR), using anterior and lateral fluoroscopy to verify needle positioning at the time of the procedure. All that is required is a urinary catheter at the time of the MR, to allow for urethral localization on the images. As with CT, intra-operative fluoroscopy could be used to implement a plan based on MR images. For investigators contemplating MR-based implants, the method described here would offer a simple way to do them, without the need for an MR scanner in the operating room.

ADDING TRUS

TRUS can be used simultaneously with CT-based implants, to give added confidence as to the proper needle positioning. When CT-based implant methodology was being perfected by K. Wallner, D. Nori and others during the early 1990s, supplemental TRUS was commonly used as a check on proper needle positioning.

YOU SHOULD WATCH THIS BEING DONE

The CT method described here is not as intuitive as TRUS-based methods. If you are considering adopting it in some form, it would be wise to observe it at one or more of the institutions where it is used routinely.

CT-BASED IMPLANTS HAVE STOOD THE TEST OF TIME

CT-based implants strike some as primitive compared to TRUS-based methods. But they are not. The results have stood the test of time, including a low risk of impotence and relatively high rates of biochemical tumor control.[Wallner 1996] In experienced hands, the procedure can be completed within 30-40 minutes, from the time the patient is anesthetized.

REFERENCES

1. Nori D, Donath D, Hilaris BS, et al. Precision Transperineal Brachytherapy in the Treatment of Early Prostate Cancer. Endo/Hypertherm 1990; 6:119-130.

2. Wallner KE, Chiu-Tsao S, Roy J, et al. An Improved Method for Transperineal Prostate Implants. J Urol 1991; 146:90-95.

3. Wallner KE, Roy J, Harrison L. Tumor control and morbidity following transperineal I-125 implantation for Stage T1/T2 prostatic carcinoma. J Clin Oncol 1996; 14:449-453.

4. Wallner KE, Roy J, Zelefsky M, Fuks Z, Harrison L. Fluoroscopic visualization of the prostatic urethra to guide transperineal prostate implantation. Int J Radiat Oncol Biol Phys 1994; 29:863-867.

Chapter 10

Evaluation

Prostate brachytherapy is often tricky. Factors such as prostate motion, TRUS imaging artifact, and sliding of radioactive sources in the needle tracks can lead to errors in carrying out a computer-generated plan. Some form of quality assurance is needed to provide feedback to the brachytherapy team regarding the adequacy of their implants, and to guide efforts to improve. Unfortunately, no generally accepted and verified system to evaluate implant quality exists.

Parameters commonly used to evaluate implant quality include total activity implanted, matched peripheral dose (MPD) and CT-based dosimetry (**Table 10-1**). In the past, total activity implanted and matched peripheral dose were the standard criteria for evaluating and reporting the quality of permanent implants. Both

Table 10-1. Ways to evaluate the technical adequacy of prostate brachytherapy.

Method	Pros	Cons
Total activity	Simple	Meaningless, except in extreme cases
MPD	Widely used in past	Misleading, almost meaningless
CT-based	Can relate sources to target	Uncertainty of prostate margins Proper timing uncertain Expensive

are crude indices, at best. CT-based evaluations hold the greatest promise for meaningful implant appraisal because CT shows both the sources and the prostatic margins, but there is still no generally accepted criteria to interpret post-implant CT scans.

TOTAL ACTIVITY

The simplest way to describe an implant is to state the total amount of radioactivity implanted. Total activity is a very crude indication of quality, because it gives no indication of the spatial relationship between dose levels and the prostate margins. If the amount of activity is similar to what is normally used, it does not mean much. However, the total amount of activity implanted can be telling if it is far from the norm. If thc total activity is very low, it is likely that the prostate is not covered adequately (unless the gland is very small). If the total activity is very high, a patient may be at higher risk of radiation complications (unless the gland is very large)

The total activity used for prostate brachytherapy has increased over the years. The total used in older, retropubic series was approximately half of what is currently used for transperineal brachytherapy (**Figure 10-1**). Higher activity in transperineal series probably reflects more accurate determination of prostate volume and shape with TRUS or CT imaging, and a better match of isodose lines to the prostate periphery than was achieved using, crude, nomogram-derived activity calculations with retropubic implants.

MPD

The matched peripheral dose (MPD) is an ingenious concept devised by Lowell Anderson at MSKCC, before the wide availability of CT-based dosime-

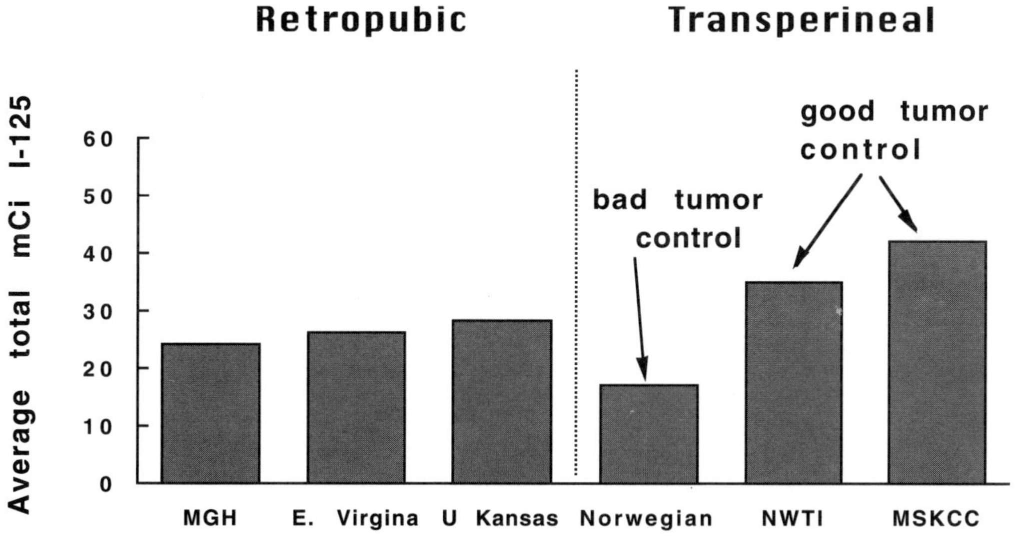

Figure 10-1. Total activity used for retropubic and transperineal implants. Clinical results from the Norwegian Radium Hospital were abysmal. (Waehre 1992) *A very low amount of I-125 was used, and there was apparently no quality assurance system in place. With such low amounts of activity, the target coverage would almost certainly have been poor. (MGH=Massachusetts General Hospital, E. Virginia=Eastern Virginia Medical School, Norwegian=Norwegian Radium Hospital)*

try.(Anderson 1993) The MPD is the dose for which the isodose contour volume equals the volume of an ellipsoid having the same orthogonal dimensions as the target volume. To calculate the MPD, source position is reproduced in three dimensions using isocentric or stereo-shift films. Dose to a lattice of points throughout the implant volume is determined by summing the contribution from each source, using computerized dose look-up tables. Several isodoses and their corresponding volumes are graphed. The MPD, corresponding to the ellipsoidal volume estimation y-axis), is taken from the x-axis of the graph (**Figure 10-2**). The MPD isodose line can be drawn in relation to the sources, on the original set of post-implant radiographs (**Figure 10-3**). Points outside the MPD volume receive less than the MPD dose. The actual isodose volumes, calculated from source positions on orthogonal films, are accurate. However, without CT-derived

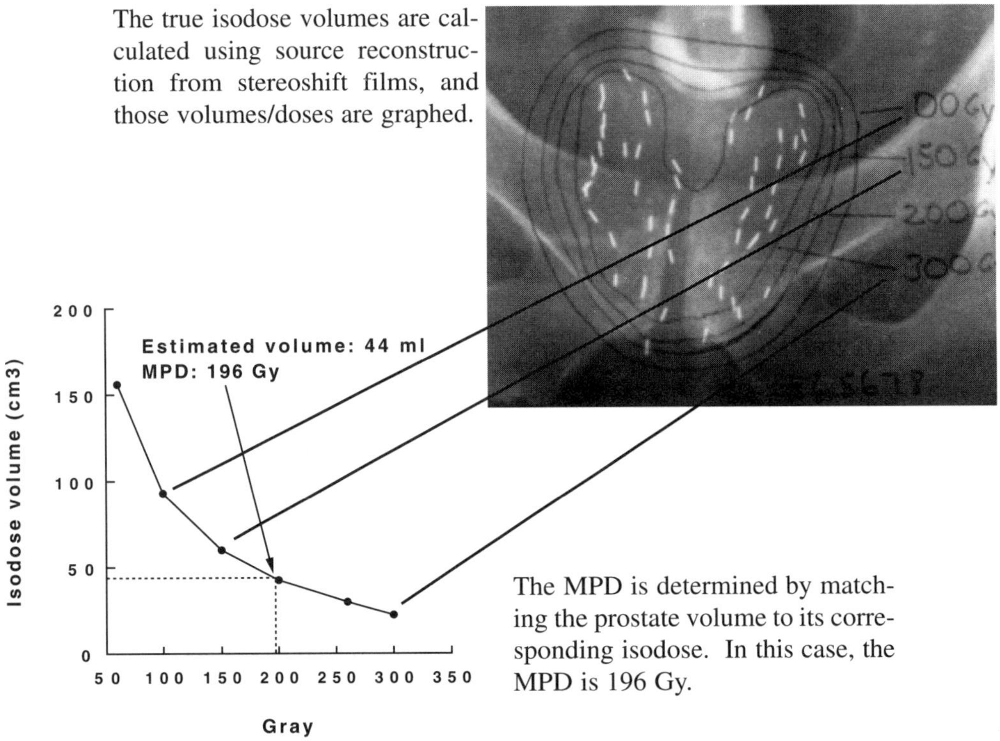

Figure 10-2. Schematic illustration of the MPD calculation. The volumes encompassed by several isodose lines are graphed against the isodose levels. The dose to the approximation of the prostatic volume is taken from the graph, going from the y-axis to the x-axis. The target volume can be estimated from orthogonal dimensions, or determined from planar reconstruction of CT, TRUS or MRI images. (JCha)

prostate definition, one cannot accurately compare the isodose volumes with the prostate margins.

Because MPD calculations use orthogonal dimensions to estimate the prostatic size (and shape), the MPD is an approximation of the dose to an approximation of the prostate volume. The true dose to the prostatic margins is not accurately reflected. This limitation of the MPD in defining what is an adequate implant is obvious from comparing MPDs of a retropubic implant (1980) to a CT-based transperineal implant (1996) (**Figure 10-3**). The MPDs for both implants are similar, but it is obvious that the transperineal implant conforms more closely

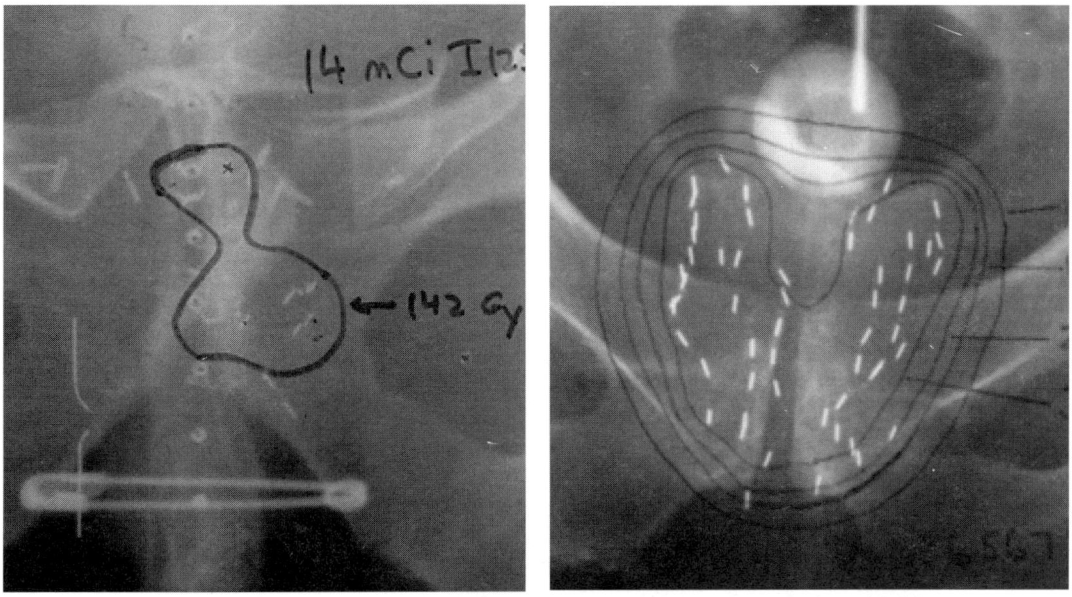

Figure 10-3. On the left is an anterior view of a 1980 retropubic implant, for which the calculated MPD is 142 Gy. On the right is a transperineal implant by K. Wallner (1996), with a similar MPD (196 Gy). These two implants are obviously of vastly different quality, even though the MPD calculations are similar.

to the prostate margins. From the MPDs alone, one would conclude erroneously that the implants are technically comparable.

Despite the inherent inaccuracy of the MPD calculation, some correlation between higher MPDs and higher local control rates has been reported.[Fuks 1991] While these data would suggest the MPD is a useful concept, the data are very suspect, as it is based on vague definitions of local failure. More importantly, the quality of the retropubic implants on which it is based is so poor by today's standards that such data is of historical interest only.

The MPD has outlived its usefulness for implants where CT definition of the target is now possible. However, it is important to understand what the MPD means because it has been widely reported in the literature. There is presently no generally accepted alternative method to report implant quality. Refinement of CT-based evaluation procedures may change that.

WHY CT-BASED DOSIMETRY?

To perform meaningful dosimetry, the source and target location must be identified in relation to each other, so the two can be compared. Post-implant CT images can identify the prostatic margin and the location of individual sources. Although a variety of CT issues still need to be worked out, CT currently offers the most practical dosimetric imaging.

MR may be a practical imaging alternative, but it is not currently widely used.(Moerland 1997) TRUS is not a practical alternative, since the image is degraded by the sources themselves, making individual sources difficult to clearly visualize.

CASUAL INSPECTION

For individual cases, much can be learned by simple inspection of a post-implant CT scan, even without sophisticated dosimetric analysis. One can determine, for instance, if sources are routinely placed too superiorly or posteriorly. Sources placed too posteriorly increase the likelihood of a rectal complication (**Figures 10-4 and 10-6**). Sources placed too close to the urethra increase the likelihood of urinary morbidity (**Figure 10-5**).

AN ABUNDANCE OF QUANTITATIVE DATA

Rigorous use of CT scanning for quality assurance will require a standardized method of dose quantification. Post-implant CT scans can be used to calculate many dosimetric parameters, including the minimum prostatic dose, the volume of prostate that receives less than the prescription dose, and urethral and rectal doses. Examples of some of these parameters are shown in the next several pages, but the brachytherapy community is still far from reaching a consensus as to which are most meaningful.

CT SHOWS WORSE TARGET COVERAGE

The MPD generally overrates implant quality. By comparing traditional MPD calculations with CT-based dosimetry for patients implanted at MSKCC, it is obvious that MPD often fails to identify instances of inferior target coverage. In nine out of ten cases at MSKCC, the MPD of greater than 150 Gy would be judged indicative of adequate dose to the prostate. However, by CT-based dosimetry, minimum target doses are far less than those measured by the MPD (**Figure 10-7**). The initial findings with CT-based post-implant dosimetry came as an unpleasant surprise.(Roy 1993)

QUANTIFYING TARGET COVERAGE

CT data can be used to generate a dose-volume histogram (DVH) of the target coverage (**Figure 10-8**). The DVH shows what percent of the target is covered by any given isodose. Unfortunately, this information cannot be easily summarized in a single number. Ideally, 100% of the target should be covered by the pre-

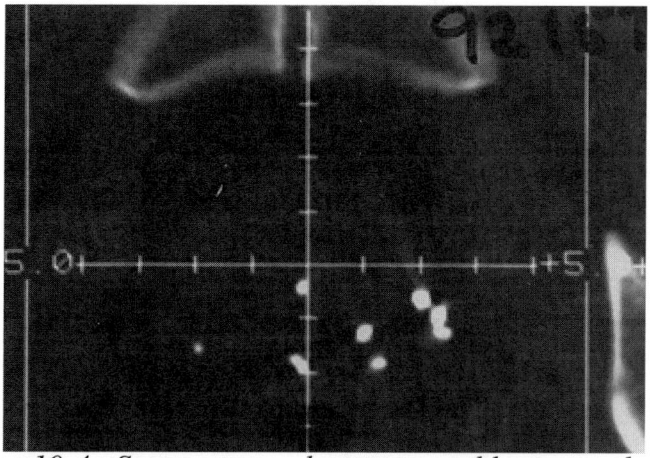

Figure 10-4. Some source placement problems are obvious on CT scan, even without sophisticated dosimetric evaluation. Multiple sources near the anterior rectal wall are obvious. This patient developed a rectal ulcer, which healed spontaneously.

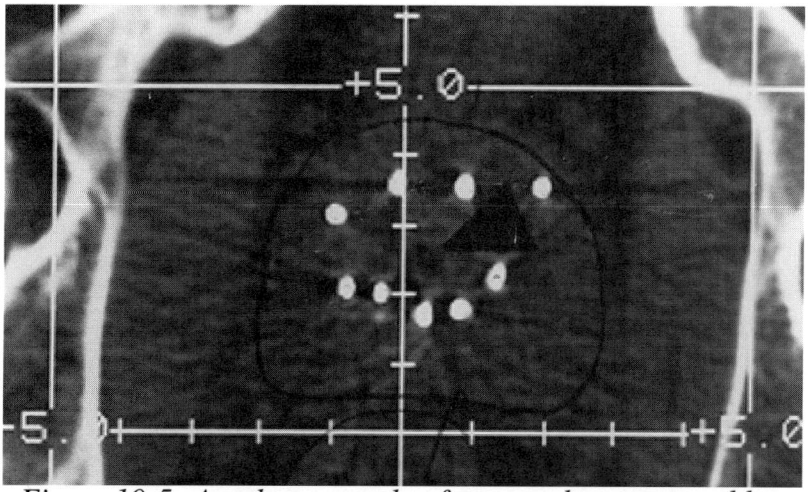

Figure 10-5. Another example of source placement problem obvious on CT, even without sophisticated dosimetric analysis: multiple sources are too close to the urethra (arrowhead). This patient experienced severe dysuria, which resolved spontaneously approximately two years afterwards.

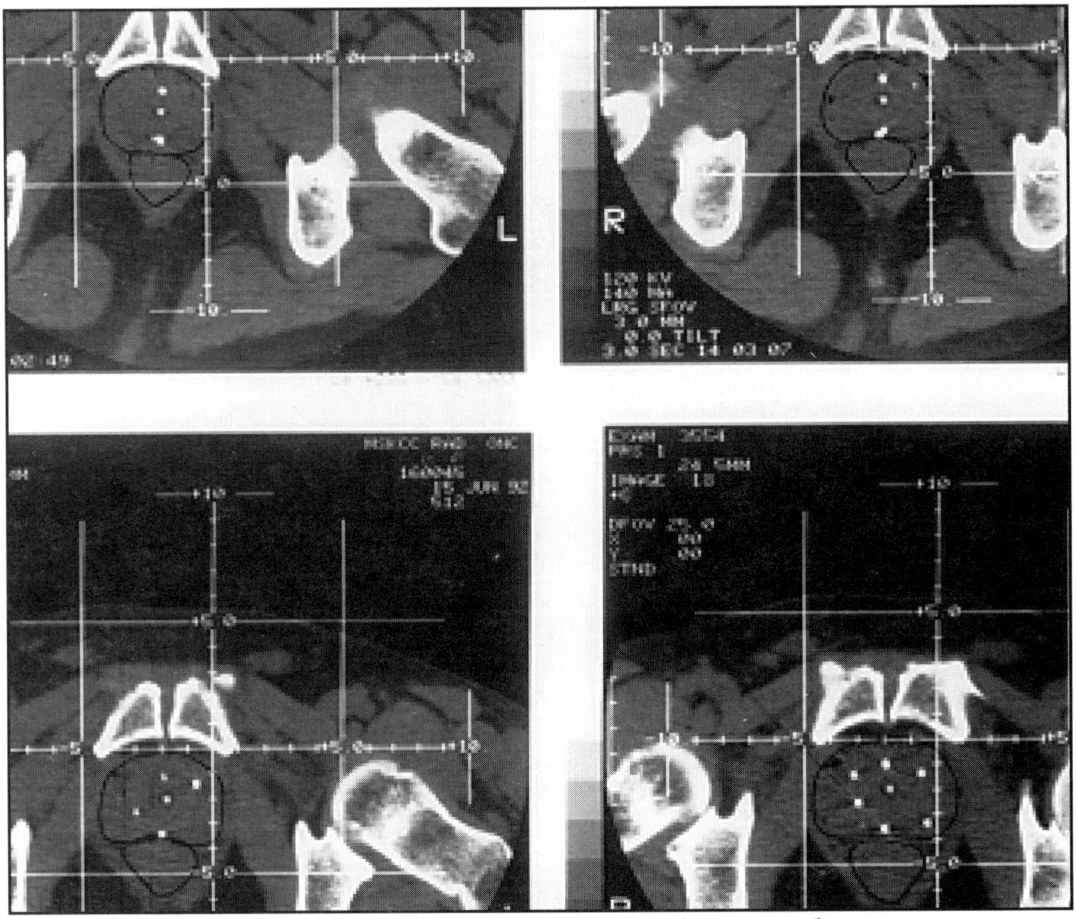

Figure 10-6. Post-implant CT showing that several sources from a single needle were placed 2 to 3 mm too posteriorly, in the rectal mucosa. This patient developed a rectal ulcer.

scription dose, without substantial areas receiving doses far in excess of that. In reality, some of the target will be underdosed and much of the prostate will receive doses far in excess of the prescription dose, due to high dose areas near the sources. An acceptable level of high dose areas has not been determined for prostate brachytherapy.

WHAT IS A GOOD IMPLANT?

Currently no generally accepted guidelines to determine what is adequate target coverage exist. Typical target coverage by the prescription dose is approximately 80 to 90% for an implant done by experienced hands (**Figure 10-9**). It is clear there is still some underdosage of the target volume, which is probably

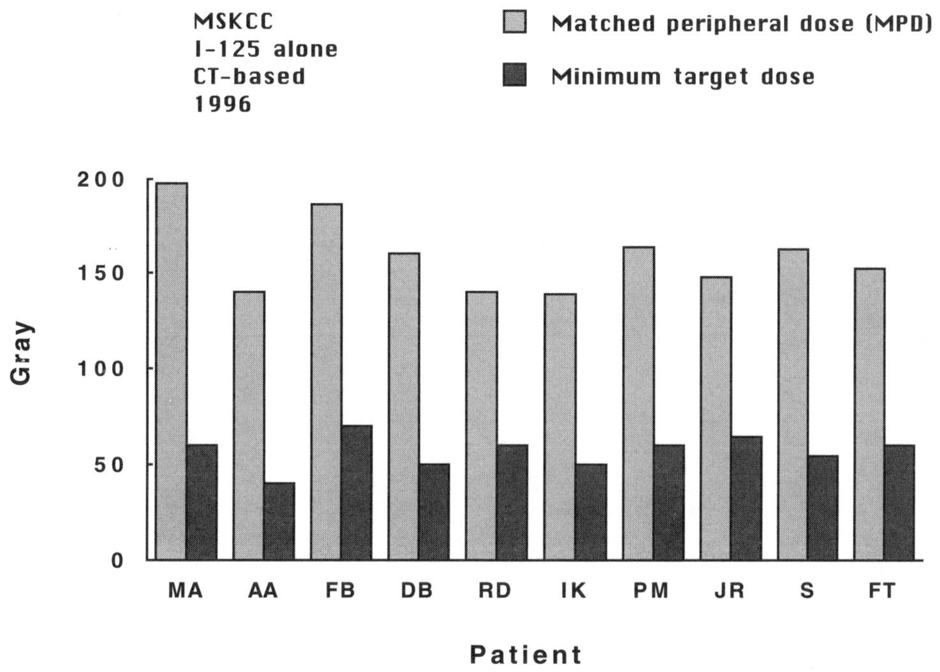

Figure 10-7. MPD versus minimum target dose, based on CT imaging. The minimum target dose is nearly always far lower than the MPD. Because of the irregular target shape, portions extend outside of an elliptical estimation of the target, as used to calculate the MPD.

acceptable (see below). **Figures 10-10 a through g** show several post-implant evaluations. Those shown are fairly representative, and were not chosen because they were the best.

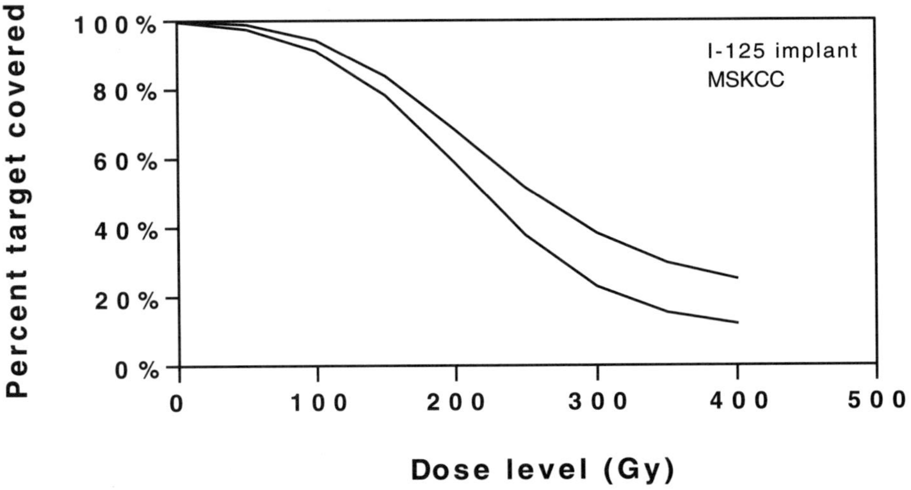

Figure 10-8. Dose volume histogram for two cases by K. Wallner. Target coverage by the prescription dose of 150 Gy was 78% and 83%.

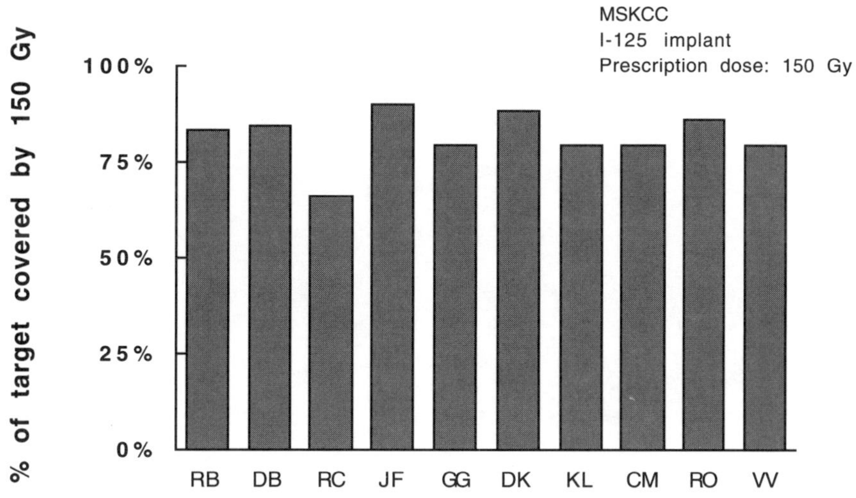

Figure 10-9. Percent target coverage by the 150 Gy iso-dose line. At MSKCC, greater than 80% coverage has been considered adequate, because some of the calculated underdosed volume is due to temporary, post-implant prostatic swelling. That volume due to temporary swelling will diminish or disappear when the swelling subsides.

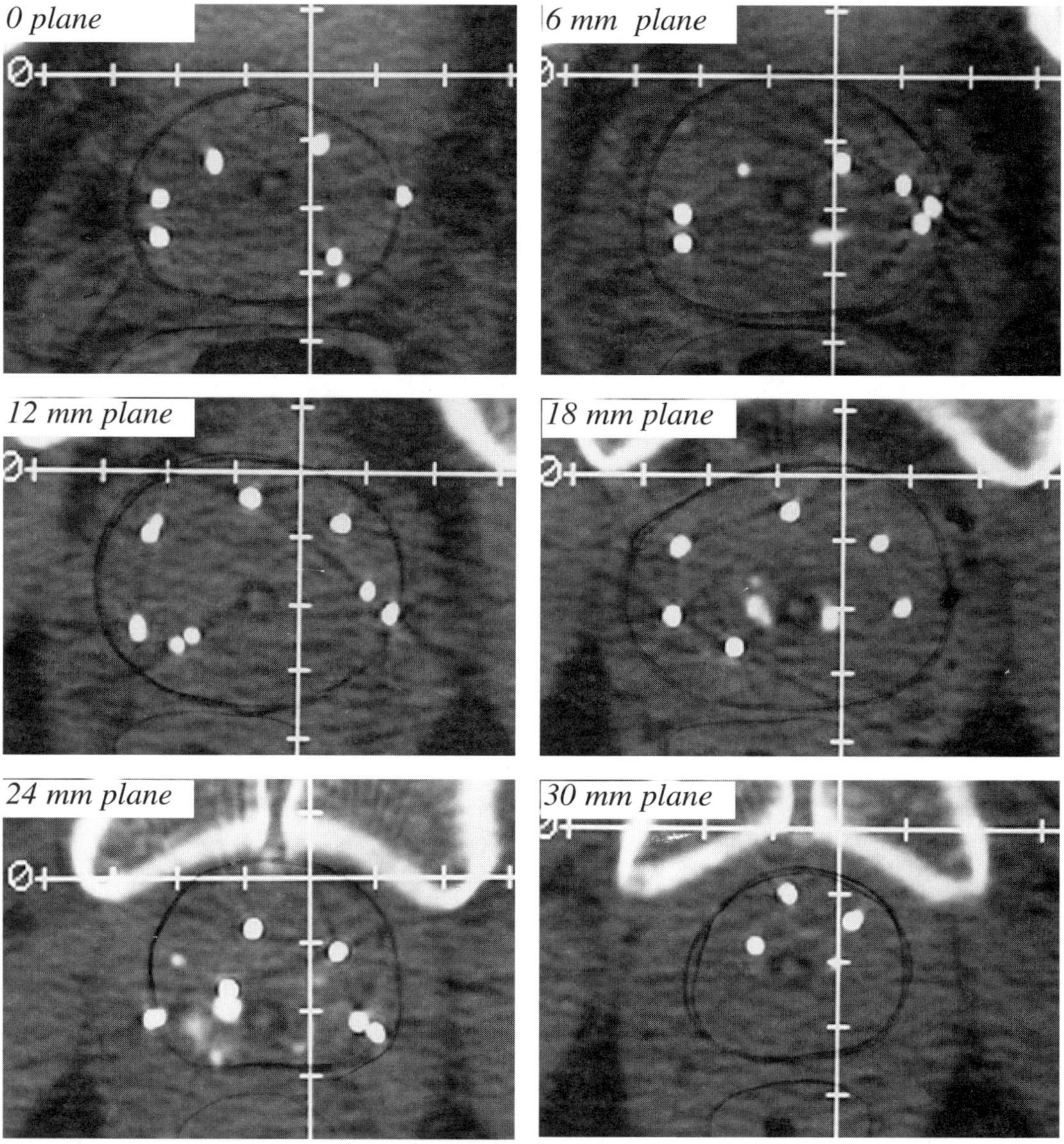

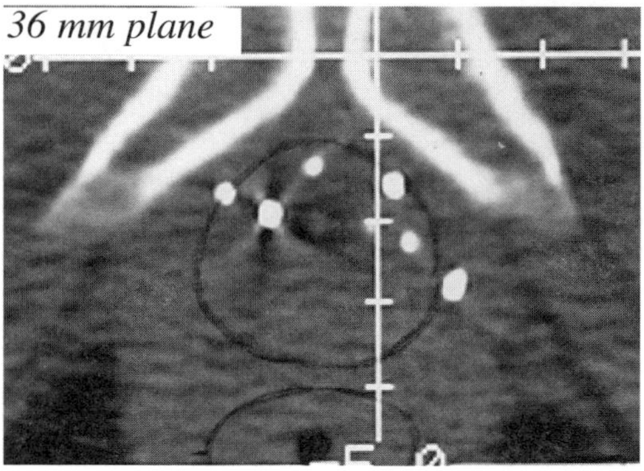

Figure 10-10a. Post-implant CT images of I-125 implant by K. Wallner (150 Gy), taken at 3 mm intervals (only alternate slices are shown here). Dilute contrast has been placed in the bladder to help delineate the bladder from the prostate. A catheter is placed in the rectum to help differentiate the rectum from the prostate and the pelvic floor, especially at the prostatic apex which blends into the pelvic musculature. (JCha)

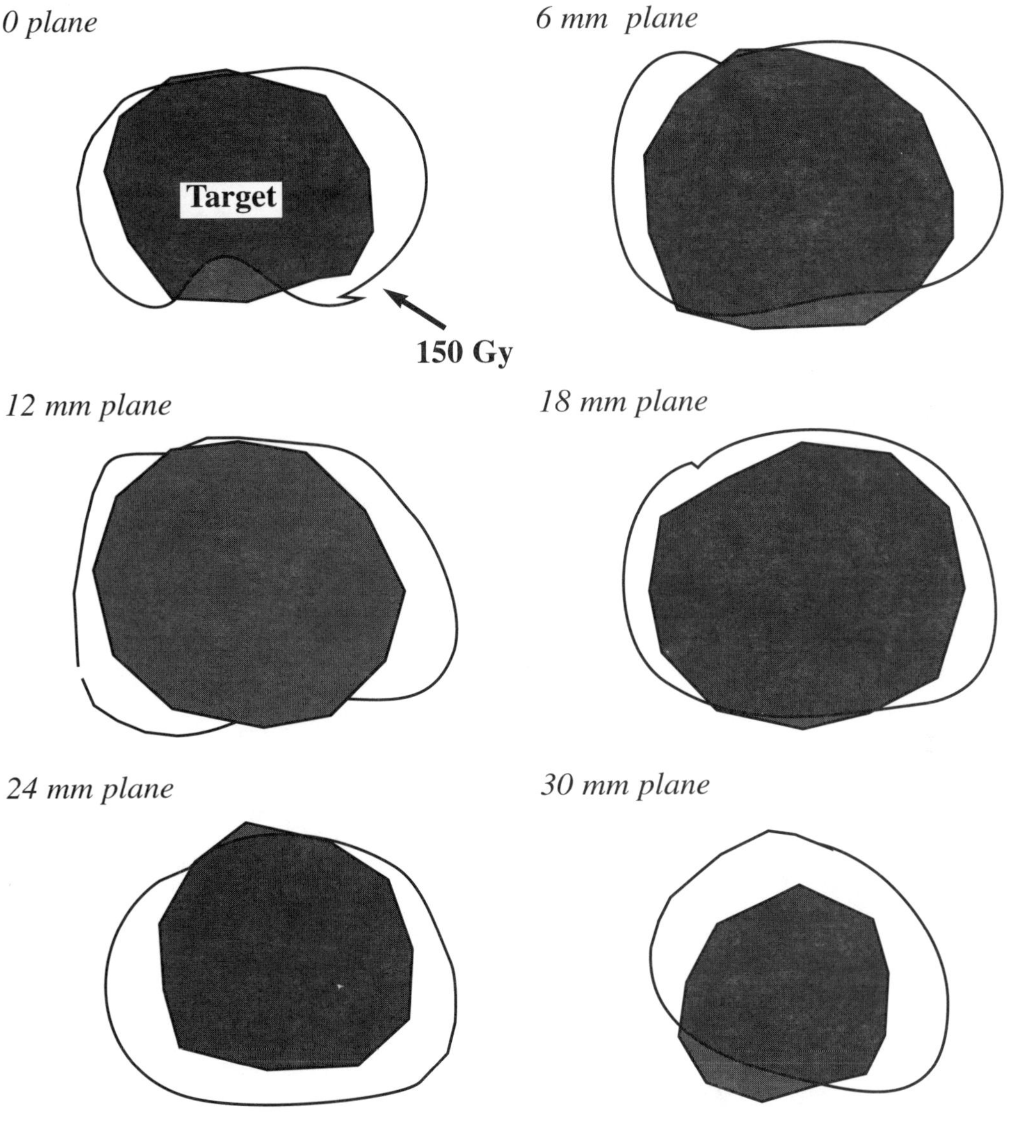

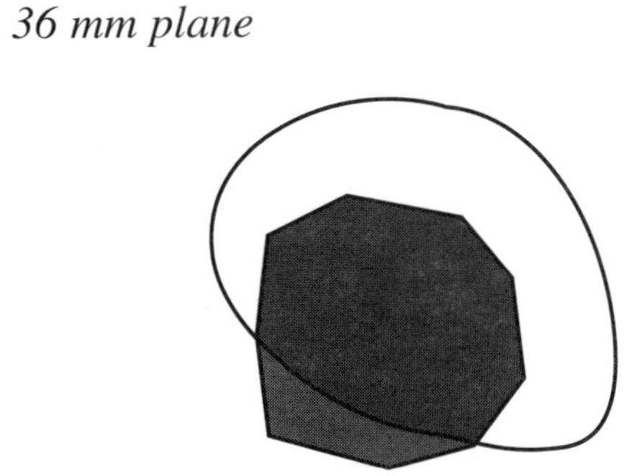

Figure 10-10b. Target coverage for patient from Figure 10-10a. 90% of the target is covered by the prescription dose. This implant would be considered satisfactory. Target coverage of greater than 80% by the prescription dose, based on post-implant CT scan done within four hours of the procedure, is considered satisfactory.

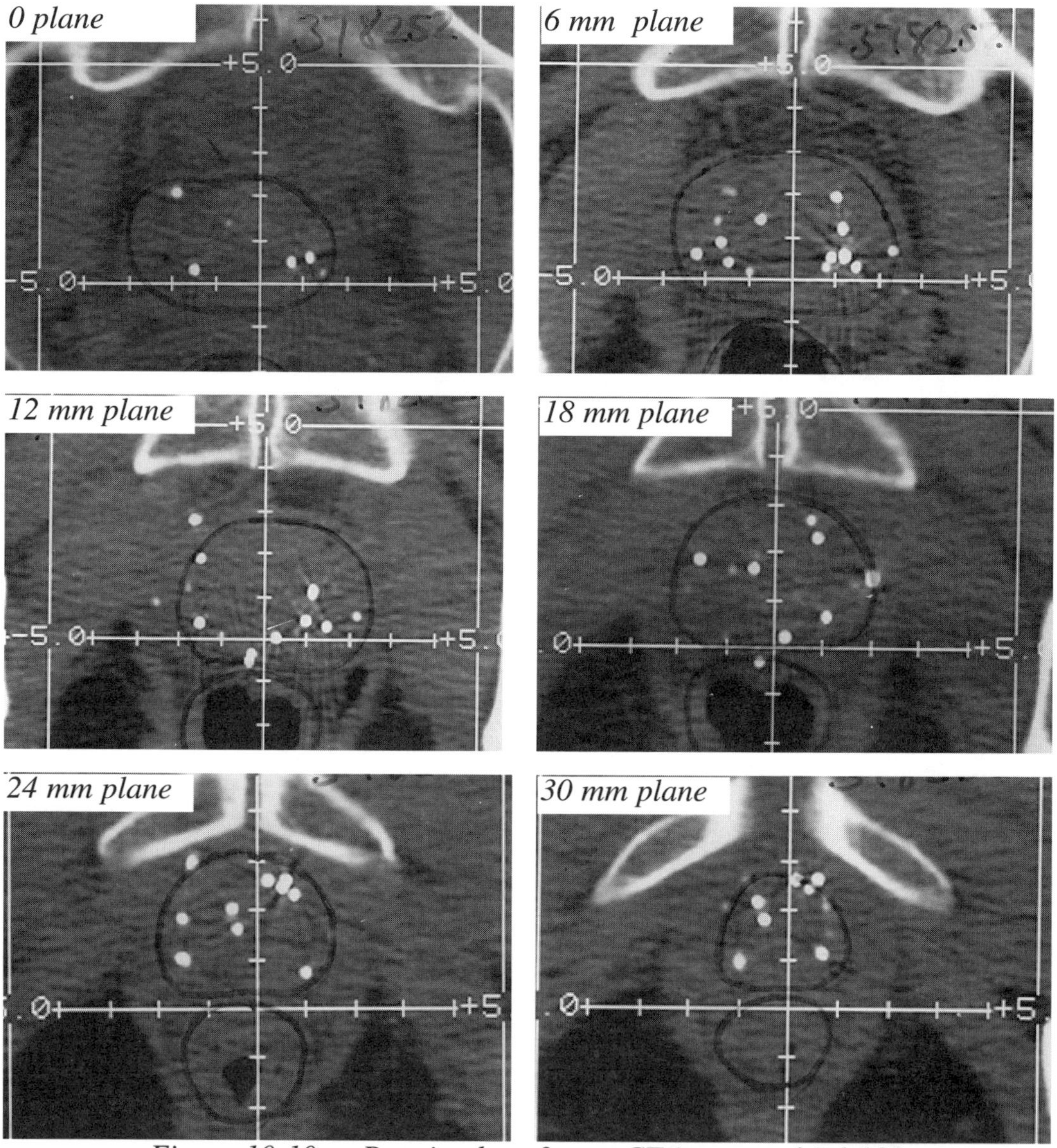

Figure 10-10c. Post-implant 3 mm CT images of Pd-103 implant (110 Gy) by K. Wallner (only alternate slices are shown here). (MSwa)

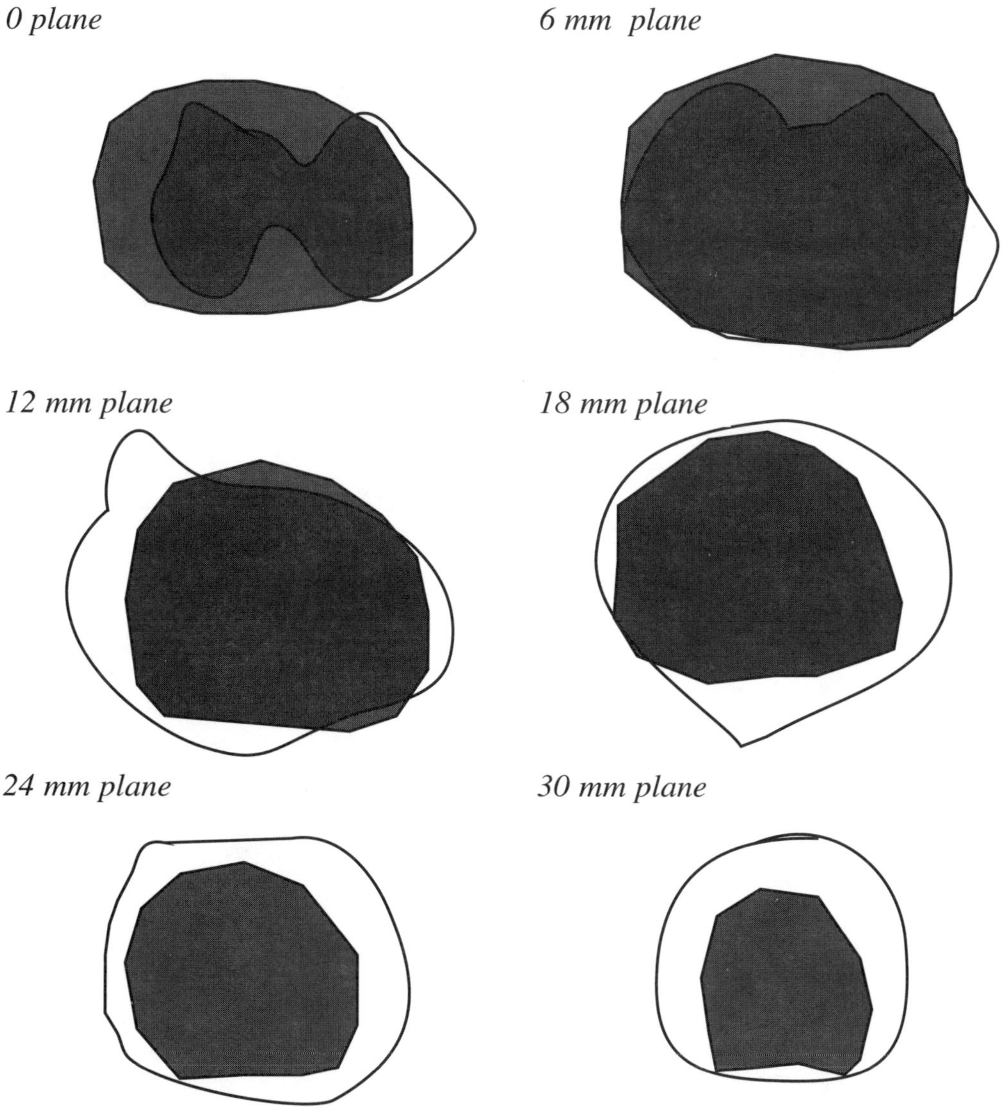

Figure 10-10d. Target coverage with Pd-103 implant for patient from Figure 10-10c. 90% of the target is covered by the prescription dose. This implant would be considered satisfactory, based on the degree of target coverage. As is the case for I-125, greater than 80% target coverage by the prescription dose by Pd-103 is considered satisfactory.

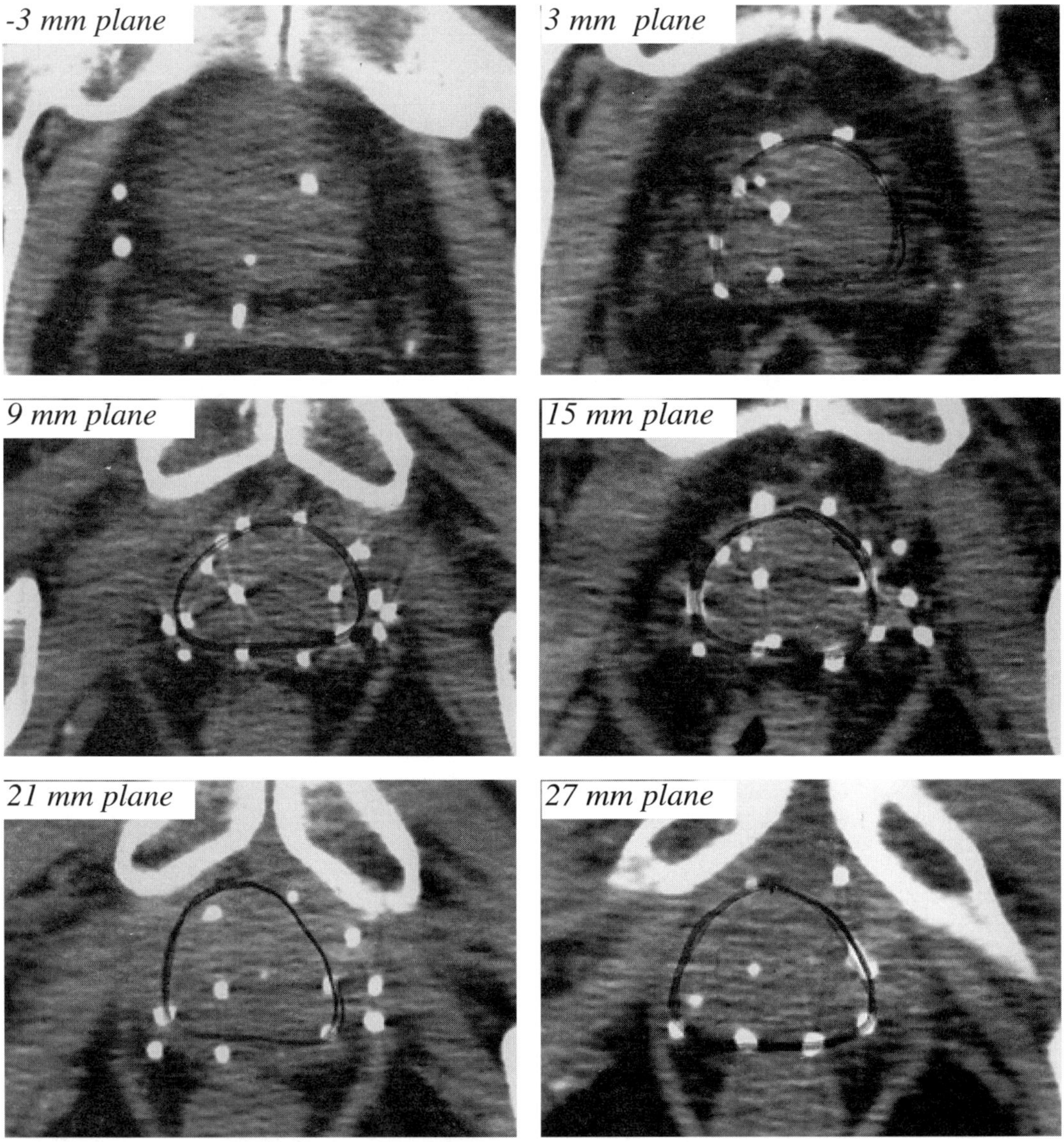

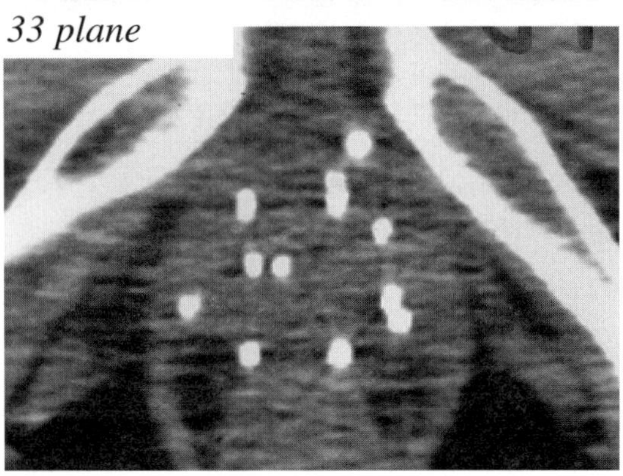

Figure 10-10e. Post-implant 3 mm CT images of Pd-103 implant (115 Gy) by M. Dattoli (only alternate slices are shown here). 104 sources of 1.4 mCi each were placed. (Fabr)

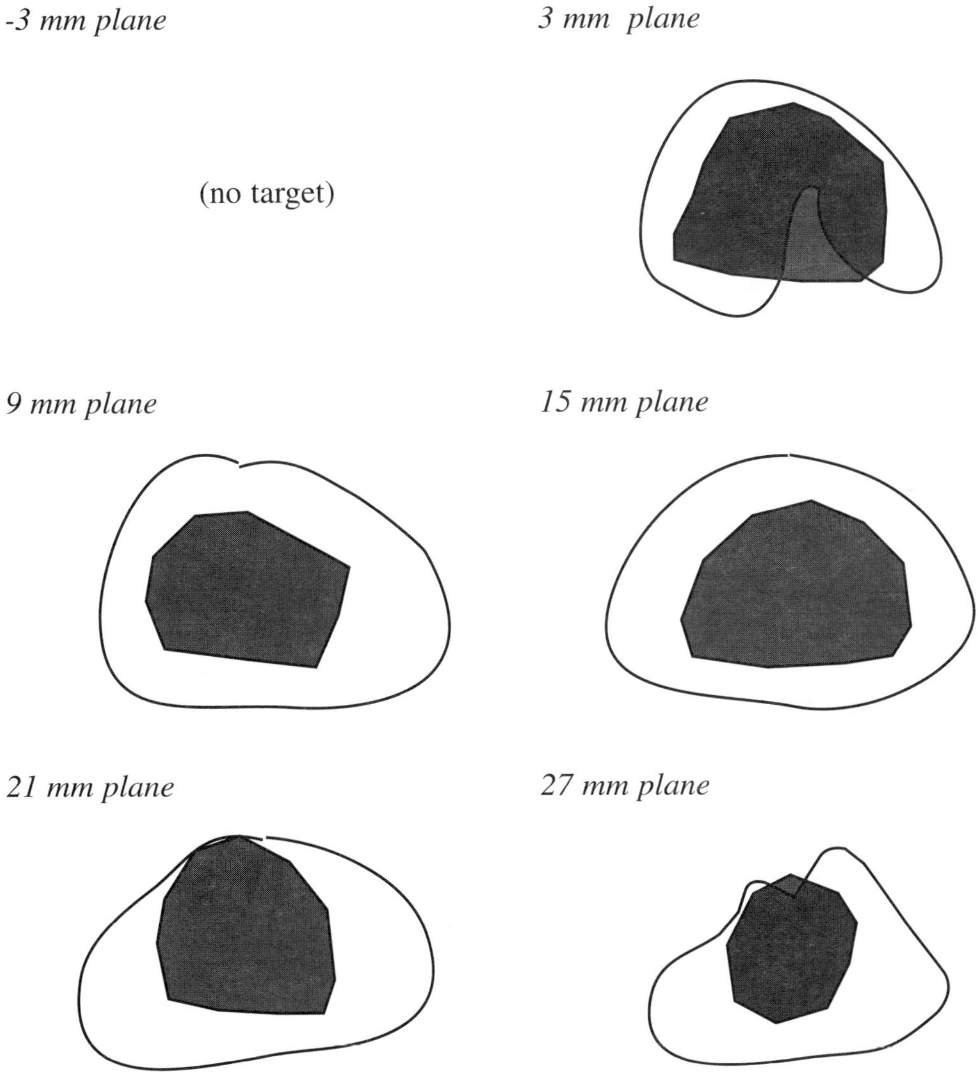

Figure 10-10f. Target coverage for patient from Figure 10-10e. 96% of the target is covered by the prescription dose of 115 Gy.

PROBLEMS WITH CT-BASED DOSIMETRY

While CT-based dosimetry is a substantial improvement over MPD, it still has shortcomings. Potential sources for error lie in the way the target volume is drawn on the post-implant scan, in determining when to get the scan and in the dynamics of prostate size changes following implantation.

Drawing targets

The prostatic margins are not sharply delineated on CT scan, and there is substantial subjectivity in defining them. Especially difficult is delineating the prostatic apex, as it blends with the pelvic floor musculature. Also, the lateral margins can be difficult to distinguish from the puborectalis muscles. Inclusion of the puborectalis in the target volume, or overly generous drawing of the prostatic apex, could lead to a falsely low prostatic dose calculation (See Figure 4-3).

When to get the scan

When the dosimetry scan should be obtained is not clear. If it is performed immediately after the implant, it will show swelling of the prostate due to needle trauma. The prostate volume will have increased by approximately 10 to 20% on the post-implant CT scan, compared to the pre-implant scan (**Figure 10-11**). Temporary post-implant swelling will falsely increase the target volume, making target coverage look inferior to what would be calculated if a dosimetry scan had been taken later, after the acute swelling had subsided.

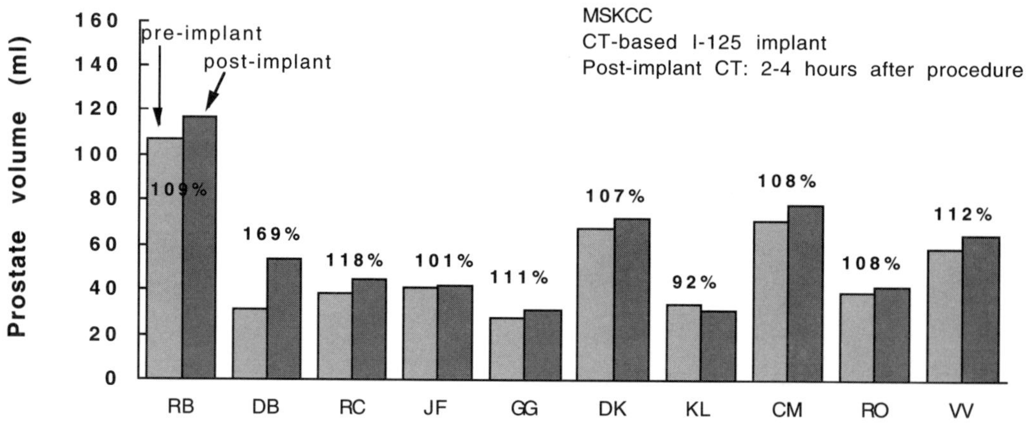

Figure 10-11. The prostate is usually swollen by approximately 5 to 20% on a CT scan taken 3 to 5 hours after the implant.

For convenience, at MSKCC scans have routinely been done the day of the procedure, three to four hours after the implant. This policy has been followed primarily because many patients come from out of state, and getting them back for a follow-up scan is sometimes impractical. By doing the scan two to four hours after the implant, the urinary catheter is still in place to allow urethral dose calculations.

Target volumes -- a moving target

In an effort to define post-implant prostate volume changes, serial scans were done for patients implanted at MSKCC. The target volume decreased by approximately 10 to 15% at two months after the day of the implant, and target coverage increased by about 15% (**Figures 10-12 and 10-13**). If the scan is done two months after the implant, the target coverage appears better than it does on the day of the implant. Unfortunately, it is not practical to use a correction factor for volume changes over time, because volume changes are not consistent from one patient to the next. Volume changes two and six months following implantation were quite variable.

What the best time is to do the evaluation CT scan is unclear. It should probably be done sooner rather than later, in case the coverage is suboptimal and more sources need to be placed. Whatever the timing, it should be consistent from one patient to the next.

Planned with TRUS, evaluated by CT?

Perhaps the biggest conceptual problem with CT-based dosimetry is that it is not the same imaging modality generally used to plan implants. One could make an argument that whatever modality is used to plan an implant should also be used to assess it. Otherwise, peculiarities of the dosimetric image modality may falsely affect conclusions drawn from the dosimetric evaluation. The most obvious example of a problem with using different imaging modalities is the tendency to derive larger prostate volumes from CT scan, than from TRUS. If the TRUS image is more accurate, using CT to assess TRUS-based implants would lead to a falsely low calculation of the degree of target coverage. In fact, the accuracy of TRUS vs CT is still unclear (See Chapter 3), and the effect of crossing imaging modalities is uncertain.

ASSESSING THE DOSE TO THE TUMOR ITSELF

Although it seems desirable to determine the dose to the tumor itself, current imaging techniques do not allow accurate delineation of cancer within the prostate. Even if it were possible, it would be best to continue to treat the entire prostate, to maximize the likelihood of eradicating microscopic synchronous cancers.

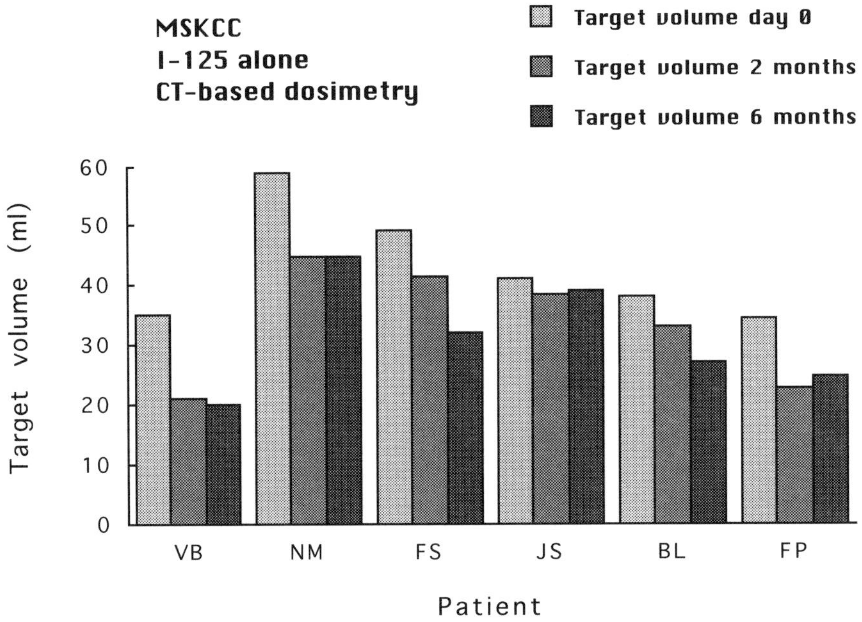

Figure 10-12. Prostate size on the day of the implant and two and six months later for patients implanted with I-125 in 1996 at MSKCC.

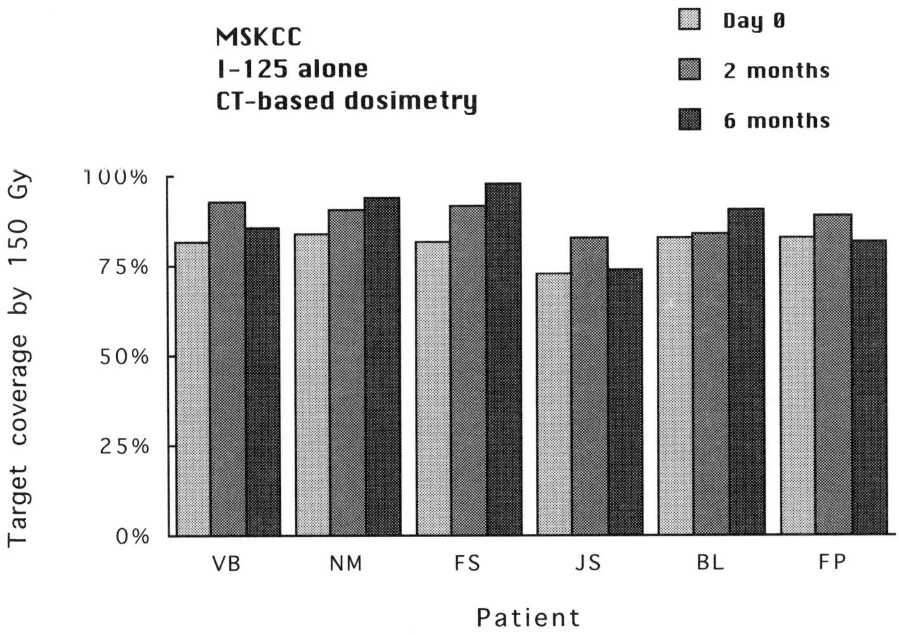

Figure 10-13. Target coverage on the day of the implant, two and six months later for patients implanted with I-125 in 1996 at MSKCC.

WHAT TO DO WHEN TARGET COVERAGE IS LESS THAN IDEAL

Uh-oh. Regardless of one's experience, there will be cases where target coverage appears insufficient. Although there are no clearly established criteria for determining adequate target coverage, there will be cases in which an implant is clearly suboptimal by one's usual standards.

When an implant seems inadequate the first thing one might do is to review the site of the positive pre-treatment biopsies. If the involved portion of the prostate is covered well by the prescription dose, and the biopsies are negative elsewhere, tumor control may not be compromised by underdosage of the apparently uninvolved portion (**Figure 10-14**). Of course, this assumes that those portions of the prostate with negative biopsy tissue truly are free of cancer. This is a certain leap of faith, especially in a patient with a substantially elevated PSA, in whom more extensive cancer would be expected.

If the prescription dose coverage is suboptimal, and one is having trouble deciding on the adequacy of an implant, it may help to run the coverage at slightly lower dose levels such as the 120 Gy and 100 Gy isodose lines. The full 150-160 Gy is likely not needed to eradicate cancer and coverage of the cancerous regions by the 120 or 100 Gy isodose line is probably adequate.

In cases where prostatic coverage is deemed deficient, one must decide how to supplement the dose delivered by the implant. There are two choices: either add some external beam radiation (EBRT), or return to the operating room to add more radioactive sources.

Adding EBRT is probably the most practical solution, but it should be approached with caution. It is one thing to add supplemental EBRT dose to a prostate that has been treated with a relatively homogeneous implant. It is another to add EBRT to a prostate that has received a full therapeutic dose to some areas, and less to others. Bringing the therapeutic dose to acceptable levels in the most underdosed regions may mean over-treating other regions, and possibly risking complications. Using sophisticated treatment planning to supplement just a portion of the gland is probably not realistic.

A second way to supplement an inadequate implant is to return to the operating room and add more sources to the underdosed region. One should first use a post-implant CT to determine the dose to be delivered by the sources already implanted, and then prepare a plan to adequately supplement the underdosed regions, without exceeding rectal or urethral tolerance.

Admittedly, there is no data to support or refute the above guidelines -- and there probably won't be for a long time.

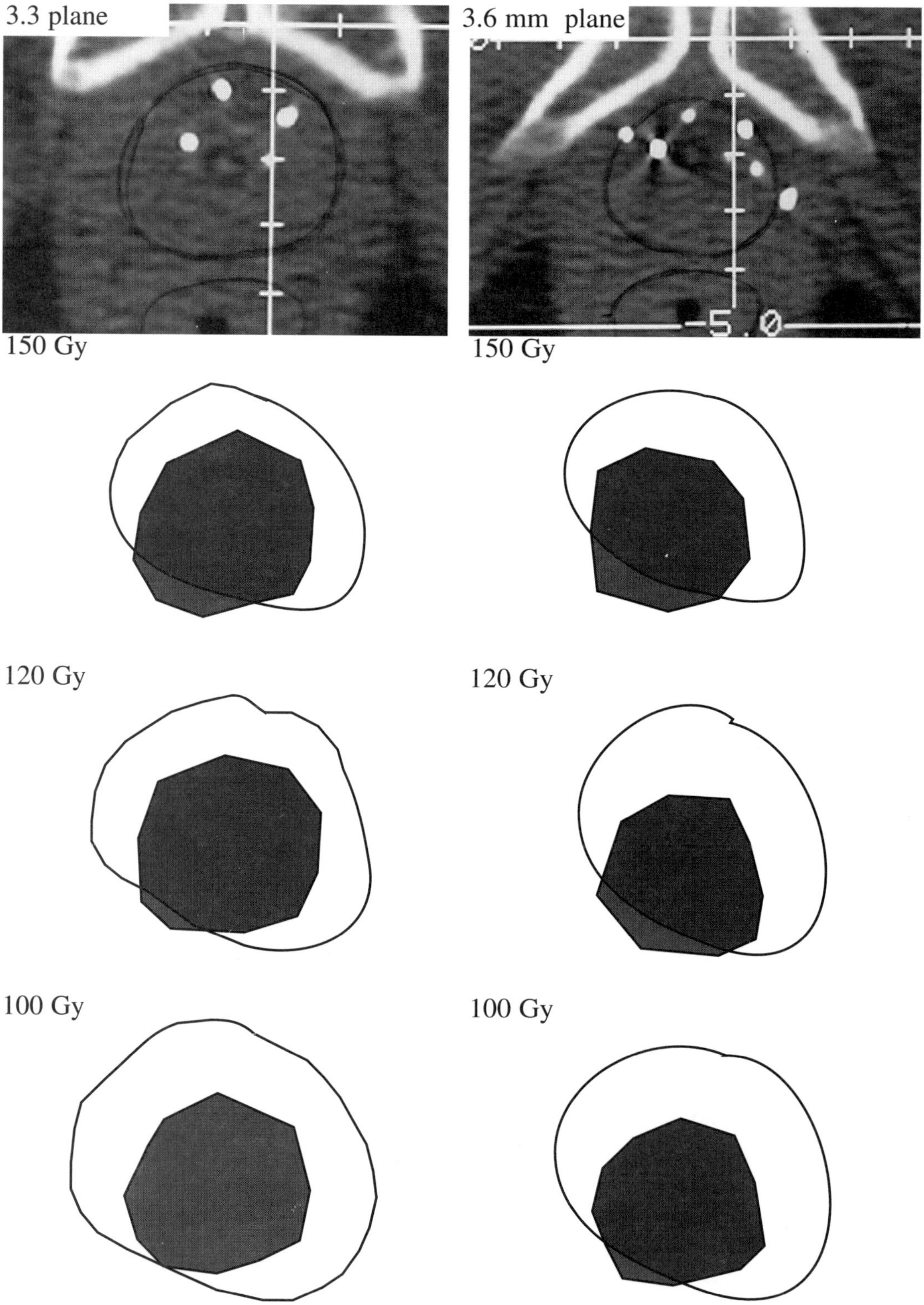

10.22

Figure 10-14. (opposite page). Example of suboptimal target coverage on post-implant evaluation scan (I-125). This patient had a positive biopsy in the right apex, which was not completely covered by the prescription dose (150 Gy). When faced with this situation, we look at the 120 and 100 Gy isodose lines. If the target is adequately covered by the lower isodoses, we may leave the implant as is. In this case, the lowest slice (3.6 plane) probably was below the prostate apex. Even though it was not well covered, the 3.3 slice was, and it was decided not to re-implant the patient. (JCha)

URETHRAL DOSES

The central urethral dose can be calculated by leaving a Foley catheter in place to identify the urethra. In patients implanted at MSKCC, it was found that urinary morbidity in the first year correlated with the maximal central urethral dose. Patients with a maximum urethral dose of less than 400 Gy were less likely to develop substantial urinary morbidity. More sophisticated calculations, including the length of urethra that received greater than 400 Gy, were no more useful for predicting morbidity than the simple parameter of maximum dose.

With a peripheral loading pattern, the central urethral dose can usually be kept well below 400 Gy with an I-125 implant (160 Gy) (**Figure 10-15**). However, because of constraints imposed by prostate size and the necessity for a given number of sources, keeping the urethral dose as low as desirable is not always possible (See Chapter 5). Until 1994, no special effort was made at MSKCC to limit the urethral dose with peripheral loading.

The desirable urethral dose limit for Pd-103 is presumed to be approximately 250 to 300 Gy, though Pd-103 doses have not been rigorously studied.

The desirable maximal urethral dose when brachytherapy is combined with EBRT has also not yet been documented. However, it should be kept as low as possible, consistent with achieving the prescribed dose at the prostate periphery.

RECTAL DOSES

A dose-surface area histogram of the rectum can be calculated to help identify patients at high risk of rectal complications. Rectal bleeding or ulceration are associated with irradiation to doses in excess of 100 Gy at the rectal wall (See Chapter 5). Causes of excessive rectal doses include errors in source placement, and ad hoc placement of additional sources not called for in the plan. If an implant

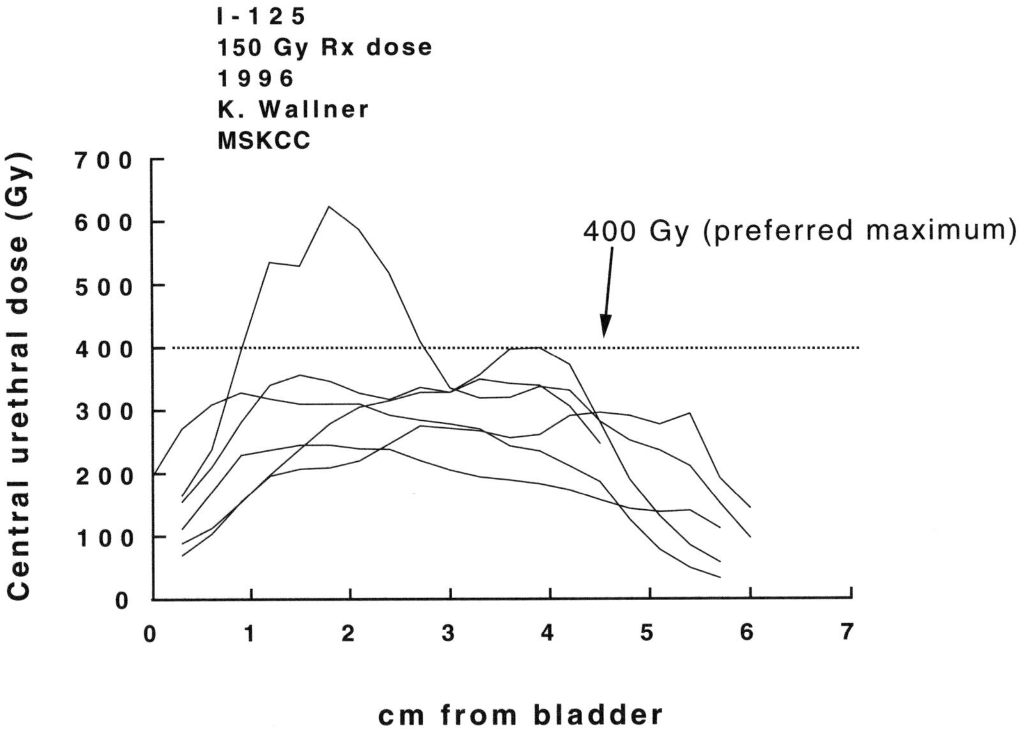

Figure 10-15. Urethral doses for six patients implanted with I-125 by K. Wallner in 1996. Urinary morbidity is less likely in patients whose maximum urethral dose is kept below 400 Gy (I-125).

is executed properly, the full prescription dose to the entire prostate volume can be achieved safely, drawing the target volume at the posterior edge of the gland as it appears on TRUS or CT.

Higher rectal complications reported in early MSKCC transperineal experience were only partially explained by the higher rectal doses delivered. Some patients who developed ulcerations did not appear to have received excessive rectal wall doses. There were, apparently, other unexplained factors that contributed to the higher incidence of rectal ulceration early in the MSKCC experience.

At current prescription doses, rectal complications are very uncommon with implants performed by experienced teams, suggesting that the prescription doses could be increased safely. However, local tumor control rates appear adequate and there may be no reason to increase the dose to the prostate.

SOURCE LOSS

Concern is often raised about the possibility of source loss from the prostate after the procedure. Sources not placed inside the prostate can migrate into the retroperitoneum or lungs. Distal migration to the perineum does not seem to occur.

Sommerkamp and colleagues reported that 90% of patients implanted retropubically lost an average of two sources, usually within the first month of implantation.(Sommerkamp 1988)

In patients recently followed up with two and six month CT scans at MSKCC, source loss was minimal. From the time of the implant, these patients lost an average of one source in the first two months, and only one of six patients lost an additional source between two and six month follow-up (**Figure 10-16**).

Sporadic reports of source migration to the pulmonary vasculature have appeared.(Steinfeld 1991) There is no known ill effect from one or more pulmonary sources, and the possibility is no reason to do routine follow-up chest x-rays.

Sources placed within the prostate should not move. However, it is common practice to draw target volumes well beyond the margin of the prostate, as

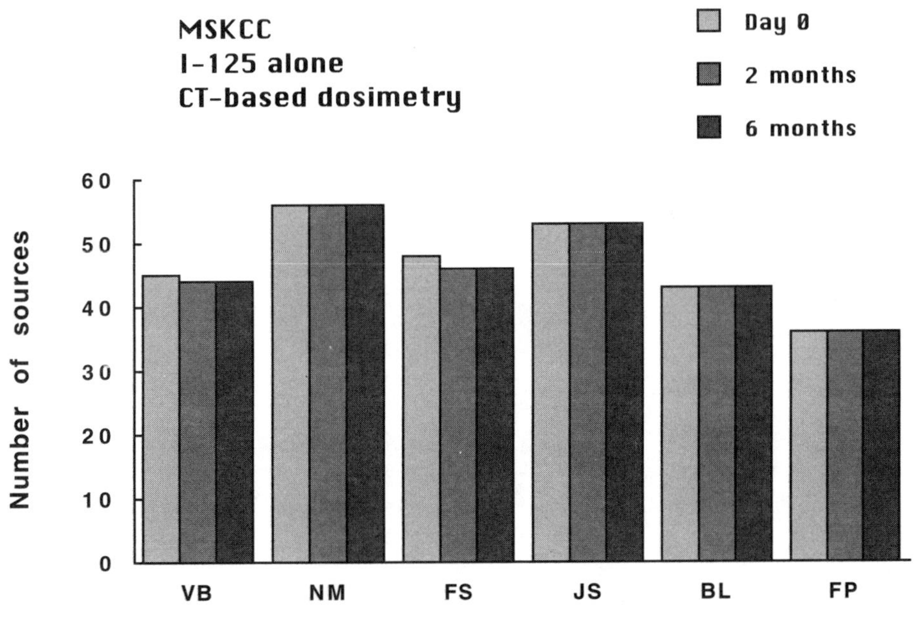

Figure 10-16. Source loss at two and six months after I-125 implantation in six patients treated by K. Wallner in 1996. Source loss over the active life of the implant was minimal.

visualized on TRUS. The intention is to add some margin, to accommodate early extracapsular extension. Adding too generous a margin on the planning target will increase the likelihood of source migration, because sources will be placed outside of the prostate parenchyma.

REAL LIFE DOSIMETRY

With currently available software, dosimetric analysis is time-consuming and expensive. However, the price of quality assurance is still small compared to the overall cost of other modalities. Target coverage should be routinely checked in every patient. If it is inadequate, corrective action can be taken to assure the highest likelihood of cure.

In the early part of one's brachytherapy experience, it would be prudent to do more extensive dosimetric analysis including urethral and rectal doses, to be assured that the implants meet generally acceptable guidelines in regards to complications and target coverage.

Once you are confident that urethral and rectal doses are being kept within acceptable limits while still achieving adequate target coverage, some corner-cutting is in order. In contrast to target coverage, routine calculation of urethral and rectal doses in every patient is probably not necessary. Detailed dosimetric studies that correlated dosimetry with urinary and rectal complications are valuable, in that they helped establish dosimetry guidelines. In practice, however, rectal and urinary complications are very low if implants are executed by the general guidelines outlined in Chapter 5. Accordingly, it seems reasonable to limit routine dosimetric analysis to the degree of target coverage.

REFERENCES

1. Anderson LL, Moni JV, Harrison LB. A nomograph for permanent implants of palladium-103 seeds. Int J Radiat Oncol Biol Phys 1993; 27:129-135.

2. Moerland MA, Wijrdeman HK, Beersma R, Bakker CJG. Evaluation of permanent I-125 prostate implants using radiography and magnetic resonance imaging. Int J Radiat Oncol Biol Phys 1997; 37:927-933.

3. Roy JN, Wallner KE, Harrington PJ, Ling CC, Anderson LL. A CT-based evaluation method for permanent implants: Application to prostate. Int J Radiat Oncol Biol Phys 1993; 26:163-169.

4. Sommerkamp H, Rupprecht M, Wannenmacher M. Seed loss in interstitial radiotherapy of prostatic carcinoma with I-125. Int J Radiat Oncol Biol Phys 1988; 14:389-392.

5. Steinfeld AD, Donahue BR, Plaine L. Pulmonary embolization of iodine-125 seeds following prostate implantation. Urol 1991; 37:149-150.

6. Waehre H, Amellem O, Stenwig AE, et al. Deoxyribonucleic acid cytometry and histological findings before and after 125-Iodine implantation of primary prostate cancer. J Urol 1992; 148:838-842.

Chapter 11

Post-operative care

Post-operative care for transperineal brachytherapy is generally simple, and complications are infrequent. There are many ways to manage patients post-operatively, and little data to support one approach over another. The pages ahead summarize our own experiences and biases regarding post-operative care.

SKIN CARE AFTER IMPLANTATION

After withdrawal of the needles, the perineum should be cleaned with a damp cloth. A 10% povidine-iodine solution can be used for this, but is probably not necessary. Application of a perineal dressing is impractical and unnecessary.

Patients are instructed to shower with soap upon returning home several hours after the implant.

CATHETER REMOVAL

To help locate the urethra and the top of the prostate, many brachytherapists place a urinary catheter for the implant procedure. The optimal time to remove the catheter is unknown. If it is removed within several hours of the procedure, there is a 10 to 15% likelihood of developing urinary retention on the evening of the implant (see Chapter 16).

Acute retention is more likely in older patients, those with large prostates, more sources, and those patients with substantial pre-implant obstructive symptoms (see Chapter 16). Prostate size, a patient's age and the number of sources are interrelated, so that the importance of one factor over the other is unclear.

The likelihood of post-operative urinary retention might be reduced by leaving the catheter in overnight to allow the acute inflammation to subside. While this policy is well-meaning, it is probably unnecessary. There is no data showing that leaving the catheter in overnight will decrease the likelihood of urinary retention. Also, retention usually resolves by the next morning anyway, so that leaving the catheter in overnight may not decrease the time that they have to wear a catheter. This would, however, increase the percent of patients who have a catheter overnight from 10% to 100%.

In those patients who require catheter re-insertion for post-implant retention, it can usually be successfully removed the next morning. If a patient still cannot urinate within several hours, the catheter is re-inserted for three days. Patients can be started on alpha-1 blockers prophylactically during this time, though its activity in acute urinary retention has not been studied. Prophylactic non-steroidal inflammatory agents might decrease the likelihood of acute urinary retention.

As an alternative to re-catheterization, patients can be instructed in self-catheterization. For patients willing to give self-catheterization a try, it is generally better tolerated than an indwelling catheter. Intermittent self-catheterization avoids irritation from the constant presence of a catheter, and allows a more normal lifestyle. Additionally, it allows patients to urinate spontaneously as they improve, rather than their having to wait for "voiding trials," as is the case with indwelling catheters.

When faced with urinary retention, surgical intervention, including TURP, transurethral incision of the prostate (TUIP), or suprapubic tube should be avoided, in favor of using longer term intermittent self-catheterization or an indwelling Foley catheter. Most patients' retention will resolve spontaneously. Surgical intervention is usually unnecessary and invites long-term urinary incontinence (see Chapter 16).

Some physicians have advocated placing a prophylactic suprapubic catheter in some or all patients, to be removed several weeks later. However, since the incidence of urinary retention is low and usually of short duration, it is difficult to justify a suprapubic procedure. It would be an invitation for iatrogenic morbidity, and a waste of money.

HEMATURIA

Most patients have some post-implant gross hematuria, which can last for one to fourteen days. Occasional patients will pass clots longer. The amount of bleeding is usually minimal, but patients occasionally pass larger amounts, probably from a urethral tear or bladder injury. When this happens, a Foley catheter can be placed and irrigated until clear. Clinically significant post-implant bleeding is rare.

For patients who develop persistent heavy bleeding, it would be reasonable to perform a cystoscopy to identify the cause. Alternatively, a catheter could simply be placed for several days, to tamponade the urethra. More aggressive, surgical intervention, should not be necessary.

DYSURIA IN THE FIRST POST-OPERATIVE WEEK

Patients usually experience substantial dysuria in the immediate post-operative period, presumably due to needle trauma. The initial trauma-related dysuria usually resolves substantially within 24 hours and is usually gone within 2-3 days. Taking non-steroidal anti-inflammatory drugs (NSAID) within several hours after implantation can help with acute discomfort. In K. Wallner's experience, patients have had no bleeding problem despite immediate use of NSAIDs. Alpha-1 blockers can be routinely prescribed during the immediate post-operative period. Narcotics generally do not help alleviate the acute dysuria.

Patients are instructed not to drink extra fluids during the first 12 hours following implantation, because this can exacerbate their already troublesome urinary problems. They are instructed to start drinking extra fluids the morning after the implant, and to continue doing so for three days. Extra fluids may decrease the likelihood of a urinary infection. Post-implant urinary tract infections are unusual, but should be treated appropriately if verified by urine culture.

GOING HOME

A patient can be sent home after recovery from anesthesia. Patients are usually asked to stay within a one-hour drive of the hospital, unless arrangements can be made for them to be seen in a local emergency room if an acute problem develops. If a patient lives more than an hour away, it is probably best that he stay close to the hospital, with friends/relatives or in a hotel.

Ideally, a medical person should contact the patient several hours after discharge to check that he has been able to urinate. Often patients will pass a small stream immediately after catheter removal, but this does not guarantee that they will not develop urinary retention over the next 24 hours. If a patient passes a stream (more than a few drops) several hours after the implant, he almost certainly will not develop retention, although his urination may be frequent and uncomfortable.

If a patient has not urinated within six hours of catheter removal, he will usually need to return to be catheterized. Some patients, depending on fluid intake and bladder capacity, may not need to urinate until the next morning. The decision to catheterize after an implant should be individualized.

One way to earlier determine the need for a catheter would be to instill fluid into the bladder prior to removing the Foley catheter. This policy is not generally followed, however, because several hours might be needed to recover from possible retentive effects due to anesthesia and trauma. It is probably wiser to send patients home with an empty bladder, and give them several hours to recover before assessing them for urinary function.

SCROTAL BRUISING

Patients commonly develop scrotal bruising several days after the procedure. It resolves spontaneously, but should be mentioned beforehand, as its unexpected appearance can be disconcerting. Application of an ice pack to the perineum immediately following the implant might decrease the likelihood and severity of bruising.

INFECTION

Post-operative infections are uncommon (see Chapter 7). Late infections occur occasionally, and should be treated appropriately, after a culture is obtained.

PAIN

Post-operative pain (apart from dysuria) is usually limited to minor perineal discomfort. More significant post-operative pain is unusual. Narcotic analgesics need not be routinely prescribed. If narcotics are needed, the situation should be carefully assessed for some unusual circumstance.

DYSURIA AFTER THE FIRST WEEK

Nearly all patients experience symptoms of radiation prostatitis, including dysuria, daytime urinary frequency and urgency to urinate (see Chapter 16). Radiation-related symptoms generally start two to three weeks following I-125 implantation, and one to two weeks after Pd-103 implantation.

About 50% of patients have few urine symptoms and do not want medication. The other half have enough frequency, nocturia, or dysuria that they want something to alleviate the discomfort. Selective alpha-1 adrenergic blockers are by far the most effective treatment for radiation prostatitis. Either terazocin (Hytrin™) or doxazocin mesylate (Cardura™) will usually relieve symptoms within several hours of use.

The usual starting dose with either drug is one or two mg at night. As noted in the package insert, there is a risk of hypotension when first starting the medication, and this risk must be respected. Hypotensive episodes are probably more likely in older, thin patients, but all patients should be warned to get up slowly, especially at night, when first starting the medication.

Some patients do well taking the drug as directed, once a day. Although both drugs are said to have a 24-hour action, patients often do better if they split the daily dose into two or more doses. Patients who do not get 24-hour relief with a single daily dose, are instructed to take the pills twice a day or even more often. In general, the total daily dose should be kept below 10 mg, because at 10 mg/day, patients commonly experience fatigue.

Radiation prostatitis begins to remit within several months of implantation, and then, at some point, alpha blockers will not be needed. When symptoms begin to remit, patients can try stopping or reducing their medication for one or two days. If radiation prostatitis symptoms persist, alpha blockers can be re-started and then stopped again in a month or two. There is much variability in responses to medication, so patients and physicians should be flexible about their usage.

EXERCISE

Patients are instructed to avoid strenuous physical activity for two days following implantation. This is considered prudent, due to anesthesia after-effects and the possibility of bleeding. After two days, all restrictions are lifted.

Physical activity generally alleviates urinary obstructive symptoms, the mechanism for which is unclear. Regular exercise should be encouraged as a treatment for obstructive urinary symptoms (and because it is generally good for people).

SEXUAL ACTIVITY

No published data exists regarding any ill effects resulting from sexual activity in the post-implant period. Surprisingly, some patients engage in sex the night of the implant, and none have reported a problem apart from some discomfort with ejaculation (see Chapter 17).

Theoretically, one or more sources could be passed with the ejaculate and therefore it seems prudent to recommend condom use for six months after I-125 implantation and two months after Pd-103. However, there has never been a report of sources being expelled with ejaculation.

RECTAL BLEEDING

Patients may have a small amount of bright red blood rectally in the immediate post-operative period, presumably due to inadvertent piercing of the rectal mucosa during the procedure, or to irritation of hemorrhoids. Bleeding due to radiation itself would generally not occur for several months.

RADIATION PRECAUTIONS

After an implant, radiation detectable at the skin surface is low. The dose rate at the skin surface immediately following a full dose I-125 implant is approximately 2 to 10 mR/hour. The typical exposure at skin surface with full dose Pd-103 implant is 1 to 5 mR/hour.

There is no data regarding the risk of these exposure rates to humans. Extrapolating from much higher dose rates, regulations have been advanced limiting the total annual radiation dose to 0.1 mR for the general public. Accordingly, the "safe" total exposure time at the anterior skin surface would be approximately 20 hours for I-125 and 50 hours for Pd-103. Of course, the "safe" exposure times would increase with each radionuclide half life that passes after the implant.

Exposure to others can be decreased with increased distance from the patient. The exposure at one meter from the pelvic skin surface is virtually undetectable with a conventional clinical ionization chamber.

If desired, exposure to others can be eliminated by the patient's wearing a lead apron, which can be fabricated from lead-lined sheeting or purchased from a radiology supply company. We do not consider this a requirement.

PSA DETERMINATIONS

The proper timetable for post-implant PSA (prostate specific antigen) determinations is still unclear. Until recently, it was common to get the first follow-up PSA one month after the procedure. However, PSA values taken before two years should not be used to make a clinical decision, because commonly the readings will rise between one and two years after an implant, and then fall again. Even if a PSA were continuously rising, a follow-up biopsy would not be recommended until two years, because of the higher rate of false positives before that time (see Chapter 14). One could even make an argument for waiting for a PSA until two years have passed. Understandably, patients are anxious to know their results sooner, but any PSA taken before two years will not be of much value. And if the PSA happens to bounce up, the patient will suffer considerable anxiety while waiting for the next value.

In contrast, patients with markedly elevated pre-treatment PSA or elevated prostatic acid phosphatase should probably be monitored more frequently, because they are at higher risk of having metastatic disease. If their PSA were rising rapidly, a bone scan should be obtained to look for rapidly advancing bone metastases that might warrant early hormonal ablation or radiation.

A reasonable compromise between a patient's desire for information about his course and the fact that an early PSA doesn't mean much, would be to get the first PSA reading at six months following the procedure and then every six months thereafter. If at two years or more following implantation the PSA is greater than 1.0 ng/ml, a repeat reading should be obtained one month later. If the PSA is consistently greater than 1.0 more than two years after implantation and is not decreasing, a repeat prostate biopsy should be performed if the patient is a potential candidate for salvage therapy.

POST-OPERATIVE CARE IS USUALLY EASY

In general, there is minimal need for physician intervention in the post-operative period. However, occasionally patients will develop problems. It is important that patients have easy access to a physician or nurse clinician for advice on how to cope with post-implant symptoms. Tincture of time is the best remedy for most urinary problems. Surgical intervention is rarely required. Second and third opinions should be sought before seriously considering surgical intervention for seemingly intractable problems.

Chapter 12

Implant versus implant+EBRT

From an oncologic perspective, nearly all early stage prostate cancer patients can be appropriately treated with brachytherapy, either with an implant alone or an implant combined with external beam radiation (EBRT). Surprisingly, there is general agreement on guidelines for choosing the proper combination of modalities, despite the lack of rigorous data comparing implant alone versus implant plus supplemental EBRT. Some patients are not considered candidates for brachytherapy, based on general health considerations or urologic conditions (see Chapter 13).

LOW RISK VERSUS HIGH RISK CANCER

Patients are divided into two categories - low risk and high risk, based on their pre-treatment PSA, Gleason score and on more subtle pathologic features of the pretreatment biopsy tissue. Patients are placed into low and high risk groups based on a correlation between PSA and Gleason score with the likelihood of extracapsular extension (ECE). Patients with a higher likelihood of ECE may fare better with combination treatment of implant and supplemental EBRT.

In fact, patients could be classified into far more than two categories. However, the purpose of classifying patients for brachytherapy is simply to provide a logical way decide who should be given supplemental EBRT -- high risk patients get it and low risk patients do not.

EXTRACAPSULAR EXTENSION (ECE)

The most common form of extraprostatic disease is the penetration of the prostate capsule. The capsule itself is a collection of fibrous layers, without a dis-

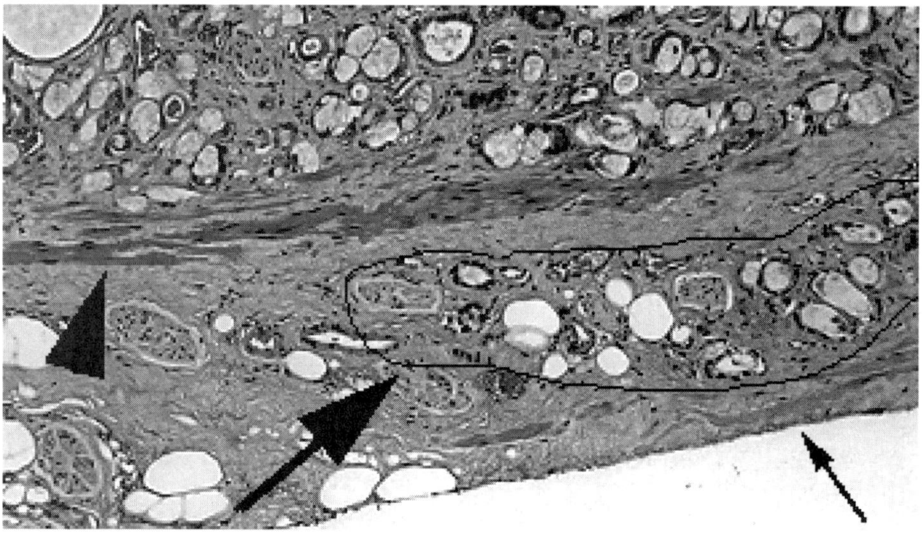

Figure 12-1. Early ECE: the extracapsular cancer is enclosed within the fine black line (large arrow). Cancer has penetrated capsule (arrowhead), and is approximately 2 mm outside of capsular margin. The cancer is still within the margin of resection (small arrow). This degree of ECE would be included within the cancericidal isodose volume of an implant alone (see Figure 12-3).

tinct margin. Cancers can achieve varying degrees of ECE prior to diagnosis. ECE can be as little as one millimeter (mm), or far more (**Figure 12-1**).

With locally effective therapy, it is the degree of cancer extension beyond the capsule that determines curability. Those patients with minimal capsular penetration are still curable, assuming the cancer is specimen confined or is covered by a cancericidal radiation dose (**Figure 12-2**). A greater degree of extraprostatic extension means that there is a lower likelihood that the cancer is confined to the prostatectomy specimen or the cancericidal isodose volume of an implant; thus the likelihood of cure is also lower (**Figure 12-3**).

WHY BRACHYTHERAPY MAY BE MORE EFFECTIVE THAN SURGERY

Prostate cancer's potential for capsular penetration extending beyond the surgical margins provides theoretical appeal to brachytherapy. Patients with capsular penetration beyond the likely surgical margin may have a higher likelihood of cure with wider therapeutic margin achieved with brachytherapy (with or without supplemental EBRT, and assuming that there is no systemic disease) (**Figure 12-4**).

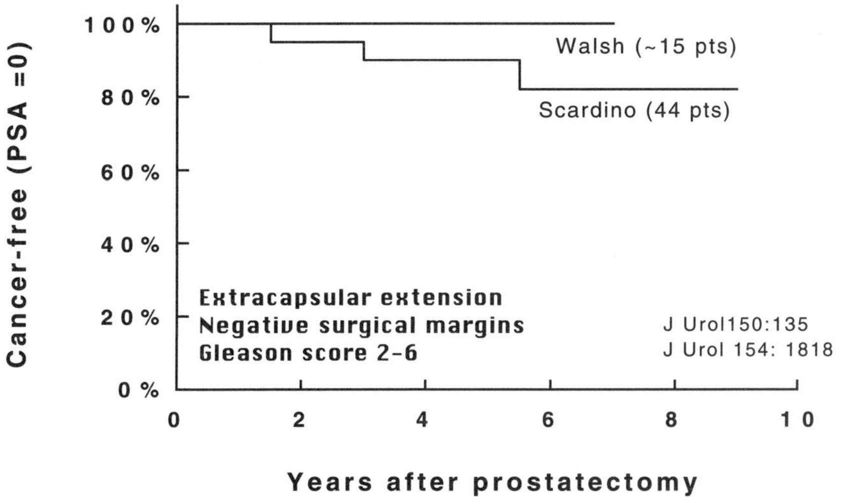

Figure 12-2. Disease-free survival for T1/T2 prostatectomy patients, with limited ECE and negative margins on the surgical specimen. Such patients are still highly curable surgically, despite the presence of ECE.

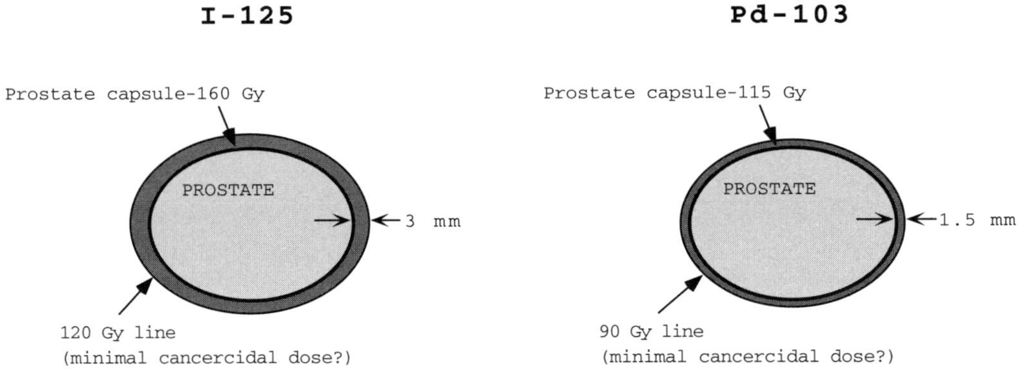

Figure 12-3. Therapeutic margin with I-125 or Pd-103 implant. The prescription doses of 160 Gy or 115 Gy are assumed to be at the prostatic margin. If the cancericidal dose is assumed to be 120 Gy for I-125 and 90 Gy for Pd-103, the therapeutic margins are approximately three mm and two mm, respectively.

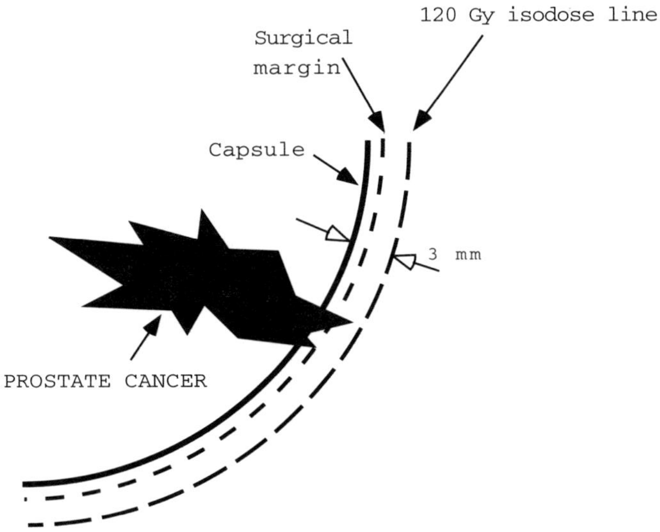

Figure 12-4. Schematic, microscopic view of extracapsular extension. Limited extraprostatic disease might receive adequate irradiation from implant alone, even if the ECE were beyond the potential surgical margin.

RATIONALE FOR SUPPLEMENTAL EBRT

Because of rapid dose fall-off, brachytherapy alone can adequately treat intracapsular disease, but only minimal ECE. Supplemental EBRT gives a larger cancericidal margin around the prostate. The magnitude of the extra margin depends on what the cancericidal dose is. There is a dose gradient away from the edge of the prostate, some point at which the combined dose falls below the cancericidal level. The magnitude of the cancericidal margin will vary depending on the brachythcrapy dosc and EBRT dose delivered.

We do not know precisely how wide the extra cancericidal margin achieved with supplemental EBRT is. It is probably a matter of several mm, which could make a substantial difference in the likelihood of cure. Presently, no amount of speculation or computer modeling can tell us what the therapeutic margin really is, because we don't know what the cancericidal doses really are.

> *Why the Partin Tables are unduly frightening*
>
> The "Partin Tables" summarize the likelihood of ECE versus PSA, Gleason score and stage. They are widely quoted both by physicians and patients. However, the Partin Tables have been misinterpreted by both physicians and patients to mean that patients with ECE are not curable. In fact, a large percentage of patients with ECE are still curable, surgically or with brachytherapy, provided that the ECE is still within the surgical margins, or within the cancericidal dose range. This should be stressed to patients, who may otherwise believe that their high likelihood of ECE is synonymous with a high likelihood of treatment failure.

Patients with a high risk of ECE that extends further from the prostatic margin than it does for patients at lower risk of ECE, should receive supplemental EBRT. PSA, tumor differentiation, and pathological features are the primary selection factors in determining the risk of ECE. Stage is less important, due to the subjectivity of the digital rectal exam and that the vast majority of patients diagnosed currently have early stage disease.

Treatment selection guidelines come largely from prostatectomy series, where the incidence of extracapsular extension, and seminal vesical or lymph node invasion has been correlated with pre-surgical clinical parameters. Many reports detail comparisons between pre-operative clinical parameters and findings from the resected prostatic margins, the most widely quoted reports being those from Partin, Walsh and colleagues at Johns Hopkins University.[Partin 1997]

PROSTATE SPECIFIC ANTIGEN (PSA)

PSA is the single most important parameter in determining the curability of early stage disease.[Pisansky 1997] Progressively higher PSA levels are associated with a progressively higher likelihood of ECE (**Figure 12-5**). Accordingly,

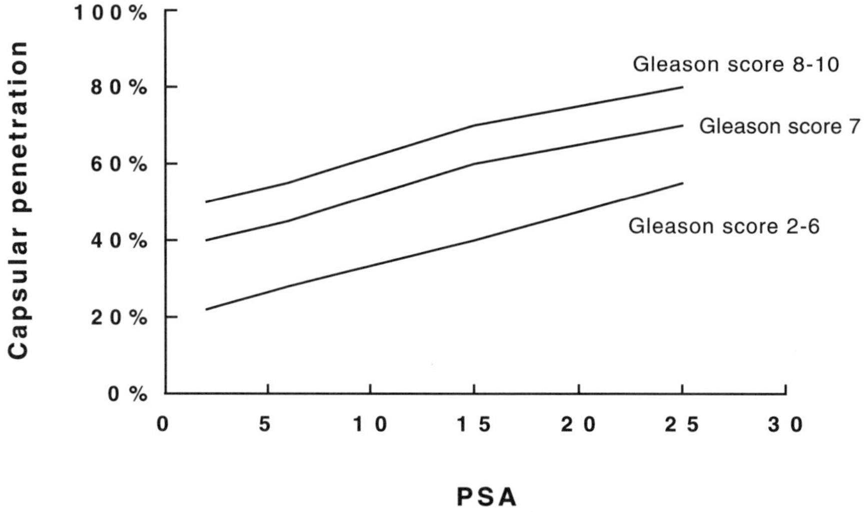

Figure 12-5. Likelihood of capsular penetration in patients with Stage T1c-T2a tumors, versus Gleason score and PSA, based on data from Johns Hopkins University.

patients with higher PSA levels are more likely to demonstrate early biochemical failure, regardless of their treatment modality.

There is commonly a 10 to 25% variability in results from the same lab on the same day, due to patient or laboratory-related factors.(Oesterling 1991) Several PSA values should be obtained on separate days in the course of a work-up, especially if the "watchful waiting" option is entertained.

One disadvantage of using PSA as a staging tool is that it lacks specificity. Other factors, including infarction and subclinical infection can raise the PSA. However, the incidence of subclinical infarction or subclinical infection that persistently elevate the PSA is low.(Nadler 1995)

Another disadvantage of PSA is its limited specificity in determining the likelihood of ECE. Some patients with advanced cancer can have low PSA values, so that a low PSA does not guarantee against substantial ECE.(Oesterling 1991) However, even for patients with high Gleason score, the likelihood of ECE is markedly lower in patients with a low PSA.

PSA categories

The risk of ECE and treatment failure is a continuum as the PSA rises (**Figure 12-6**). PSA categories of 0-4, 4-10, and 10-20 are generally used to classify patients into prognostic categories for radiation or prostatectomy. The choice

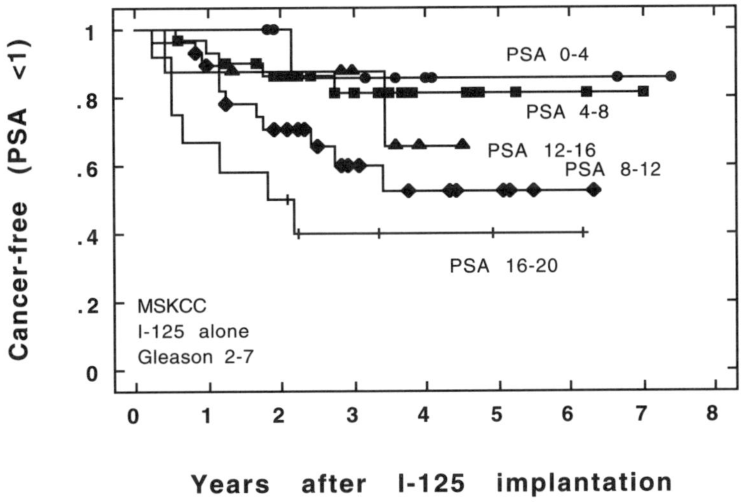

Figure 12-6. Freedom from biochemical failure following I-125 brachytherapy for Stage T1/T2 disease, with progressively higher pre-treatment PSA.

of PSA risk categories is arbitrary. There is nothing special about these categories, beyond the fact that they are generally used.

Where to draw the PSA line

Patients with a PSA less than 10 have a low likelihood of substantial ECE and should be curable with the narrow margins of an implant alone. The PSA-based tumor control rates with implant alone for low risk patients appear as good as those achieved with any other modality, including implant plus supplemental EBRT. To date, no convincing data shows that such patients will do better if treated with supplemental EBRT (**Figures 12-7 & 12-8**).

Patients with PSA greater than 10 have a higher likelihood of ECE, with a higher chance that some cancer extends beyond the 2 to 3 mm therapeutic margin of an implant alone. These patients should receive supplemental EBRT to have a wider therapeutic margin around their prostate.

It makes sense that supplemental EBRT will add to the therapeutic efficacy of an implant alone in patients at high risk of ECE, and available data regarding implant plus supplemental EBRT appears superior to that reported with implant alone or EBRT alone (**Figures 12-7 & 12-8**). Although superiority of combined modality therapy for higher risk patients has not been substantiated in a controlled trial, it seems reasonable to treat higher risk patients with supplemental

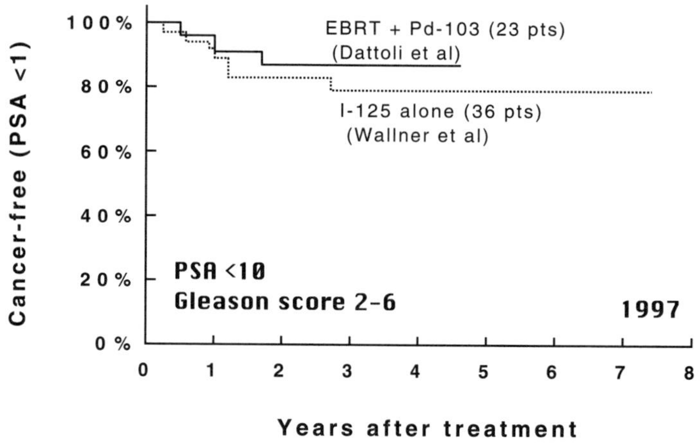

Figure 12-7a. Disease-free survival after implant alone versus implant plus EBRT for patients with Gleason 6 or less, and PSA below 10. (This is not adjusted for stage.) There is no obvious advantage to adding supplemental EBRT for these patients at low risk of substantial ECE. The combined modality group includes T3 patients, whereas they have been excluded from the I-125 alone group.

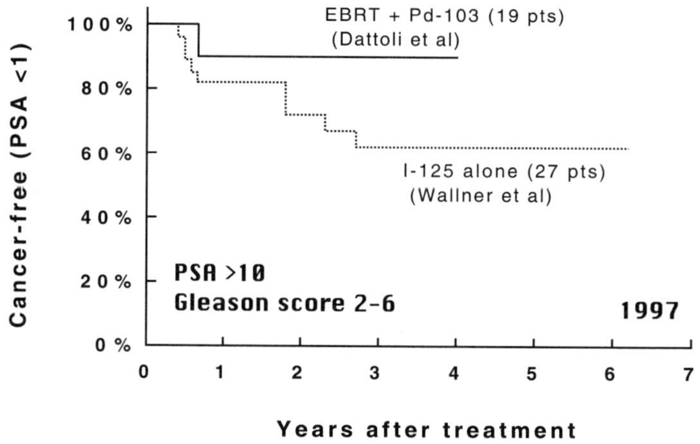

Figure 12-7b. Disease-free survival after implant alone versus implant plus EBRT for patients with Gleason 6 or less, and PSA above 10. Although this is a retrospective comparison of uncontrolled series, there appears to be an advantage to adding supplemental EBRT to these patients at higher risk of substantial ECE. This is not adjusted for stage. The combined modality group includes T3 patients, whereas they have been excluded from the I-125 alone group.

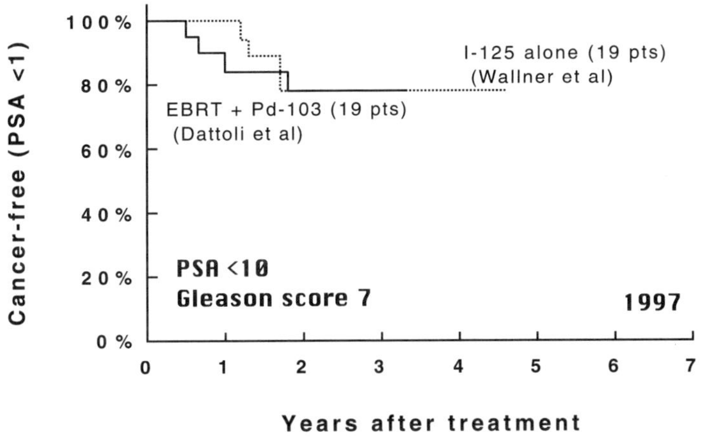

Figure 12-8a. Disease-free survival after implant alone versus implant plus EBRT for patients with Gleason 7 and PSA below 10. There is no obvious advantage to adding supplemental EBRT for these patients at a lower risk of substantial ECE. This is not adjusted for stage. The combined modality group includes T3 patients, whereas they have been excluded from the I-125 alone group.

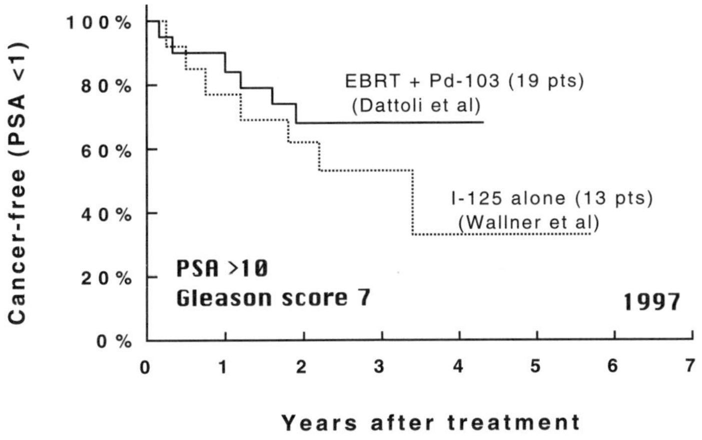

Figure 12-8b. Disease-free survival after implant alone versus EBRT plus implant boost for patients with Gleason 7 and PSA above 10. Although this is a retrospective comparison of uncontrolled series, there appears to be an advantage to adding supplemental EBRT to these patients at higher risk of substantial ECE. This is not adjusted for stage. The combined modality group includes T3 patients, whereas they have been excluded from the I-125 alone group.

controlled trial, it seems reasonable to treat higher risk patients with supplemental EBRT until data to the contrary is published.

PROSTATIC ACID PHOSPHATASE (PAP)

Prostatic cancer cells lose their orientation with the basement membrane and secrete prostatic acid phosphatase away from the acinar lumen, into the stroma. Therefore, more advanced tumors are more likely to secrete PAP into the stroma, from where it can reach the general circulation. An elevated PAP level correlates with a very high likelihood of ECE and with a high failure rate after surgery.(Salo 1988) Until the widespread adoption of PSA testing, acid phosphatase was a routine part of staging.

PSA has a greater sensitivity for early ECE than does PAP, but there is no absolute PSA value that definitely indicates extraprostatic disease. In contrast, nearly all patients with elevated PAP have extracapsular extension.(Salo 1988) PAP is the best predictor of early biochemical failure in patients with otherwise high risk features and it therefore may be a more accurate indicator of micrometastatic disease than PSA.(Dattoli 1996) PAP has little correlation with Gleason score or PSA (**Figure 12-9a and b**).

Its value for lower risk patients, generally treated with implant alone, has not been studied. Nevertheless, it probably should be checked routinely for all patients, as it may be a good screen for micrometastatic disease in patients with relatively low PSA and Gleason score.

Patients with elevated PAP should probably receive supplemental EBRT. Although their biochemical failure rate with supplemental EBRT is high, it would likely be even higher with implant alone.

Patients with markedly elevated PAP are at extremely high risk of both substantial ECE and of disseminated disease (see **Figure 15-8**). Their chances of cure with EBRT alone or implant alone are probably near zero if the enzymatic PAP is greater than 10 (normal : 0 to 2). Prostatectomy is unlikely to be any more effective than implant plus supplemental EBRT because of the high likelihood of ECE and distant disease. Patients with an elevated PAP reading need effective adjunctive therapy. Hormonal deprivation is one consideration. Although there is currently no convincing evidence that hormonal ablation or any other adjunctive therapy will increase the cure rate, adjunctive therapy should be considered for all patients with an elevated PAP, preferably as part of a controlled study.

GLEASON SCORE

The Gleason score has become the standard pathology grading system for prostate cancer in North America. The use of the Gleason score, however, is complicated by the fact that its interpretation has not been uniform. In the past few years, there has been an upward migration of the scores. Reasons for upward

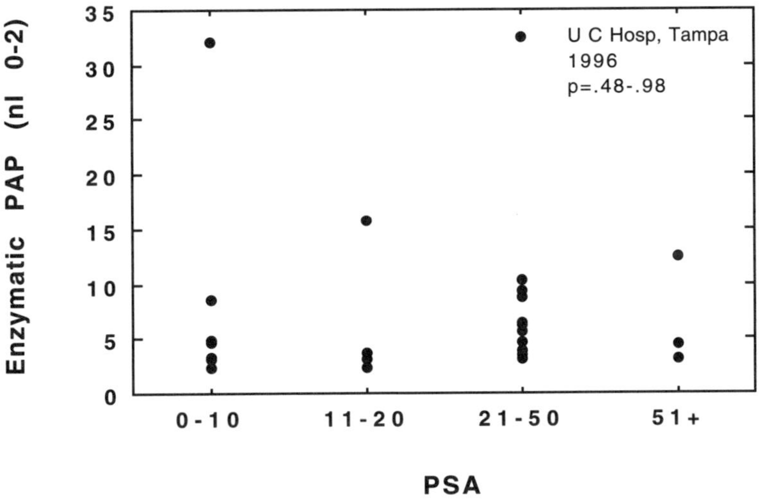

Figure 12-9a. There is little correlation between PAP and PSA. In multivariate analysis, PAP is an independent predictor of failure.

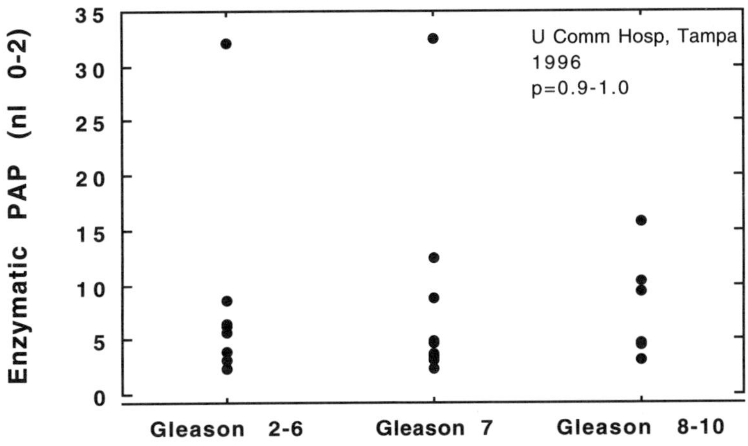

Figure 12-9b. There is little correlation between PAP and Gleason score. In multivariate analysis, PAP is an independent predictor of failure.

migration include the decline in TURPs for diagnosis, since transitional zone cancers tend to be better differentiated. Also, the Gleason scale is today being applied differently than when it was first introduced.(Epstein 1996, Ca 78:350) The way the scale is currently being applied, nearly all tumors are scored as a Gleason 6 or higher. Very few tumors are Gleason 2 to 5 and only about 10% are scored 8-10.(Partin 1997) The scale is now less useful since most tumors fall within a limited part of it.

Higher Gleason scores are associated with a higher probability of ECE (**Figure 12-5**). However, the Gleason score is of far less prognostic importance than PSA or PAP.(Pisansky 1997)(Dattoli 1996) The relatively low prognostic significance of the Gleason score is apparent when perusing Figures 12-5 and 12-11, in which the curves for increasing Gleason score are quite close to each other.

Patients with Gleason scores of 2 to 6 are generally at low risk of ECE or biochemical failure after treatment, as long as their pre-treatment PSA was low. If that PSA was high, a Gleason score of 2 to 6 is less reassuring. There are several explanations as to why a low Gleason score is not predictive of a good outcome in patients with higher PSA levels. Higher PSAs are generally associated with larger tumors, which are less likely to be sterilized with radiation. The high failure risk in patients with low Gleason scores but high PSA levels is also partly explained by sampling error. Biopsies provide only a small fraction of cancerous tissue and since prostate cancers are frequently heterogeneous, at least 50% of tumors are seen to contain higher Gleason score regions when the entire prostate is available for review.(Ohori 1994)

Gleason score 7

Gleason score 7 tumors have a component of "pattern 4," defined as a fusing of the neoplastic glands (**Figure 12-10**).(Gleason 1974) For Glcason score 7 patients, the likelihood of ECE climbs to 50% overall, and the post-prostatectomy or post-EBRT prognosis falls substantially.(Partin 1997)(Zeitman 1994) Patients with Gleason score 7, regardless of their PSA are generally treated with a combination of implant plus EBRT. Despite this nearly universal practice, the necessity of supplemental EBRT in patients with low PSA levels is not clearly established.

At MSKCC, Gleason score 7 patients have frequently been treated with implant alone. Their prognosis differed markedly depending on their pre-treatment PSA.(Grann 1998) For those patients with a PSA less than 10 ng/ml, the prognosis was similar to that of patients with lower Gleason scores. The results for such patients were similar to that for Gleason 7 patients treated with implant plus EBRT at University Community Hospital, Tampa (UCHT)(**Figure 12-8**). Based on comparison of the MSKCC and UCHT experience, patients with Gleason scores 7 and PSA under 10 appear to do as well with implant alone as with implant plus EBRT. Therefore, the addition of supplemental EBRT might be avoided in

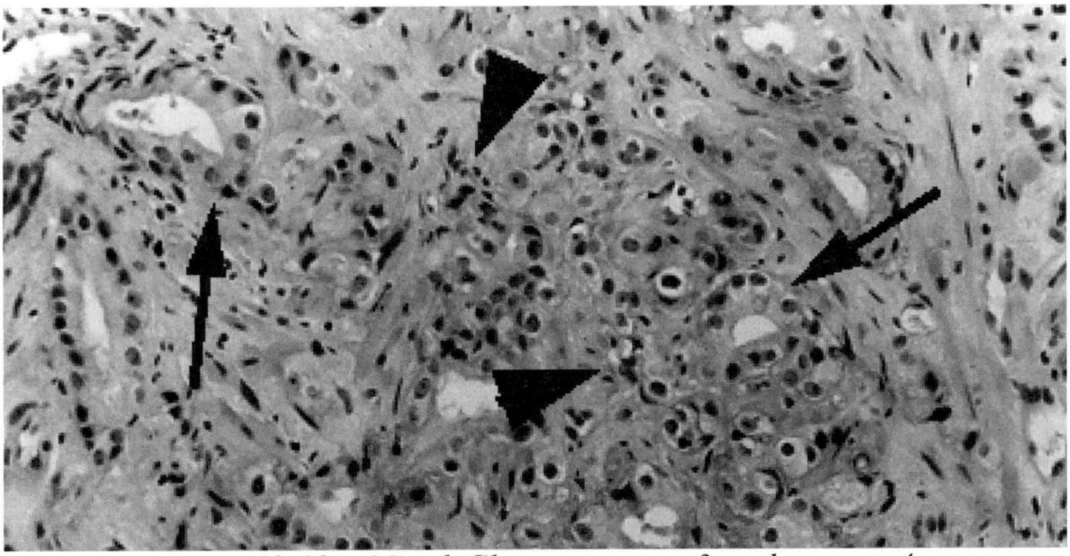

Figure 12-10. Mixed Gleason pattern 3 and pattern 4. Pattern 3 includes glandular structures (arrows). The pattern 4 area has a loss of glandular structure (arrowheads), indicative of poor differentiation, consistent with a worse prognosis for patients with Gleason scores 7 versus 6.

patients with Gleason 7 and PSA under 10, as it costs more and may carry a greater risk of complications. However, the data on which this is based should be considered preliminary, and longer follow-up is needed to make a firmer recommendation in this regard.

For patients with Gleason 7 and PSA above 10, the argument for administering supplemental EBRT is more compelling, as these patients appear to do better with combined modality therapy than with implant alone. The results with implant alone at MSKCC were dismal. Over 50% had biochemical failure within 3 years, and there was no clear plateau on the disease-free curve. In contrast, the biochemical tumor control rates with implant plus EBRT were still above 50% (**Figure 12-8**). Unless data to the contrary emerges from other series, the use of supplemental EBRT for patients with Gleason score 7 and PSA above 10 should probably be considered standard.

Gleason 8-10

Patients with Gleason scores of 8 to 10 have generally done poorly after surgery or conventional EBRT.[Zeitman 1994] While the prognosis for such patients is not good, those with low pre-treatment PSA may still do well. Data regarding the treatment outcome for patients with high Gleason score but low pre-treatment

PSA is still very limited. Roach and colleagues showed that the early biochemical failure rate is only approximately 20% following treatment with conformal EBRT, provided that the patient's pre-treatment PSA was less than 20.(Roach 1996)

Patients with high Gleason scores but low PSA levels probably still have a low tumor burden, and can be cured with effective local therapy. They might even do well with an implant alone, as have patients with Gleason score 7 and PSA less than 10 who were treated with I-125 alone at MSKCC. For the time being, however, the nearly universal recommendation of supplemental EBRT for patients with Gleason scores of 8 to 10 seems prudent.

STAGE

Statistically, the clinical stage of the cancer has far less prognostic importance than the PSA level, in part because of the subjectivity of the digital rectal exam (DRE) and because palpable abnormalities of the prostate are often not cancerous.(Pisansky 1997) Patients with clinical Stage T2b disease are at a slightly higher risk of ECE and are generally treated with supplemental EBRT (**Figure 12-11**). However, because of the relatively weak association of clinical stage with ECE, an argument could easily be made, in the presence of low PSA and Gleason score, to ignore stage. Even determining the presence of gross ECE (clinical stage

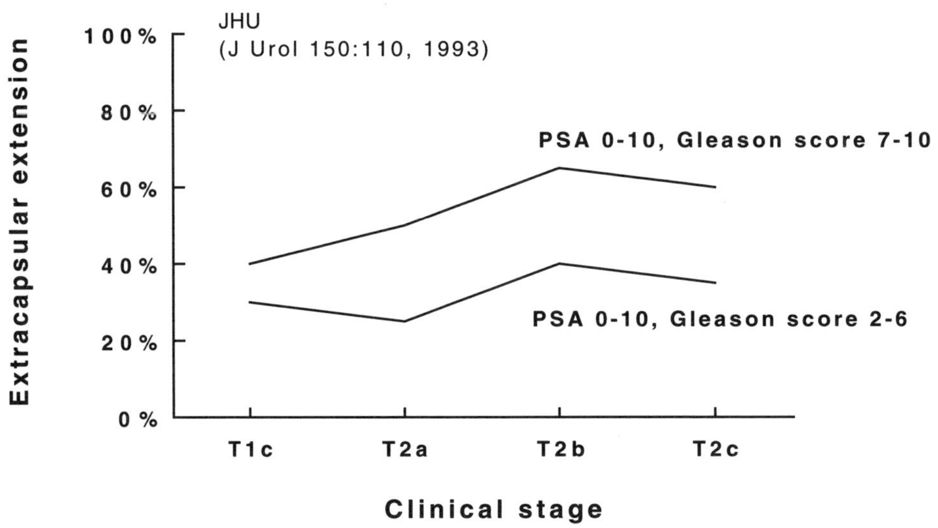

Figure 12-11. Minimal effect of clinical stage on the likelihood of ECE. The subjective nature of the digital rectal exam diminishes the prognostic importance of clinical staging.

T3) is wrought with subjectivity, although it would seem prudent to treat any patient with stage T3 on DRE with supplemental EBRT.

Patients considered to have T3 disease by what is believed to be seminal vesicle involvement on digital rectal exam should receive supplemental EBRT. In these cases, seminal vesicle biopsy to verify the digital exam is probably warranted.

PSA and Gleason score should be added to the staging system

Even though both PSA level and Gleason score are better determinants of patient's curability than DRE, neither is included in the clinical staging system. Dumb. PSA and Gleason score should be added to the staging system soon, to make it more relevant.

SEMINAL VESICLE INVOLVEMENT

Spread of cancer to the seminal vesicles is correlated with PSA and Gleason score (**Figure 12-12**). Patients with a PSA above 20 and Gleason score of 7 or more are at high risk of seminal vesicle involvement, and some researchers have argued that a pre-treatment biopsy in these patients is warranted.(Stone 1995) However, patients with markedly elevated PSA or Gleason scores would receive supplemental EBRT covering the seminal vesicles regardless, so that seminal vesicle biopsy results would generally not change the treatment approach.

Cancerous invasion of the peri-vesicle tissue or the muscular wall of the seminal vesicle is associated with a high likelihood of post-surgical cancer recurrence (**Figure 12-13**). (Epstein 1993) However, judging from prostatectomy series, some patients with seminal vesicle involvement may still be surgically curable. It is reasonable to assume that similarly, some are curable with radiation, though the likelihood of cure is probably quite low.

The seminal vesicles cannot be treated adequately with brachytherapy alone, due to a rapid dose fall-off from the prostate edge. Sources cannot be reliably placed in the seminal vesicles because the vesicles move when pushed by a needle tip, and because sources tend to migrate after being ejected in their vicinity. It is possible (but unlikely) that suture-mounted sources could allow more reliable source placement in the seminal vesicles. Iridium-192 sources inside stiff after-loading needles may be placed in the seminal vesicles, but the dosimetry to the seminal vesicles would still be questionable as the seminal vesicle are irregular structures which change their position as the bladder expands and contracts. In patients suspected or proven to have seminal vesicle involvement, supplemental EBRT should be used to offer a reasonable likelihood of adequately radiating the seminal vesicles. This point is moot, however, since most patients with seminal vesicle involvement would receive supplemental EBRT based on other factors anyway (PSA above 10 or Gleason of 7 or higher).

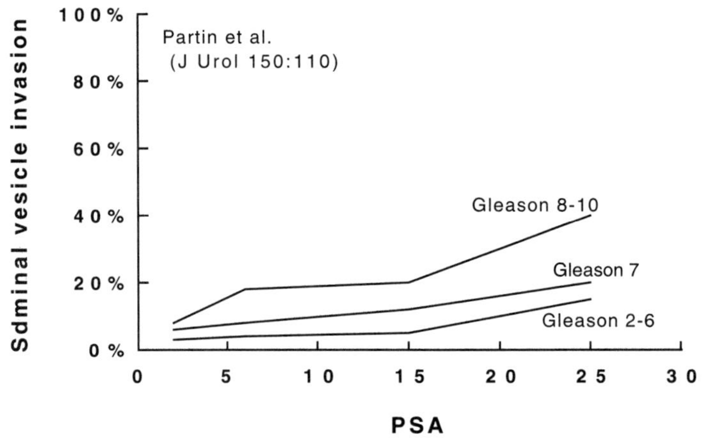

Figure 12-12. Likelihood of seminal vesicle invasion in patients with Stage T1c-T2a tumors, versus Gleason score and PSA. readings.

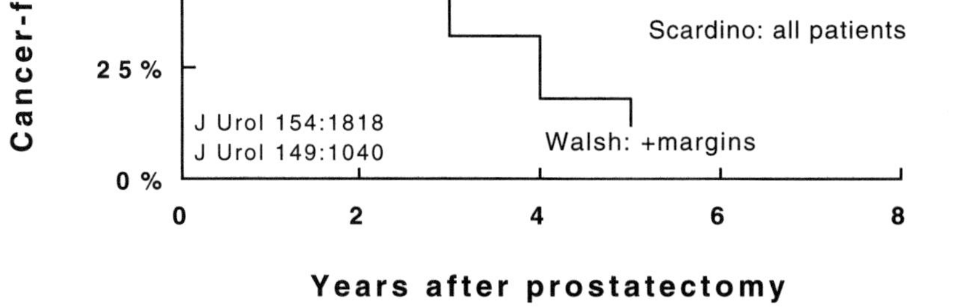

Figure 12-13. Freedom from failure for patients with seminal vesicle involvement and negative lymph nodes. There is some evidence of curability (plateau of the disease-free curves) in these series, if the lymph nodes and surgical margins are negative.

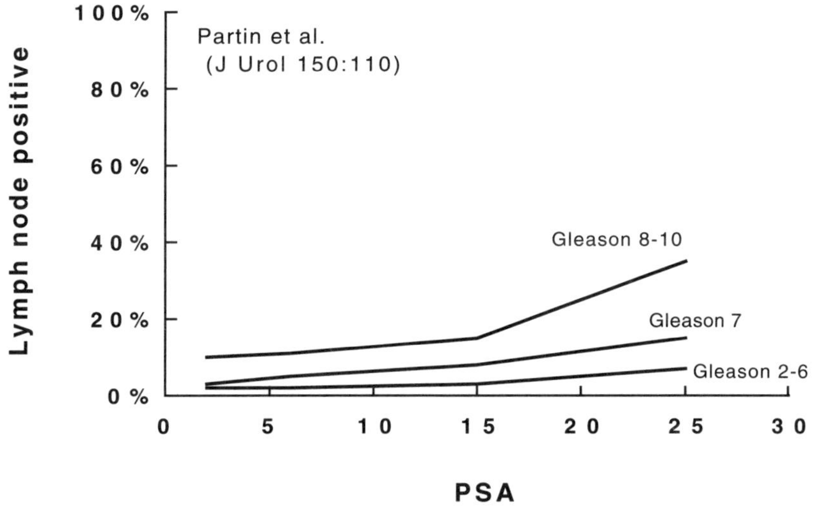

Figure 12-14. Likelihood of lymph node invasion in patients with stage T1c-T2a tumors, versus Gleason score and PSA.

LYMPH NODE DISSECTION

Patients with PSA below 20 and Gleason score of 7 or less have a very low likelihood of having cancerous lymph node invasion. Routine staging lymph node dissection is generally not warranted (**Figure 12-14**). If brachytherapy alone is considered for patients at a higher risk of lymph node or seminal vesicle invasion, a pre-implant biopsy of both sites is justifiable. A finding of lymph node involvement is generally a contraindication to brachytherapy, in favor of observation or EBRT with hormonal blockade.

OTHER PATHOLOGICAL FEATURES

The Gleason score is the most widely used prognostic biopsy feature. However, other pathological features have been more closely correlated with extraprostatic disease, and perhaps with prognosis. The most widely studied pathological features are the extent of tumor in the biopsy specimen, and perineural invasion.

Extensive disease in biopsy specimens

Extensive tumor in the pre-treatment biopsy sample is loosely correlated with a higher likelihood of larger primary tumors and ECE, based on analysis of

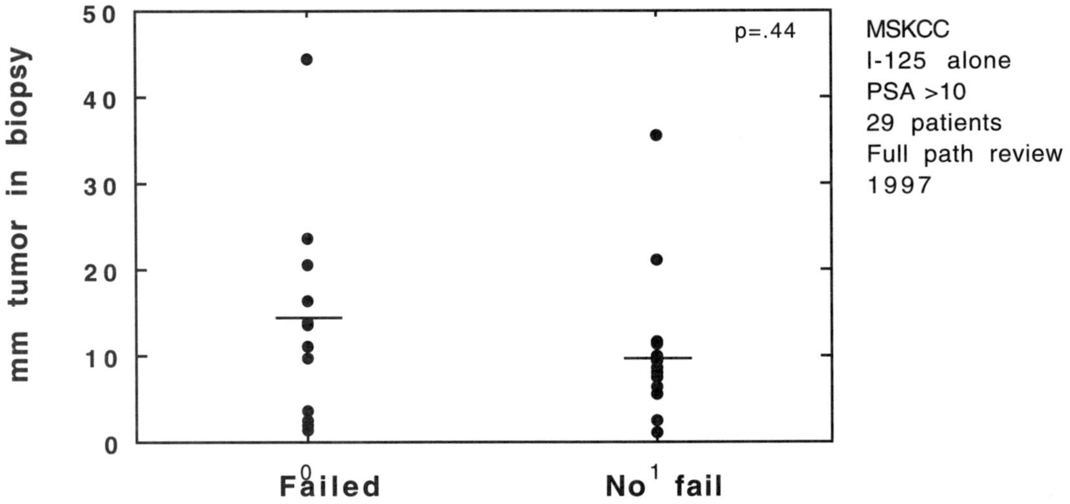

Figure 12-15. mm tumor in the biopsy specimen for patients with or without biochemical failure. There is a non-significant trend of a higher failure rate in patients with more extensive tissue involvement.

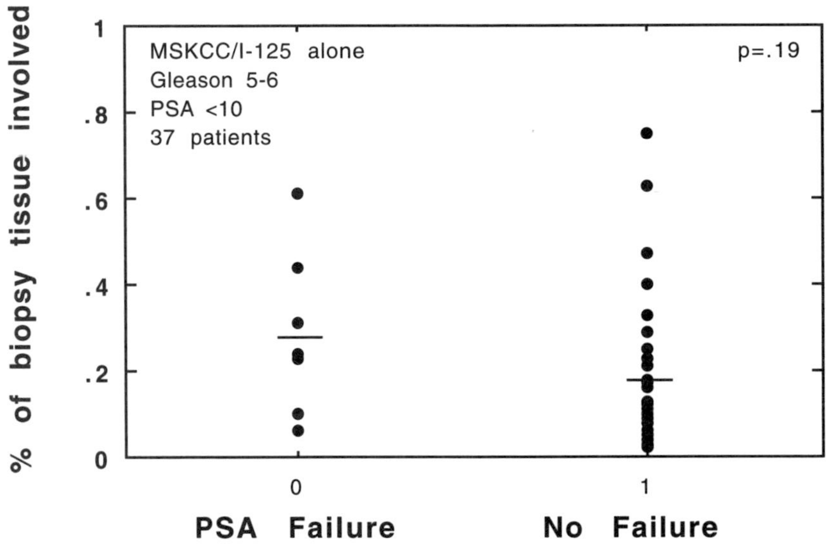

Figure 12-16. Extent of tumor in biopsy specimen in patients with or without biochemical failure. There is a non-significant trend of a higher failure rate in patients with more extensive tissue involvement.

prostatectomy specimens.(Cupp 1995) The amount of tumor can be quantified by the number of involved cores, the length of cancer in the specimen, or the percentage of the specimen involved. Each parameter is a reflection of the same factor: how much of the prostate is involved by cancer.

In patients treated with I-125 implant alone at MSKCC, the total linear tumor length was only a weak prognostic indicator (**Figure 12-15**). The percentage of the biopsy tissue replaced by tumor was also only weakly correlated with risk of failure (**Figure 12-16**).

The use of quantitative tumor measurements on needle biopsy to predict prognosis or to choose treatment should be done cautiously. While extensive tumor correlates with advanced pathological stage, a finding of only limited amounts of cancer (less than 10 mm) does not guarantee a lack of extracapsular extension or a good prognosis. Investigators have generally agreed that pathological parameters reflective of tumor bulk have shown some relevance statistically, but that there is considerable overlap between failing and non-failing patients.(Goto 1996)(Cupp 1995) The sampling error inherent in the biopsy procedure makes the validity of tumor quantification for an individual patient subject to chance. Nonetheless, statistically tumor quantification may be more predictive than Gleason score, and probably should be used more often to guide treatment decisions. It seems reasonable to add supplemental EBRT for patients with more than 10 to 15 mm tumor in their total biopsy tissue (assuming six cores were taken) or if greater than 20% of the total biopsy tissue is replaced by cancer.

Bilateral positive biopsies

Bilateral positive biopsies indicate a higher likelihood of ECE.(Davieli 1992) As with extensive tumor in the biopsy specimen, substantial room for sampling error exists, and the presence of a bilateral positive biopsy in itself cannot be reliably used to make a decision regarding the treatment modality. However, it should enhance one's enthusiasm for using supplemental EBRT.

Perineural invasion

The clinical relevance of perineural invasion in the biopsy sample is still unclear. Villers and colleagues reported that perineural invasion in the prostatectomy specimen was frequently associated with transcapsular extension and that perineural invasion was one mechanism for transcapsular spread. (Villers 1989) Johns Hopkins University investigators showed that patients with pre-surgical biopsy specimens showing perineural invasion had a 97% likelihood of extracapsular extension on the prostatectomy specimen.(Bastacky 1993) The researchers concluded that finding perineural invasion was a very poor prognostic sign. However, they failed to present any clinical data to show that patients with perineural invasion actually had a less favorable clinical course.

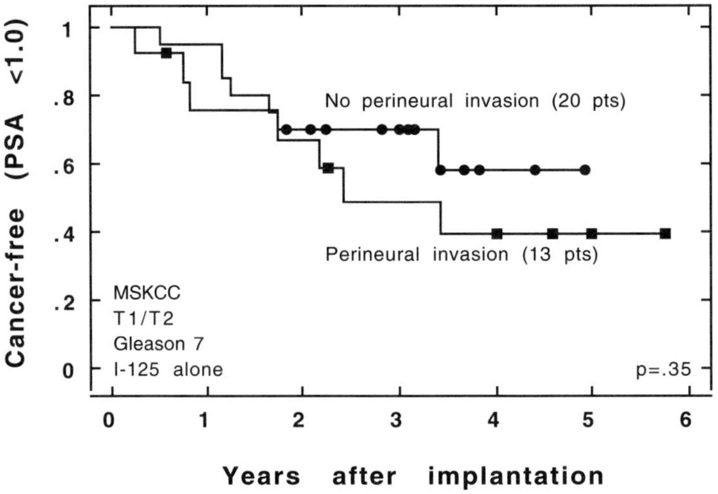

Figure 12-17. Freedom from biochemical recurrence for patients with Gleason 7 tumors, with or without perineural invasion.

In patients treated with implant alone at MSKCC, the presence of perineural invasion did not substantially affect prognosis (**Figure 12-17**). The lack of clearly inferior clinical outcome for patients implanted at MSKCC is still consistent with findings from Stanford and JHU, in that patients with perineural invasion may well have a higher likelihood of early ECE. Such patients are apparently still highly curable, however, providing that the extracapsular disease has not extended more than a few mm from the prostatic margin. If it has not, implant radiation can still eradicate all the cancer. Patients with more extensive ECE are not curable, but their incurability has probably already been reflected in a higher PSA level or Gleason score, and is not any better identified by the presence of perineural invasion.

Like other higher risk pathological features, the presence of perineural invasion, because of the greater likelihood of extensive ECE, might make one more likely to recommend supplemental EBRT. However, if other factors are favorable, perineural invasion alone should not be an indication for supplemental EBRT.

ARE IMAGING STUDIES USEFUL?

After stage, PSA and biopsy pathology are considered, there is substantial uncertainty about the presence of ECE and curability. The ability to stage patients more accurately is paramount, because supplemental EBRT, which may increase the cure rate and definitely increases the cost, could be used more judiciously. Computerized tomography (CT) and magnetic resonance (MR) are commonly used in the hope of staging patients more accurately. Unfortunately, both tests are of questionable value.

CT scanning

The value of a CT scan as a staging tool is highly questionable. No controlled study has determined the accuracy of CT scanning in determining nodal status or ECE in prostate cancer. CT scanning is a waste of time and money in lower risk patients, for whom the likelihood of finding enlarged lymph nodes is negligible. The chance of showing subtle ECE, that is not apparent on digital rectal exam, is probably miniscule.

Considering how commonly CT is used to stage patients, it is surprising that no rigorous studies have been done to evaluate its utility in that regard. Using CT to look for enlarged pelvic lymph nodes may be more justifiable in patients with markedly elevated PSA. A needle or laparoscopic biopsy would be needed to verify cancerous involvement of abnormally enlarged lymph nodes.

TRUS

TRUS (transrectal ultrasound) has been tested prospectively in a multi-institutional trial, which compared its findings to those of the prostatectomy specimen.[(Rifkin 1990)] TRUS was no better than chance alone in determining which patients were likely to have ECE. Its sensitivity to detect ECE was only 66%, and its specificity was only 46%. Because of its poor sensitivity and specificity, TRUS should not be used routinely to stage prostate cancer. For staging, its use should be limited to biopsy guidance.

MR

MR scanning appears to provide much more information about internal architecture and capsular penetration than CT or TRUS (see Figure 4-1). It seems logical that MR would be a more accurate staging tool, and it probably is, as MR can detect ECE of 3 mm or greater.[(Schiebler 1993)] Patients with a small degree of ECE (less than 3 mm) are still potentially curable with implant alone, so that if MR does not reveal ECE, an implant should be sufficient. Patients with greater than 3 mm ECE are less likely to have cancer beyond the cancericidal isodose line (120 Gy?), and should receive supplemental EBRT.

D'Amico and colleagues have made considerable effort to define which patients are most likely to benefit from MR staging.[(D'Amico 1996)] Patients with PSA below 10 and Gleason score 6 or lower are candidates for treatment by implant alone. It is in these patients that imaging studies could be useful in deter-

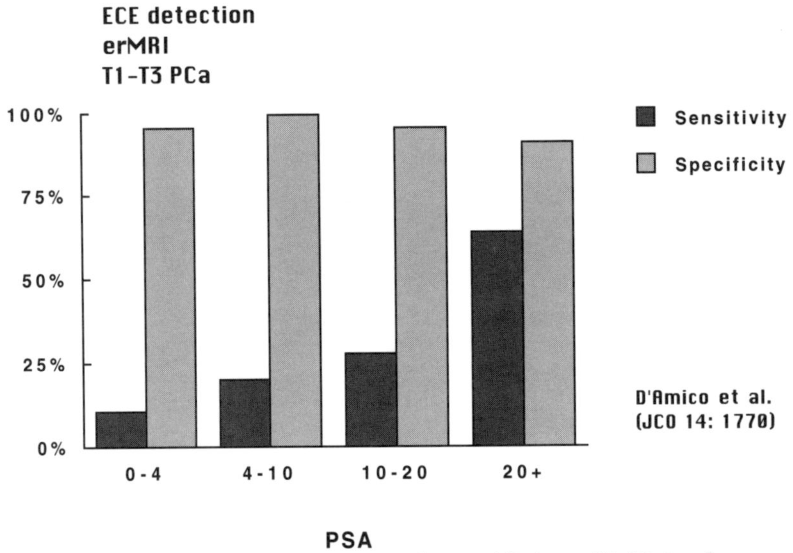

Figure 12-18a. Sensitivity and specificity of MR in detecting ECE, based on pre-treatment PSA. In low PSA patients, there is little likelihood of detecting ECE, which would presumably be of minimal extent anyway. Although MR sensitivity is greater at higher PSA, those patients would routinely be treated with supplemental EBRT anyway.

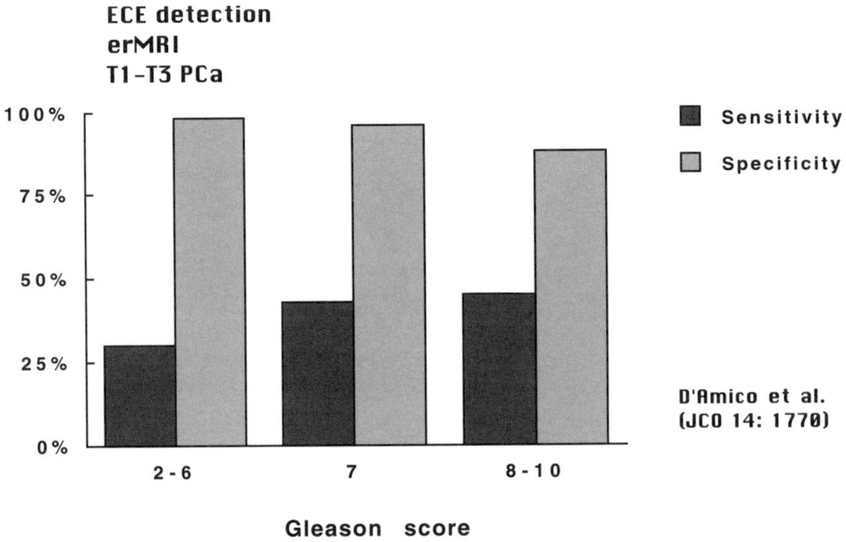

Figure 12-18b. Sensitivity and specificity of MR in detecting ECE, based on pre-treatment Gleason score. At low Gleason score, there is little likelihood of detecting ECE. Although MR sensitivity is greater at higher Gleason score, those patients with higher scores would routinely be treated with supplemental EBRT anyway.

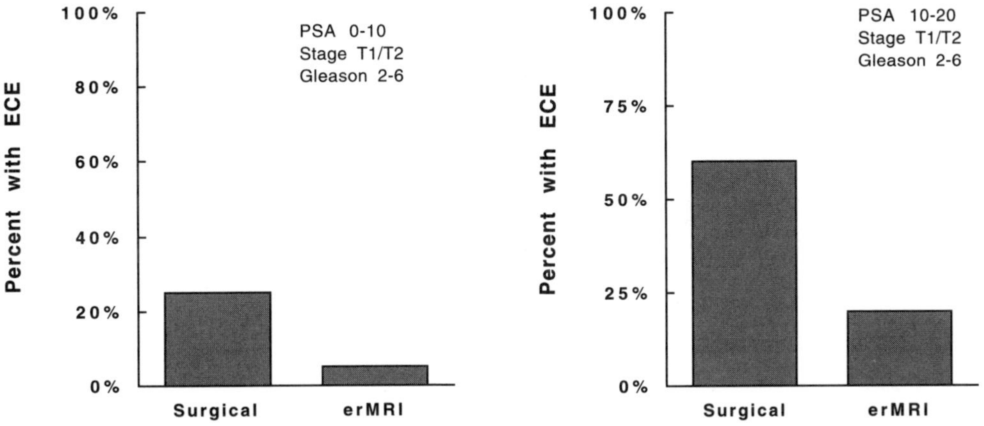

Figure 12-19. Sensitivity for detecting ECE in T1/T2, low risk prostate cancer. In patients with PSA below 10, the likelihood of detecting ECE with endorectal MR (erMR) is so small that its routine use is questionable. The likelihood of detecting substantial ECE is higher for patients with PSA above 10, but those patients would generally receive supplemental EBRT based on PSA levels alone anyway -- MR would not influence the treatment decision.

mining which patients already have extraprostatic disease, calling for supplemental EBRT.

The problem with routine MR scanning in low risk patients is that only a tiny percentage of them will have their treatment altered by the test findings. The incidence of ECE is only 20 to 30%, and of those, only approximately 10% will have ECE detected by MR (**Figures 12-18 and 12-19**). The low sensitivity of MR in low risk patients makes its routine use questionable.

MR has a higher sensitivity in patients with high grade cancers or high PSA levels. However, patients with Gleason scores of 8 or more, or PSA levels of 10 or higher are at such high risk of ECE or seminal vesicle invasion that they should receive supplemental EBRT regardless of imaging studies.

The use of MR to screen for pelvic lymphadenopathy in low stage, low PSA patients is especially dumb. In the prospective NCI staging trial, only 1 of 23 stage T1 or T2 patients with cancerous pelvic lymph nodes was detected by MR.(Rifkin 1990)

CRITERIA FOR IMPLANT ALONE - IN PLAIN ENGLISH

The generally accepted criteria for treatment with implant alone are PSA levels of 10 or lower, Gleason score of 6 or less and clinical stages T1-T2a (**Table**

Table 12-1. Criteria for adding supplemental EBRT to brachytherapy.

<u>Generally accepted criteria</u>:	PSA >10 Gleason ≥7 Clinical T2c/T3
<u>Less certain criteria</u>:	Extensive tumor in biopsy (>10 mm) Bilateral positive biopsies Perineural invasion ECE by MR

12-1). Patients with stage T2b-c lesions which are associated with low PSA and Gleason scores should be equally good candidates for treatment by implant alone. Finding limited tumor in the biopsy sample and absence of perineural invasion should increase the comfort level in treatment with implant alone, but these factors should not be, in themselves, criteria for treatment selection.

SUPPLEMENTAL EBRT - IN PLAIN ENGLISH

Patients with a high risk of ECE include those with PSA levels above 10, Gleason scores of 8 or more or T3 tumors determined by digital rectal examination (**Figure 12-20**). They have a high risk of biochemical failure with any modality (**Figure 12-21**). Supplemental EBRT allows for wider coverage of periprostatic disease and seminal vesicles, theoretically giving a higher likelihood of cancer eradication. This strategy has produced results that compare favorably with prostatectomy or EBRT alone.(Dattoli 1996)

WHEN IS BRACHYTHERAPY A WASTE OF TIME?

Distant metastases

Patients with documented distant metastases will generally not benefit from aggressive local therapy. Brachytherapy is not usually a consideration in their care. as only a small percentage of them will suffer symptomatically from local disease.

Positive (cancerous) lymph nodes

Patients with known pelvic lymph node involvement are generally considered incurable, although there are some more encouraging reports.(Sands 1995) If a patient with known lymph node involvement is treated for cure, brachytherapy would generally not be given. However, if such patients are potentially curable

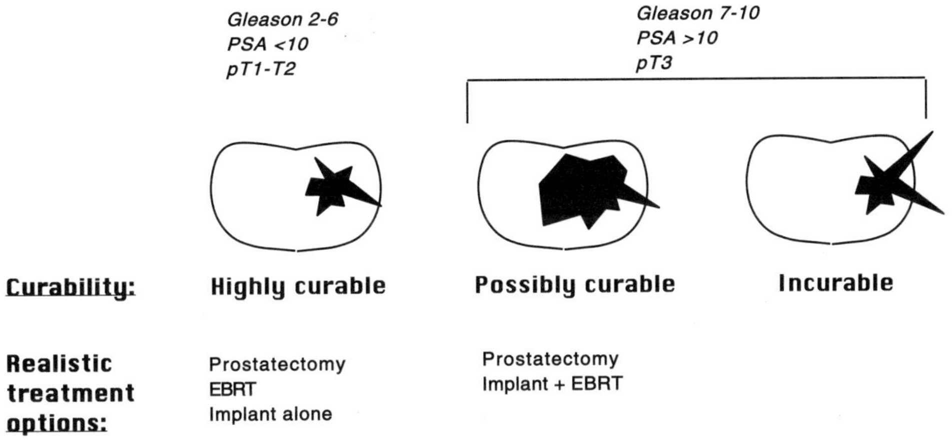

Figure 12-20. Low risk versus high risk prostatic carcinoma. Given current published data, patients with high risk carcinoma are infrequently curable with EBRT alone. Their potential for cure is probably higher with prostatectomy or brachytherapy-based radiation, though this has not been proven in a controlled trial.

(i.e: without distant metastases), aggressive brachytherapy-based local therapy might help.

Bad numbers

Patients with very high PSA levels, Gleason scores or elevated PAP have a very high likelihood of failing treatment, whether due to substantial ECE, lymph node involvement, or distant disease. Although their chances of cure are low, surgical series and brachytherapy series usually show some evidence of a plateau on the freedom from failure curve, indicating that some finite percent of such patients are curable. Accordingly, if a patient otherwise has a life expectancy of more than 5 years, aggressive brachytherapy-based treatment is warranted. However, every effort should first be made to rule out distant metastases and lymph node metastases.

USE OF IMPLANT PLUS EBRT IN LOW RISK PATIENTS

Because there is at least a 10% likelihood of ECE even in low risk patients (those with PSA less than 10 and Gleason score below 7), it could be argued that all patients should be given supplemental EBRT. A reasonable argument, it is dif-

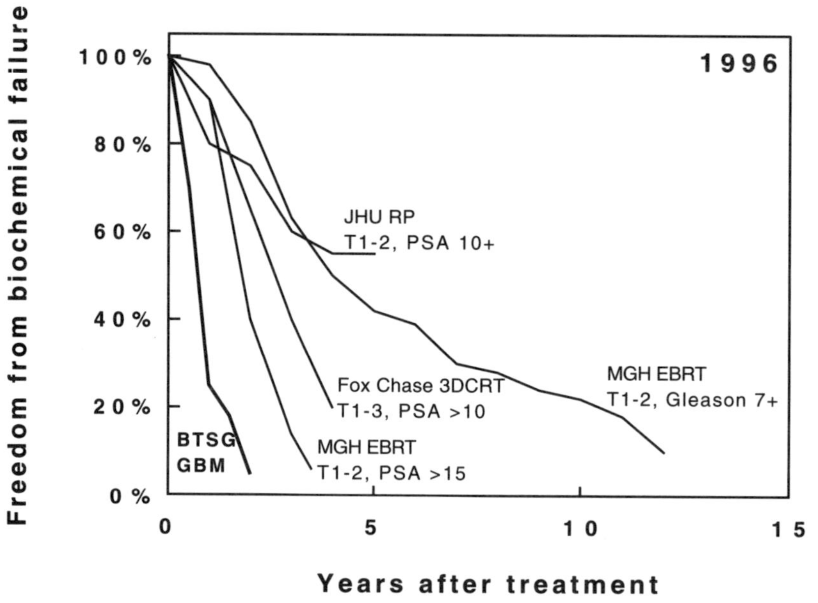

Figure 12-21. Likelihood of cure with conventional dose EBRT alone or surgery, in patients with PSA above 10 or Gleason score 7 or greater. The survival for patients with glioblastoma multiforme brain tumors (GBM) treated with EBRT+BCNU on BTSG study (J Neurosurg, 1978) is shown at the far left of the curve. Their cure rate is essentially zero. With conventional dose EBRT alone, at some of the most respected institutions, the biochemical cure rate for patients with PSA above 10 or Gleason score 7 or more has been similar to that for GBM. The freedom from failure after radical prostatectomy at Johns Hopkins University begins to level off at about 50%, suggesting that some higher risk patients can be cured surgically.

ficult to reconcile. One argument against it is that low risk patients who do have ECE will probably have only minimal ECE, that should be treated sufficiently by the dose fall-off region around an implant. A second argument against supplemental EBRT in low risk patients is that no investigator has shown better results with it, compared to what can be achieved with an implant alone. A third reason against use of supplemental EBRT in low risk patients is that it probably increases the likelihood of impotence and rectal injury.

One more reason not to use supplemental EBRT in all patients is the added cost. Although one would prefer not to use cost in making a treatment decision, it is an important issue, as prostate cancer is so common. Widespread use of additional, expensive, unnecessary therapy adds substantially to our total societal cost.

REAL LIFE CHOICES

Treatment choice guidelines are nothing more than that -- guidelines. Because of the uncertainty in PSA readings, biopsy interpretations and imaging studies, one can not tell whether or not there is substantial ECE in an individual patient, and whether supplemental EBRT is necessary. Patients have become quite savvy, often being well versed in the issues considered in treatment. In cases where the choice between an implant alone or implant plus supplemental EBRT is unclear, the situation should be explained carefully to the patient and a mutual decision reached.

REFERENCES

1. Bastacky SI, Walsh PC, Epstein JI. Relationship between perineural tumor invasion on needle biopsy and radical prostatectomy capsular penetration in clinical stage B adenocarcinoma of the prostate. Am J Surg Path 1993; 17:336-341.

2. Cupp MR, Bostwick DG, Myers RP, Oesterling JE. The volume of prostate cancer in the biopsy specimen cannot reliably predict the quantity of cancer in the radical prostatectomy specimen on an individual basis. J Urol 1995; 153:1543-1548.

3. D'Amico AV, Whittington R, Malkowicz SB, Schultz D. Critical analysis of the ability of the endorectal coil magnetic resonance imaging scan to predict pathologic stage, margin status, and postoperative prostate-specific antigen failure in patients with clinically organ-confined prostate cancer. J Clin Oncol 1996; 14:1770-1777.

4. Dattoli M, Wallner K, Sorace R. Pd-103 brachytherapy and external beam irradiation for clinically localized, high-risk prostatic carcinoma. Int J Radiat Oncol Biol Phys 1996; 35:875-879.

5. Epstein JI, Carmichael M, Walsh PC. Adenocarcinoma of the prostate invading the seminal vesicle: definition and relation of tumor volume, grade and margins of resection to prognosis. J Urol 1993; 149:1040-1045.

6. Gleason DF, Mellinger GT. Prediction of Prognosis for Prostatic Adenocarcinoma by Combined Histologic Grading and Clinical Staging. J Urol 1974; 111:58-64.

7. Goto Y, Ohori M, Arakawa A, Kattan MW. Distinguishing clinically important from unimportant prostate cancers before treatment: Value of systematic biopsies. J Urol 1996; 156:1059-1063.

8. Grann A, Gaudin PB, Raben A, Wallner KE. Pathologic features from prostate needle biopsy and prognosis after I-125 brachytherapy. (submitted) 1998;

9. Nadler RB, Humphrey PA, Smith DS, Catalona WJ. Effect of inflammation and benign prostatic hyperplasia on elevated serum specific antigen levels. J Urol 1995; 154:407-413.

10. Oesterling JE. Prostate-specific antigen: A valuable clinical tool. Oncology 1991; 5:107-122.

11. Ohori M, Wheeler TM, Kattan MW, Goto Y. Prognostic significance of positive surgical margins in radical prostatectomy specimens. J Urol 1995; 154:1818-1824.

12. Partin AW, Kattan MW, Subong ENP, Walsh PC. Combination of prostate-specific antigen, clinical stage, and Gleason score to predict pathological stage of localized prostate cancer. JAMA 1997; 277:1445-1451.

13. Pisansky TM, Kahn MJ, Rasp GM, Cha SS. A multiple prognostic index predictive of disease outcome after irradiation for clinically localized prostate carcinoma. Cancer 1997; 79:337-344.

14. Rifkin MD, Zerhouni EA, Gatsonis CA, Quint LE. Comparison of magnetic resonance imaging and ultrasonography in staging early prostate cancer. NEJM 1990; 323:621-626.

15. Roach M, Meehan S, Kroll S, Weil M. Radiotherapy for high grade clinically localized adenocarcinoma of the prostate. J Urol 1996; 156:1719-1723.

16. Salo JO, Rannikko S. The value of acid phosphatase measurements in predicting extracapsular cancer growth before radical prostatectomy. Br J Urol 1988; 62:439-442.

17. Sands ME, Pollack A, Zagars GK. Influence of radiotherapy on node-positive prostate cancer treated with androgen ablation. Int J Radiat Oncol Biol Phys 1995; 31:13-19.

18. Schiebler ML, Schnall M, Pollack HM, et.al. . Current role of MR imaging in the staging of of adenocarcinoma of the prostate. Radiol 1993; 189:339.

19. Stone NN, Stock RG, Unger P. Indications for seminal vesicle biopsy and laparoscopic pelvic lymph node dissection in men with localized carcinoma of the prostate. J Urol 1995; 154:1392-1396.

20. Villers A, McNeal JE, Redwine EA, Freiha FS. The role of perineural space invasion in the local spread of prostatic adenocarcinoma. J Urol 1989; 142:763-768.

21. Zietman AL, Edelstein RA, Coen JJ, Babayan RK, Krane RJ. Radical prostatectomy for adenocarcinoma of the prostate: the influence of preoperative and pathologic findings on biochemical disease-free outcome. Urol 1994; 43:828-833.

Chapter 13

Who can't have an implant

Some patients are not ideal candidates for brachytherapy, due to pretreatment conditions that may predispose them to morbidity. Unfortunately, there is still limited data to help determine who is most prone to post-implant morbidity. Much of the generally accepted contraindications are based on clinical impression of the treating physicians. More, objective data should become available in the next few years as many more patients are treated with brachytherapy and more studies are published.

Prior TURP, general health status, age, pubic arch interference, urinary retention risk, obesity, bowel disease, prior abdominal surgery and prior pelvic radiation are all factors that influence the decision regarding a patient's suitability for brachytherapy.

TURP

There is continued controversy regarding brachytherapy in patients with prior transurethral resection of the prostate (TURP). Blasko, Grimm and Ragde, previously of Northwest Tumor Institute (NWTI), reported that approximately 50% of such patients will develop post-implant incontinence when treated with a uniform source distribution as was done in the early days of transperineal brachytherapy (See Chapter 16). Most disturbing, the incontinence incidence of their patients has continued to climb with longer follow-up (unpublished data).

Contrary to the NWTI experience, the risk of incontinence in patients who had prior TURP and were implanted by Wallner or Dattoli has been low (5%), probably explained by their policy of peripheral loading, whereby sources are kept toward the prostatic periphery to minimize the likelihood of excessive urethral doses (see Chapter 5). Without a peripheral loading pattern, the urethral doses can easily exceed 700 Gy, versus 250 to 300 Gy with peripheral source placement.(Wallner 1995)

If brachytherapy is contemplated for a patient with a prior TURP, at least a one cm rim of tissue should remain around the TURP defect, so there is adequate tissue to hold the sources. CT and/or TRUS are used to assess the adequacy of tissue remaining. After TURP, a waiting interval of one to three months has been recommended, to allow adequate time for re-epitheliazation of the urethral lining.(Seymore 1986) The recommendation of a waiting period is based on experimental murine data rather than on human experience, but waiting seems like a prudent policy.

Patients with prior TURP should be cautioned that they could be at a higher risk of incontinence after brachytherapy regardless of the dosimetric approach, and that reports on this are conflicting. However, if excessive urethral doses are avoided, the risk of incontinence is probably low.

AGE

Lower age limit

Despite a lack of evidence that cure rates vary with age, there has been a reluctance to recommend brachytherapy for younger patients. The primary reason is the lack of long-term data to verify brachytherapy's equivalence with prostatectomy. Based on data from MSKCC and the University Community Hospital, Tampa, the biochemical failure rate after brachytherapy, with follow-up between five and ten years, is no different

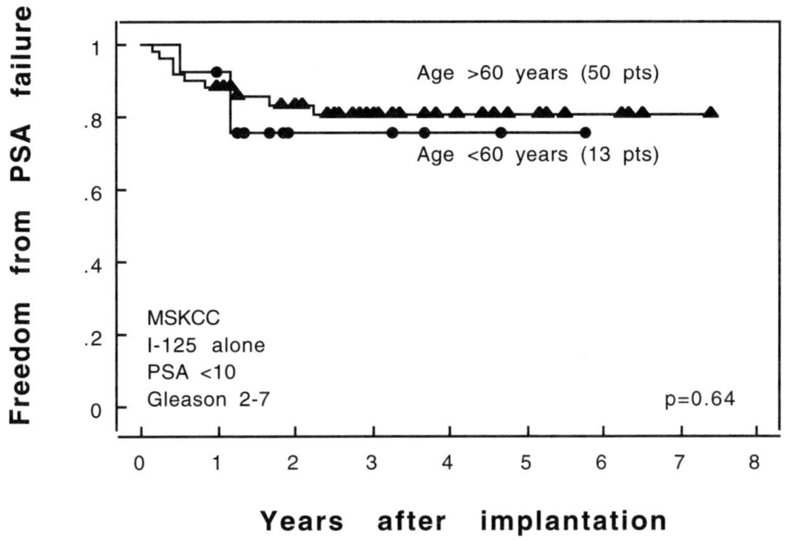

Figure 13-1. Likelihood of biochemical relapse in patients greater or less than 60 years old treated with I-125 alone for stage T1/T2 disease and pre-treatment PSA less than 10 ng/ml.

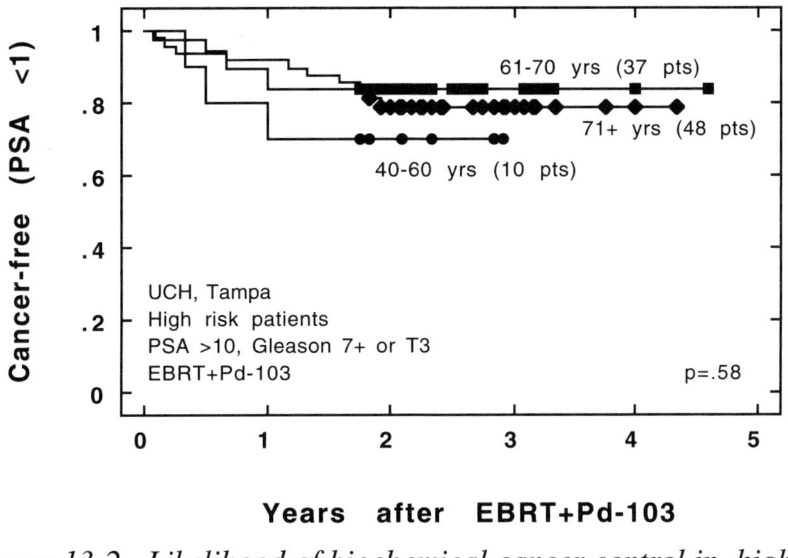

Figure 13-2. Likelihood of biochemical cancer control in high risk patients treated with EBRT plus Pd-103 boost by M. Dattoli. There is no substantial difference among age groups, but follow-up is still short.

in younger patients after I-125 implant alone or after Pd-103 plus supplemental external beam radiation (EBRT) (**Figures 13-1 & 13-2**). Similarly, age itself has no demonstrable effect on the the likelihood of cure following EBRT.(Freedman 1996) Current follow-up data appears equivalent to that of surgery, but longer follow-up would be more comforting. Despite the lack of data against use of brachytherapy in younger patients, they should be cautioned about the lack of long-term follow-up information.

There is concern that younger patients, destined to live longer in general, may be at a higher risk of secondary malignancies due to radiation exposure. No excess incidence of radiation-related malignancies has been reported following retropubic implants from the 1970s, but the number of such patients available for review is relatively low, and second malignancies may not emerge until 30 to 40 years following treatment.

Upper age limit

The major issue regarding brachytherapy for older patients is the same as for other modalities -- will the patient live long enough to benefit from the eradication of his cancer? Because of the long natural history of prostate cancer, patients with low grade cancer or low PSA levels should have a life expectancy of 10 years or more to justify treatment of their cancer. A 10-year life expectancy is used as a standard because the likelihood of a patient dying from low grade untreated prostate cancer is less than 10% at 10 years, and probably even lower for patients with an initial PSA less than 10 ng/ml.(Johansson 1997) North American men in their 70s generally have life expectancy of 10 years or more (**Figure 13-3**).

Patients with high grade cancer or high PSA at initial presentation are at risk of cancer death earlier and should be considered for treatment if their life expectancy otherwise is in excess of five years.

Although not well documented in the literature, older patients may not tolerate radiation prostatitis as well as younger men. The possibility of a more difficult post-implant course should be considered when contemplating brachytherapy for older men. Advanced age may also place them at higher risk of anesthetic problems, which should be addressed on an individual basis.

GENERAL HEALTH

Based on the previous arguments regarding expected longevity, patients with low risk prostate cancer, in generally poor health and with life expectancies of less than 10 years would probably not benefit from aggressive, brachytherapy-based therapy. Determining a patient's likelihood of

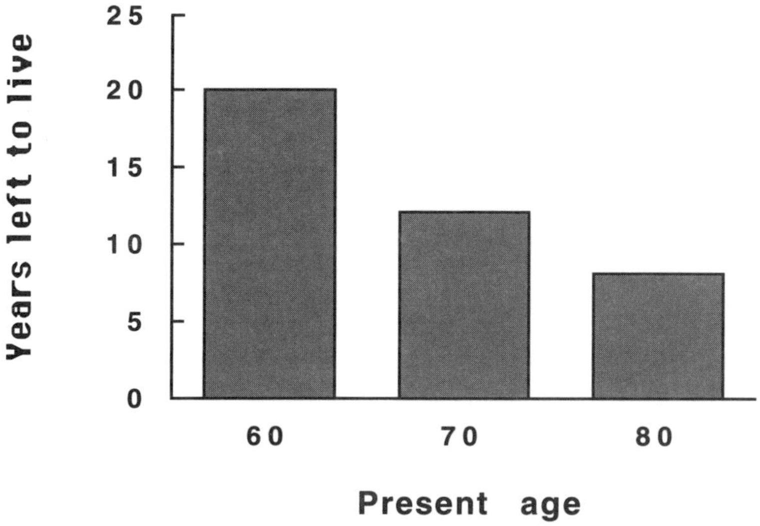

Figure 13-3. Approximate life expectancy in US males, by current age.

living more than 10 years despite cardiac, diabetic or pulmonary problems should generally be made in consultation with the primary care physician.

PUBIC ARCH INTERFERENCE

The anterior portion of the prostate can be difficult to reach with transperineal needles, due to interference by the pubic bones. Pubic arch interference is more likely in patients with larger volume glands, and in those with a narrow pubic arch. For a given patient, determining the likelihood of pubic arch interference is based on the size and shape of the prostate and the configuration of the pubic bones. As a general rule, pubic arch interference is more likely in patients whose TRUS prostate volume is greater than 60 cc.

For patients in whom pubic arch interference seems likely, a pre-implant CT scan can be used to evaluate the likelihood of interference. Once a CT scan is obtained, the largest prostate contour is overlaid on the smallest region of the pubic arch image. When there is more than one cm of overlap, pubic arch interference is likely to be a problem.

A more precise method to check for pubic arch interference is to reconstruct and image of the prostate from a CT scan and overlay the template coordinates, using appropriate software. This can be done routinely with CT-based pre-planning, but is not currently available on commercial planning systems (see Chapter 9).

One way to facilitate the implantation of a larger prostate gland is to place the patient in the extended lithotomy position (see Chapter 8). Alternatively, two to three months of androgen blockade should decrease the size of the prostate by approximately 30% to 50%, facilitating implantation of the anterior and lateral portions. Using one or both strategies, most patients can be implanted successfully.

THE RISK OF URINARY RETENTION

Urinary retention is the most common complication of prostate brachytherapy. In most cases, retention lasts only a few days and is of no real consequence. However, a small percentage of patients develop refractory retention, the hassle and discomfort of which might make the patient regret having chosen brachytherapy. Unfortunately, identifying in advance those patients destined to develop refractory retention is difficult (see Chapter 16). Prostate volume, the number of sources and the patient's age are all only loosely related to the risk of urinary retention.

American Urological Association score (AUA score), or urinary flow studies might be used to predict a patient's risk of developing retention. However, the precise relationship between AUA score or flow rate, and the likelihood of post-implant retention has not been well documented.

Big prostates

Patients with larger prostates are more likely to develop acute and refractory urinary retention. However, there is substantial overlap in prostate volume of patients who do and do not develop retention, so that size alone cannot be used as a rigorous criteria in predicting the likelihood of urinary retention.

Too much radiation activity (?)

More radiation activity, in itself, may not increase the likelihood of complications. Larger prostate glands require more total activity to cover the target, and a larger number or sources is correlated with the risk of urinary retention. However, the use of more activity may simply be a reflection of prostate size, which in itself is correlated with the risk of retention.

Obstructive symptoms

Patients with substantial obstructive symptoms are probably at a higher risk of developing urinary retention following brachytherapy. However, the relationship between pre-implant obstructive symptoms and post-implant urinary obstruction has not been rigorously studied.

Patients with substantial obstructive symptoms could be evaluated with pre-implant cystoscopy and urodynamics to determine the degree of obstruction, as presumably, patients with substantial hypertrophy and obstruction are predisposed to post-implant retention. While this policy seems logical, there are no statistics to show its efficacy.

The AUA score might be used to predict who is likely to to develop urinary obstruction. At the University of Washington, patients with a score of 16 or greater are cautioned that they could be at a high risk of developing retention, and so are advised against brachytherapy or placed on androgen ablation for 3 months prior, in an effort to improve their flow.

The value of urodynamic studies to determine a patient's likelihood of experiencing radiation-induced urinary morbidity has not been studied rigorously.

ANDROGEN DEPRIVATION TO DECREASE THE RISK OF URINARY RETENTION

Patients deemed to be at a high risk of post-implant obstruction could be treated with hormonal ablation prior to brachytherapy, with the hope of decreasing the degree of obstruction and decreasing the likelihood of developing chronic urinary retention. Such a policy seems reasonable, but there are no studies that confirm its success. The experience of the authors suggest that this maneuver is helpful in some patients.

PROPHYLACTIC TRANSURETHRAL INCISION OF THE PROSTATE (TUIP)

One way to avoid problems in patients deemed to be at a high risk of retention would be to perform a prophylactic TUIP prior to or at the time of the implant.

M. Dattoli and J. Etheridge, at University Community Hospital, Tampa have substantial experience with prophylactic TUIP or minimal TURP one month prior, or at the time of the implant. They have found a low incidence of post-implant urinary retention, without an increased risk of urinary incontinence. Blasko and Ragde have also had success with this approach in patients with high AUA scores and evidence of median lobe hypertrophy on cystoscopy. However, there has been no peer-reviewed, published summary of their experience and clear guidelines for this approach are lacking.

OBESITY

Considering the high prevalence of obesity in modern society, surprising little has been reported regarding prostate cancer treatment for obese patients. Some evidence suggests that obesity confers a better prognosis, perhaps due to hormonal influences.(Daniell 1996) However, obesity can present technical difficulties for prostatectomy and for EBRT. Obese patients are more likely to develop nearly all post-operative complications, and are therefore generally discouraged from undergoing surgery.

Obese patients are more difficult to set-up properly for EBRT, although the degree of technical problem that obesity poses has never been quantified. Difficulty with reproducibility of patient set-up would presumably increase the risk of complications, and decrease the likelihood of tumor control. Set-up problems in obese patients would be especially worrisome for conformal EBRT, where the margin for error is smaller.

Obesity poses a relatively minor problem for brachytherapy, in contrast to EBRT or surgery. Obese patients have routinely been treated with brachytherapy by K. Wallner, J. Blasko and M. Dattoli as an alternative to other modalities, with satisfactory dosimetry and no obesity-related complications. Operative set-up can take longer, with less room to maneuver between the patient's legs, but these conditions have not posed substantial problems (**Figure 13-4**).

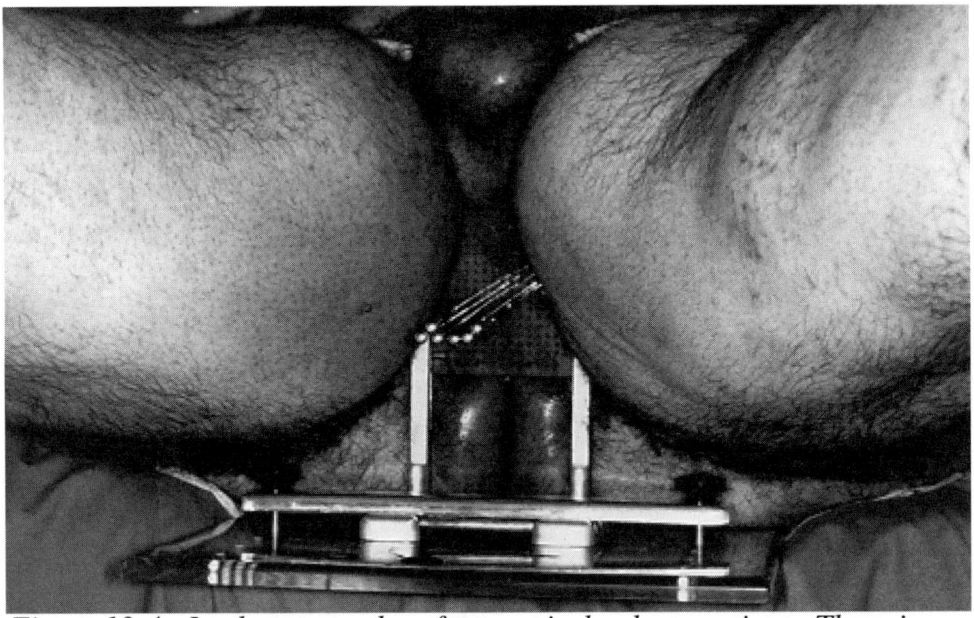

Figure 13-4. Implant procedure for massively obese patient. There is much less room to maneuver in the perineal area, and fluoroscopic images are of poorer quality due to large tissue mass.

INFLAMMATORY BOWEL DISEASE

"Inflammatory bowel disease" (IBD) includes both ulcerative colitis and regional enteritis (Crohn's disease). Both are chronic, idiopathic inflammatory disorders of the gastrointestinal tract. Based on general incidence rates, roughly 250 patients are diagnosed annually in the United States with having prostate cancer along with IBD.

There is a widespread belief that patients with IBD are at higher risk of radiation-related complications.[Hoffman 1989] However, only a single published mention of a bowel complication from EBRT in IBD patients with prostate cancer exists.[Leibel 1993] Whether EBRT truly presents a higher risk of complications in IBD patients is unknown. Presumably, many IBD patients are referred for prostatectomy due to a concern that they are at increased risk of radiation complications.

Patients with IBD might be advised to have brachytherapy, as an alternative to surgery, the rationale being that less rectal surface area would be irradiated, perhaps decreasing the likelihood of radiation complications (See Chapter 3). None of the six patients with a history of IBD treated with I-125 prostate brachytherapy for early-stage prostate cancer at MSKCC from 1991 to 1996 experienced unusual or significant gastrointestinal side effects following implantation.[Grann 1998] J. Blasko has treated four patients with documented rectal IBD involvement, with no complications at two to four years follow-up.

With the limited information available, it appears that prostate brachytherapy is a safe alternative to prostatectomy in patients with a history of IBD. Based on the single case of a rectal fistula developing after a relatively low EBRT dose reported by Leibel and colleagues, we are reluctant to add EBRT to brachytherapy in IBD patients. However, for patients who refuse surgery, implant plus supplemental EBRT would probably be safer than using full dose EBRT alone.

PRIOR ABDOMINAL SURGERY

Patients with a history of abdominal or pelvic surgery could be at a higher risk of radiation-related bowel complications. Such patients are sometimes advised against EBRT. Brachytherapy would probably be a less risky treatment in such situations, as it entails less radiation to the bowel wall (see Chapter 3). Occasional patients with prior surgery have been implanted as an alternative to full dose EBRT, and have not experienced adverse post-implant courses (data not reported). For such patients who have higher Gleason scores or PSA levels, adding 40 to 50 Gy EBRT to a brachytherapy boost would probably be safer than treating with full dose EBRT.

PRIOR RADIATION

Occasionally patients diagnosed with prostate cancer will have had prior pelvic radiation for another malignancy. If the dose to the rectal wall was greater than 40 Gy, brachytherapy would probably carry too high a risk of complications, regardless of the time since the prior radiation. Prostatectomy would be preferable in such cases, but making a therapeutic decision in these cases is difficult. Brachytherapy might still be offered, with a full explanation of the risks presented to the patient beforehand.

RELATIVE VERSUS ABSOLUTE CONTRAINDICATIONS

Prior urethral surgery, advanced age, obstructive symptoms and potential pubic arch interference should be considered *relative* contraindications to brachytherapy. Patients with such criteria may still choose brachytherapy, even if they are at a higher risk of complications. Brachytherapy may still be their best choice if it offers a better chance for cure or a lesser likelihood of incontinence or impotence. In patients with relative contraindications, it would be wise to document that their situation and the alternatives were presented and considered.

REFERENCES

1. Freedman GM, Hanlon AL, Lee WR, Hanks GE. Young patients with prostate cancer have an outcome justifying their treatment with external beam radiation. Int J Radiat Oncol Biol Phys 1996; 35:243-250.

2. Grann A, Wallner K. Prostate brachytherapy in patients with inflammatory bowel disease. Int J Radiat Oncol Biol Phys 1998; In press:

3. Hoffman M, Kalter C, Roberts W, Cavanagh D. Early cervical cancer coexistent with idiopathic inflammatory bowel disease. S Med J 1989; 82:905-906.

4. Johansson J, Holmberg L, Johansson S, Bergstrom R. Fifteen-year survival in prostate cancer: A prospective, population-based study in Sweden. JAMA 1997; 277:467-471.

5. Leibel SA, Heimann R, Kutcher GJ. Three-dimensional conformal radiation therapy in locally advanced carcinoma of the prostate: preliminary results of a phase I dose-escalation study. Int J Radiat Oncol Biol Phys 1993; 26:

6. Wallner KE, Roy J, Harrison L. Dosimetry guidelines to minimize urethral and rectal morbidity following transperineal I-125 prostate brachytherapy. Int J Radiat Oncol Biol Phys 1995; 32:465-471.

Chapter 14

Evaluating cancer status

Assessing the efficacy of treatment for early stage prostate cancer is hampered by the cancer's long natural history and by imprecise methods of assessing local tumor control. Ideally, survival should be the endpoint by which treatment efficacy is judged. However, analysis of the treatment effect on survival requires long follow-up because most men with early stage disease will not be at risk for cancer-related death until 10 years or more have passed.(Johansson 1997)

DIGITAL RECTAL EXAM

The digital rectal exam (DRE) was the most common method to evaluate treatment results, and probably the least meaningful. Determining local control following irradiation has usually been based on the regression of palpable tumor. Reliance on palpability is complicated by the subjectivity of the DRE and the fact that a large percentage of tumors diagnosed currently are not even palpable prior to therapy.

Perez and colleagues found no correlation between tumor regression determined by rectal exam, and local or distant recurrence.(Perez 1986) Patients with Stage C disease did poorly, despite a high degree of tumor regression found by DRE.

The DRE is probably most accurate in patients with stage T3 (C) disease, for which local tumor growth is more obvious and not so subject to interpretation. But such patients comprise only a small proportion of those currently diagnosed.

PROSTATE SPECIFIC ANTIGEN (PSA)

PSA has allowed a shift to a biochemical analysis of tumor control, dramatically decreasing the time it takes to detect residual disease. PSA allows for a much more objective measure of residual cancer than the DRE. It has substantially improved our ability to predict and to identify treatment failure after all forms of therapy.

Determining biochemical success following any form of radiation is not as simple as after surgery, after which the entire prostate and entire cancer are removed and the PSA should be zero. Following radiation, may variables can affect the rate of PSA decline and the absolute level attained. Among these factors are the amount of normal glandular tissue remaining, the tumor regression kinetics, and the potential for prostatitis in the post-treatment period. Although these uncertainties exist, PSA remains the best single test to measure short-term success.

WHAT HAPPENS TO PSA AFTER BRACHYTHERAPY

Following brachytherapy, the serum PSA level declines substantially in nearly all patients, reflecting local tumor regression. The rate of PSA decline is variable (**Figure 14-1**) and has not, in itself, been consistently correlated with prognosis after EBRT.(Zagars 1995)

Time for PSA to reach nadir

Consistent with the variability in the rate of PSA decline, there is a wide range of times for PSA levels to reach nadir, from one month to well over two years (**Figure 14-1**).

In patients treated with EBRT, the time to nadir has no apparent relationship to prognosis.(Pisansky 1993)(Zagars 1995) Similarly, there is no relationship between the length of time for PSA to nadir and the likelihood of late biochemical failure in patients with early stage disease implanted with I-125 at MSKCC (**Figure 14-2a & b**).

PSA nadir levels

The likelihood of subsequent chemical or clinical failure is correlated with nadir PSA values. It is well established from EBRT series that lower PSA nadirs are associated with a lower likelihood of cancer recurrence. The relationship between PSA nadir levels and disease-free status is most evident for nadirs of 1 to 4, but some relationship probably also exists at levels below 1.0 (**Figure 14-3**).(Zagars 1995)(Critz 1996)

No specific nadir PSA value guarantees against late biochemical failure. Even some patients with undetectable post-implant PSA will ultimately develop late biochemical failure.

Pre-treatment PSA holds its value

Even among patients with post-treatment PSA nadir below 1 ng/ml, the pre-treatment PSA holds substantial prognostic significance. Those patients with nadirs less than one, but with pre-treatment PSA levels less than 10 have lower late

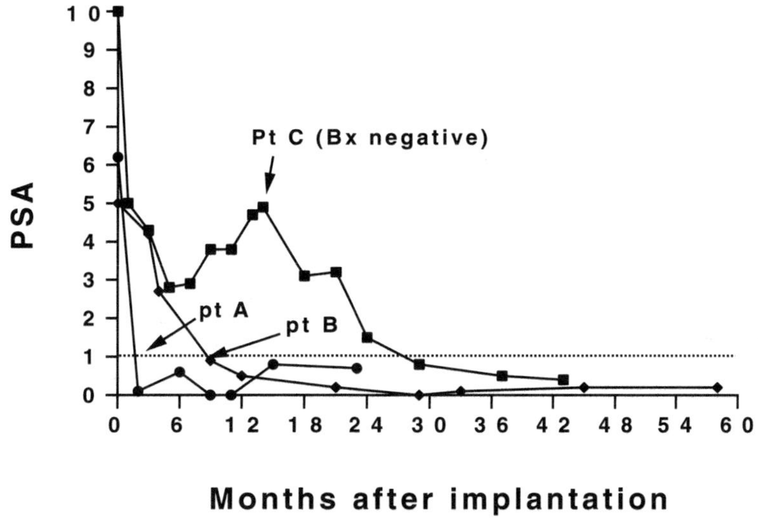

Figure 14-1. There is striking variability in the rate of PSA decline. Patients A and B dropped below 1 ng/ml at one and nine months, respectively. Patient C took 3 years to reach nadir. He was biopsied at two years (negative), and eventually fell below 1.0. His last PSA was less than 1.0, four years after implant.

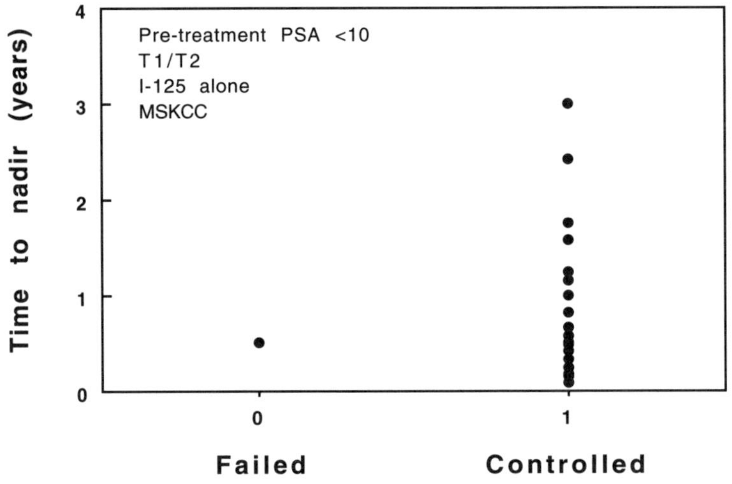

Figure 14-2a. Time to PSA nadir in patients with nadir below 1.0, and initial PSA less than 10. There was no relationship between the time to PSA nadir and the likelihood of subsequent biochemical failure.

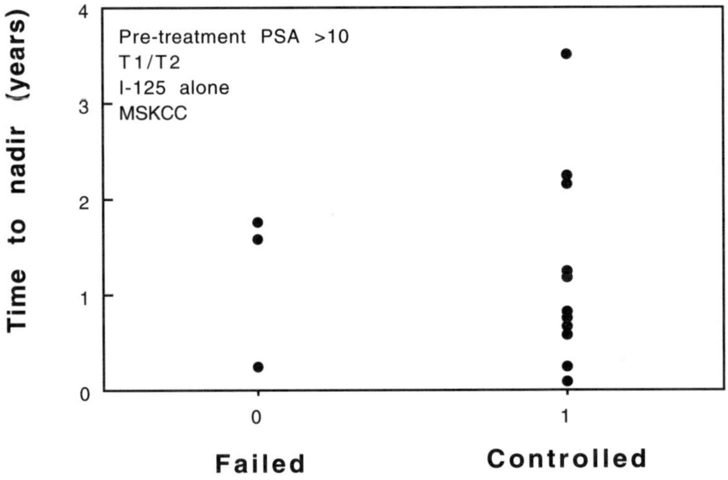

Figure 14-2b. Time to PSA nadir in patients with nadir below 1.0, and initial PSA greater than 10. There was no relationship between the time to nadir and the likelihood of subsequent biochemical failure.

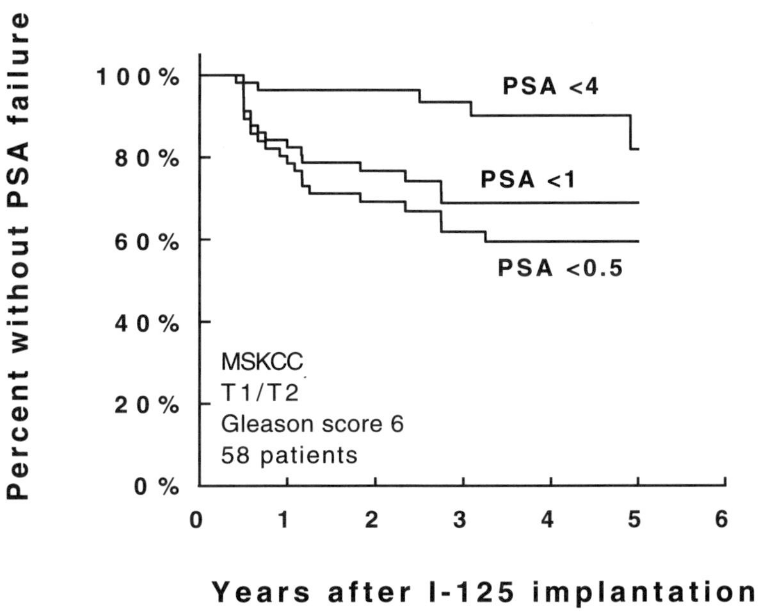

Figure 14-3. PSA-based cancer-free rates using biochemical cancer control criteria of PSA <4.0, <1.0 or <.5.0 ng/ml. The lower the PSA required to be considered cancer-free, the lower the apparent cure rate. The difference between 1.0 versus 0.5 is much less than that between 4.0 and 1.0, because most patients who nadir below 1.0 will go below 0.5.

biochemical failure rates than those with nadirs under 1.0 and pre-treatment PSA above 10 (**Figure 14-4**).

Benign PSA rises

Benign PSA rises occur commonly between 12 to 24 months following implantation (**Figure 14-5**). These late PSA rises seem to correspond to late recurrence of radiation-related urinary symptoms, and are apparently due to radiation-related tissue changes. The prognosis for such patients appears good (**Figure 14.6**). While there is currently no precise explanation for benign PSA rises after brachytherapy, their frequent occurrence is something to be aware of. Because of many patients' tendency to panic with any PSA rise, they should be warned in advance of the possibility of a benign PSA rise. Patients need to be reassured that it is not a significant event. Benign PSA rises occur in approximately one-third of

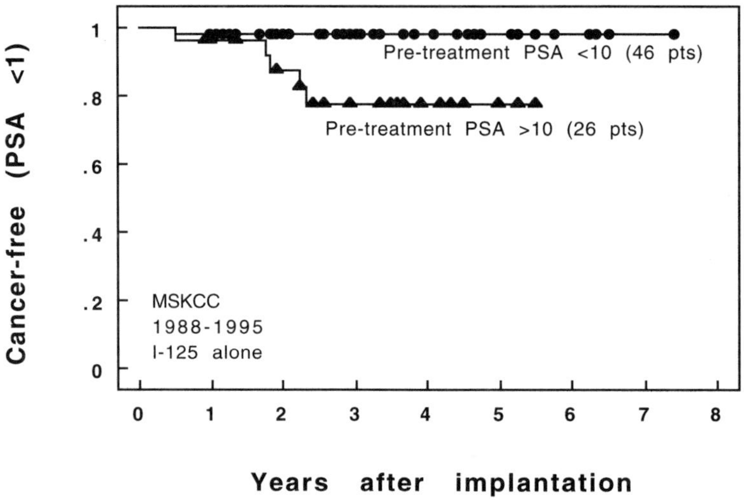

Figure 14-4. Freedom from biochemical failure in patients with nadir below 1.0 is still influenced by the pre-treatment PSA. Among patients with a nadir below 1.0, those with pre-treatment PSA greater than 10 had a higher failure rate than those with pre-treatment PSA less than 10.

patients and support the argument for a minimum 2.5 year follow-up to assess PSA response.(Shipley 1996)

Are we being too strict?

There is no single PSA nadir value that ensures that a patient's cancer will not recur. It is still not clear whether a patient with a nadir PSA above 1.0 is definitely going to recur, or if in some patients, a higher nadir PSA value is reflective of benign residual disease. It is possible that in some patients, a higher nadir PSA is due to benign prostatic hypertrophy (BPH). But if residual BPH can account for a persistently elevated PSA after radiation, the number of patients in this category is probably very small, because nearly all patients who receive pelvic radiation for other cancers have a post-radiation PSA below 1.0.(Willett 1994)

Rising PSA as an indicator of failure

A rising PSA after treatment is very likely to be followed, with a lag time of several years, by clinically evident failure. With up to four years follow-up, approximately 50% of patients with a rising PSA will develop clinically evident failure.(Kaplan 1993)(Ritter 1992) With longer follow-up, possibly all patients with a

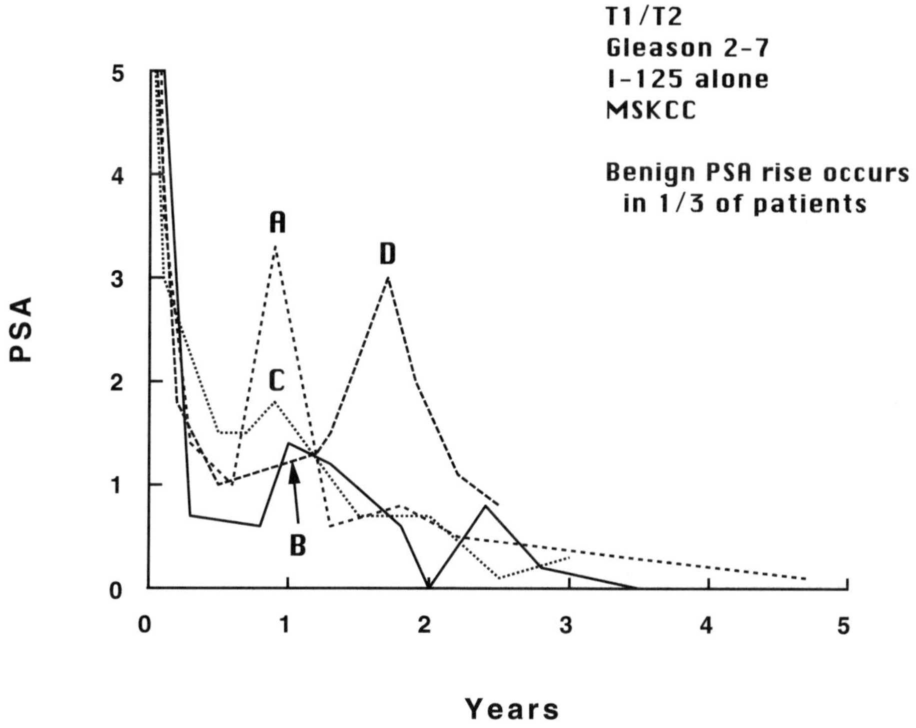

Figure 14-5. Approximately one-third of patients treated with I-125 will experience a benign PSA rise, usually between 12 and 24 months after implantation. There is no obvious correlation between benign PSA increases and subsequent biochemical failure (see Figure 14-6).

rising PSA level will ultimately develop clinical failure.

ACTUARIAL VERSUS "RAW" STATISTICS

Until the 1980s, survival rates were generally reported as the "straight" (or "raw") percentage of patients alive at a particular time. No consideration was made for the length of time patients were followed. The cure rates appeared higher because patients with shorter follow-up had not had as much time to manifest failure, but they were still included in the denominator.

Over the past 15 years, actuarial calculations have become the generally accepted method of reporting cancer-free rates. The use of actuarial statistics allows for the inclusion of patients with shorter follow-up, without favorably bias-

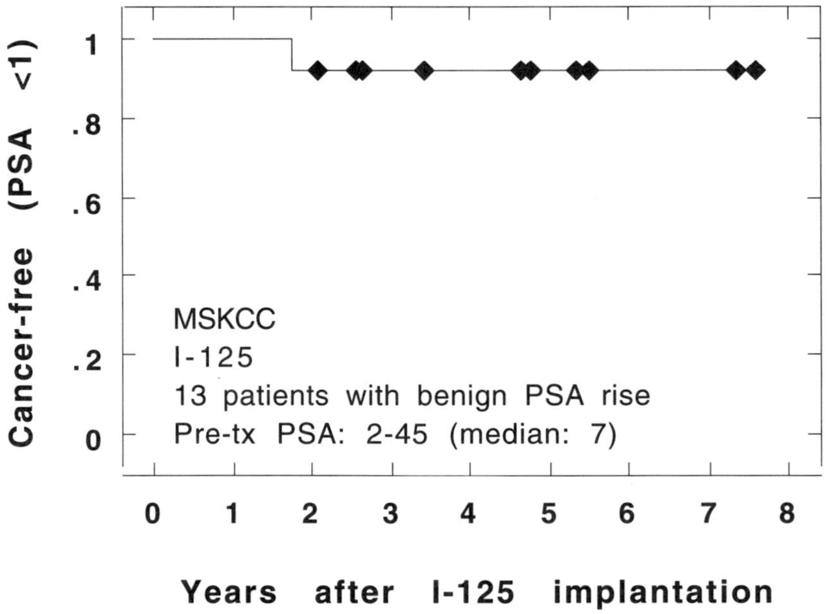

Figure 14-6. PSA-based freedom from progression in 13 patients who had a benign PSA rise between one and two years after I-125 implantation. Each patient had an initial PSA nadir of 1.0 ng/ml or less, then rose above 1.0 ng/ml between one and two years after treatment, and subsequently fell back below 1.0 ng/ml. Despite their temporary PSA rise, their overall freedom from biochemical progression has been low, so far.

ing longer-term results. In contrast to raw percentages, the denominator for actuarial calculations is continuously adjusted, to drop patients who have not been followed long. Patients are excluded from the calculations at the time of their last follow-up, a process called "censoring." Censored patients are usually marked on the graph by Xs or dots, to give a visual estimate of their follow-up times (**Figure 14-7**).

Actuarial calculation methods have several variations, the most common being the Berkson-Gage ("life table") and the Kaplan-Meier (product-limit method). The Kaplan-Meier is the most widely used in cancer research. It calculates changes in the cancer-free status whenever an event (failure) occurs, rather than at regular intervals, as is done for the Berkson-Gage calculation. The difference between the two methods is minimal.

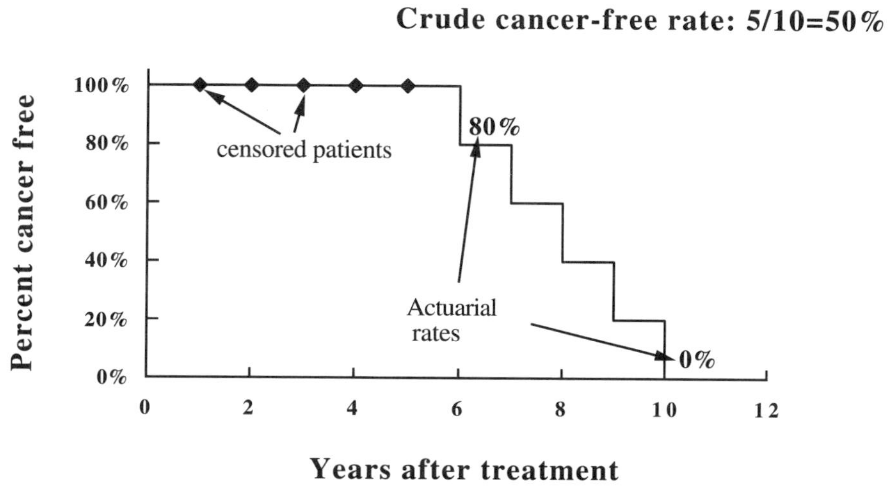

Figure 14-7. Example of freedom from biochemical failure, using crude versus actuarial calculations. In this example, five of ten patients have failed, all in the first five years of treatment. The crude freedom from failure is 50%. By actuarial calculation, the cure rate is 0%, because all patients followed beyond five years have failed. When using crude statistics, including patients with less than five years follow-up inflates the cure rate.

The statistical difference between curves can be calculated in several ways, the most common being the log-rank test and the generalized Wilcoxin. Log-rank analysis is more reflective of differences in the late portion of the curves, and is probably preferable for tracking slow-recurring cancers such as prostate cancer.

While the use of actuarial statistics is a much more realistic method than crude percentages, it can still favorably bias the data, at least for short follow-up times. Patients with short follow-up may cause the initial portion of the curve to appear very favorable, simply because sufficient time has not elapsed for patients to begin to manifest failure, whether clinical or biochemical. This favorable bias caused by patients with short follow-up has rightly lead some investigators to call for the exclusion of patients with less than 2.5 years follow-up.(Shipley 1996)

DETERMINING CURE RATES FROM GRAPHS

There is no universally accepted definition of "cure" for prostate cancer. With nearly all types of cancer, there is an initial rapid failure rate among treated

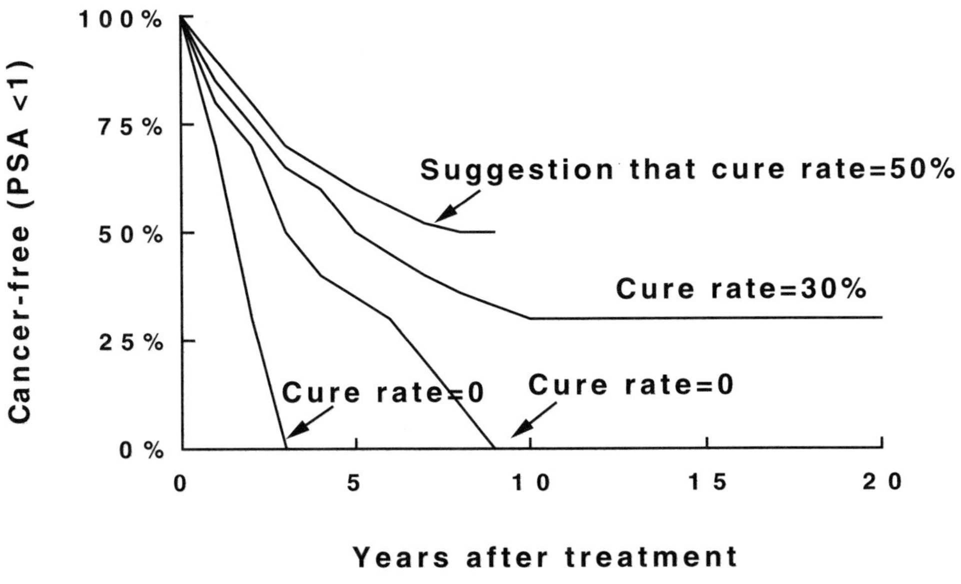

Figure 14-8. Cure rates should be determined by where the freedom-from-cancer curve plateaus. If there is no plateau, there is no evidence that any patients are cured by the treatment being studied.

patients, followed by a leveling off of the curves as the percentage of the remaining patients with persistent cancer falls. Ideally, the time point on the graph at which no further patients fail should be taken as the cure rate (**Figure 14-8**). With prostate cancer, there is probably no time point, with any treatment modality, after which no more failures will occur. Usually a small late rate of failure persists. Some late failures could be due to second malignancies within the prostate, but differentiating late recurrences from second primaries is not currently practical. From a practical view, that point at which the failure rate decelerates to near zero is generally taken as the "cure" rate. It should be qualified as the "apparent" or approximate cure rate, because a small percent of patients will fail with longer follow-up.

DEFINING BIOCHEMICAL FAILURE IN THIS TEXT

For most of the data reported in this text, biochemical failure is defined as a PSA reading of more than 1.0 ng/ml at last follow-up. Patients are censored at last follow-up if their PSA is still decreasing. Patients whose PSA level plateaus at a value greater than 1.0 are scored as failures at the time at which their PSA plateaued (**Figure 14-9**).

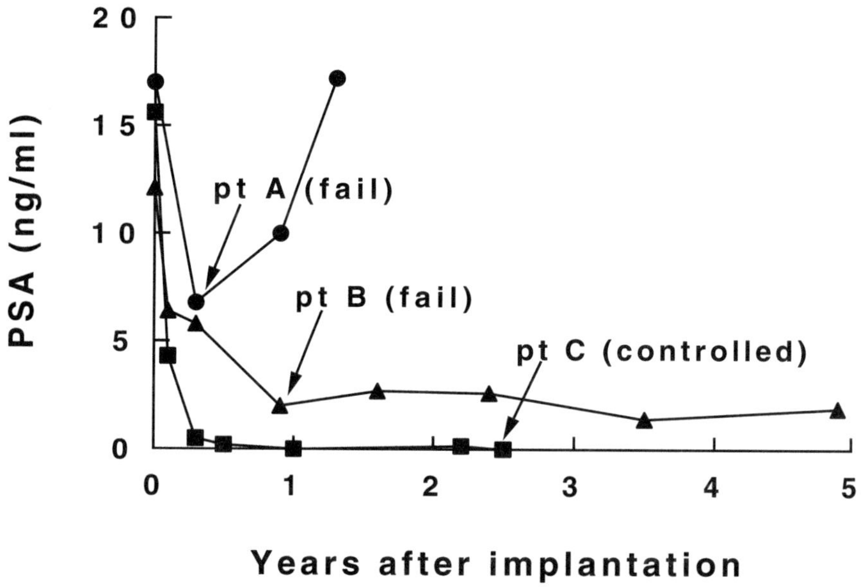

Figure 14-9. Example of how biochemical failure is defined in this text. Patient A is considered to have failed at the time his PSA rises. Patient B's PSA has reached a plateau at a value above 1.0 at 11 months following implantation, and is considered to have failed at that time, even though his PSA has not started to rise. While some may argue that this is being too strict, it probably is not.

Whatever guidelines are used to define biochemical failure, there will always be some ambiguity in individual cases. Probably the most common is with patients whose last PSAs are slightly higher than previous values, but still below 1.0. Ambiguous cases are usually only a tiny fraction of the total, and however one chooses to deal with them statistically, they should not have a substantial effect on the reported cancer-free rates. With longer follow-up, ambiguous cases should become less frequent. PSA failure is like pornography -- it is difficult to define, but you'll know it when you see it.

LOCAL VERSUS DISTANT FAILURE

A rising PSA level is a general marker of disease progression. However, it does not in itself distinguish between local and distant failure. To analyze the effect of irradiation on local tumor control, some method of distinguishing local from distant failure is needed.

Rate of PSA rise

The rate of PSA rise may help distinguish between local and distant failures. After EBRT, patients with rapidly rising PSA (doubling time less than 12 months) are more likely to have distant metastases.(Lee 1997)(Ritter 1992) However, the rate of rise is not a very specific criteria for determining local versus distant failure, because there is a large overlap between these groups. There is no reported data regarding the rate of post-brachytherapy PSA rise and the site of failure.

Post-treatment biopsies

Post-treatment biopsies have been used sporadically to determine more objectively local tumor eradication. Compared to the digital rectal exam, post-treatment prostatic biopsies always show a much higher incidence of residual tumor. In nearly all reported series, patients with histologically viable tumor have a substantially greater likelihood of developing local recurrence and distant metastases.(Kuban 1992)(Scardino 1985)

Some authors have argued that a histologically viable tumor is irrelevant. Wishful thinking. The only series that showed no adverse effect of residual histologically viable tumor was that by Cox and Kline.(Cox 1983) Their results were clouded, however, by the fact that some patients received hormonal ablation, and because the biopsies were done under digital guidance, which presumably shows a much lower incidence of positive biopsies compared to sextant TRUS-guided biopsies.(Kabalin 1989) The use of TRUS guidance along with a larger number of samples appears to result in a higher positive biopsy rate, a factor not controlled for in the past.(Kabalin 1989)

Post-implant biopsies are conceptually appealing, but their routine use is limited by the lack of effective therapy in the case of a positive biopsy, ambiguity in interpretation of biopsy samples, and the fact that biopsies are almost always negative in patients with a low PSA at the time of the biopsy.(Prestidge 1997)

While the biopsy results following EBRT are unfavorable, the results following prostatectomy are not much better. Foster and Abi-aad showed that biopsies of the anastomosis in patients with an elevated PSA level were positive in approximately 50% of patients.(Foster 1993)(Abi-aad 1992) Surgeons who perseverate on the need for post-radiation biopsies need to be constantly reminded of this work.

The majority of biopsies are clearly negative or positive. However, a small percent show residual cancer with radiation effect, and have been termed "indeterminate." With time, most indeterminate samples become negative, suggesting that substantial radiation effect is indicative of tumoricidal damage which simply needs more time to become histologically evident.(Prestidge 1997)

BONE SCAN

In the absence of a rising PSA, routine follow-up bone scans are not warranted. Bone scans are rarely positive at initial diagnosis, with a PSA of less than 20 ng/ml. The same probably holds true for recurrent tumors, but to date, little has been published in this regard.(Lee 1997) Routine repeat bone scan, as part of follow-up, should only be performed if the PSA is greater than 10 ng/ml (or higher?) or if there is clinical suspicion of bone metastases.

IS BIOCHEMICAL FAILURE RELEVANT?

PSA has emerged as the most sensitive indicator of residual disease. But we have a lot to learn yet about PSA follow-up. We know that a high nadir PSA level or a rising PSA are bad, but we don't yet know how often patients without rising PSA levels are cured. Some patients with undetectable post-treatment PSA will still fail with longer follow-up. How common those patients will be is still not known.

It is true that PSA failure in itself is not necessarily clinically significant, as patients with rising PSA levels may remain symptom-free for many years. It has been suggested that physicians and patients get too concerned about a biochemical parameter that may have little practical relevance. Only partly true. If a patient has persistent cancer after "curative" radiation, it means that treatment did not eradicate his cancer. If the patient remains asymptomatic, it is likely his cancer would have remained subclinical, even without treatment. Although a lack of symptoms is good for a patient's quality of life, the treatment itself was ineffective in eradicating his cancer, and he most likely did not need treatment in the first place.

REFERENCES

1. Abi-Aad AS, Macfarlane MT, Stein A, deKernion JB. Detection of local recurrence after radical prostatectomy by prostate specific antigen and transrectal ultrasound. J Urol 1992; 147:952-955.

2. Cox JD, Kline RW. Do prostatic biopsies 12 months or more after external irradiation for adenocarcinoma, Stage III, predict long-term survival? Int J Radiat Oncol Biol Phys 1983; 9:299-303.

3. Critz FA, Levinson AK, Williams WH, Holladay DA. Prostate-specific antigen nadir: The optimum level after irradiation for prostate cancer. J Clin Oncol 1996; 14:2893-2900.

4. Foster LS, Jajodia P, Fournier G, Shinohara K, et.al. . The value of prostate specific antigen and transrectal guided biopsy in detecting prostatic fossa recurrences following radical prostatectomy. J Urol 1993; 149:1024-1028.

5. Kabalin JN, Hodge KK, McNeal JE, Freiha FS, Stamey TA. Identification of Residual Cancer in the Prostate Following Radiation Therapy: Role of Transrectal Ultrasound Guided Biopsy and Prostatic Specific Antigen. J Urol 1989; 142:326-331.

6. Kaplan ID, Cox RS, Bagshaw MA. Prostate specific antigen after external beam radiotherapy for prostatic cancer: followup. J Urol 1993; 149:519-522.

7. Kuban DA, El-Mahdi AM, Schellhammer P. The significance of post-irradiation prostate biopsy with long-term follow-up. Int J Radiat Oncol Biol Phys 1992; 24:409-414.

8. Lee WR, Hanks GE, Hanlon A. Increasing prostate-specific antigen profile following definitive radiation therapy for localized prostate cancer: Clinical observations. J Clin Oncol 1997; 15:230-238.

9. Perez CA, Pilepich MV, Zivnuska F. Tumor control in definitive irradiation of localized carcinoma of the prostate. Int J Radiat Oncol Biol Phys 1986; 12:523-531.

10. Pisansky TM, Cha SS, Earle JD, et al. Prostate-specific antigen as a pretherapy prognostic factor in patients treated with radiation therapy for clinically localized prostate cancer. J /Clin Oncol 1993; 11:2158-2166.

11. Ritter MA, Messing EM, Shanahan TG, Potts S, Chappell RJ, Kinsella TJ. Prostate-specific antigen as a predictor of radiotherapy response and patterns of failure in localized prostate cancer. J Clin Oncol 1992; 10:1208-1217.

12. Scardino P T, Wheeler T M. Prostatic Biopsy after Irradiation Therapy for Prostatic Cancer. Urol 1985; 25:39-46.

13. Shipley WU. PSA following irradiation for prostate cancer: The upcoming ASTRO symposium. Int J Radiat Oncol Biol Phys 1996; 35:1115.

14. Willett CG, Zietman AL, Shipley WU, Coen JJ. The effect of pelvic radiation therapy on serum levels of prostate specific antigen. J Urol 1994; 151:1579-1581.

15. Zagars GK, Pollack A, Kavadi, VS. Prostate-specific antigen and radiation therapy for clinically localized prostate cancer. Int J Radiat Oncol Biol Phys 1995; 32:293-306.

Chapter 15

Cancer control

SLIM PICKINGS

There are still limited data regarding PSA-based follow-up after prostate brachytherapy. Like the situation for nerve-sparing prostatectomy, nearly all published data for tumor control rates for brachytherapy comes from a handful of physicians, and may not be truly representative of the overall brachytherapy experience.

BRACHYTHERAPY ALONE: I-125

Wallner and colleagues at Memorial Sloan-Kettering Cancer Center (MSKCC) meticulously followed a group of over 100 patients treated from 1988 through 1994. This group included the earliest patients, some of whom had what would now be considered suboptimal implants. The pathology slides were re-reviewed in 1997 (**Table 15-1**).(Grann 1998)

As with other modalities, the disease-free rate is highly dependent on the pre-treatment PSA. Using biochemical control criteria (PSA below 1), patients with a pre-treatment PSA less than 10 had an approximately 80% disease-free rate at five years, similar to that reported after external beam radiation (EBRT) alone or in experienced surgical hands (**Figure 15-1**).(Partin 1993)(Zagars 1995)

Patients with a pre-treatment PSA above 10 had a much higher failure rate. At least 50% of these patients failed within three years. The silver lining is that there is some evidence of a plateau on the disease-free curves, suggesting that some patients with larger tumor volumes can be cured with implant alone. The failure rate for patients with PSA levels above 10 appears somewhat lower than that reported for most EBRT series.

Overall, patients with lower Gleason scores did better than patients with Gleason scores of 7 (**Figure 15-2**). Patients with Gleason scores of 7 are of special interest, because conventional wisdom is that they should receive supplemental EBRT because of their higher likelihood of extracapsular extension. In the MSKCC experience, patients with Gleason scores of 7 and PSA below 10 had a 5-year disease-free rate similar to those patients with Gleason score 6 and PSA below 10 (**Figure 15-3a**). Whether or not supplemental EBRT is needed for these patients is unclear. In contrast, patients with Gleason scores 7 and PSA above 10 had a poor prognosis with I-125 alone and probably would fare better with supplemental EBRT (**Figure 15-3b**)

In multivariate analysis, the pre-treatment PSA reading was by far the most important prognostic feature, with the Gleason score of minimal statistical importance (**Table 15-2**). Pathological features from the pre-treatment biopsy (extent of tumor in the biopsy specimens and perineural invasion) had far less prognostic significance than pre-treatment PSA (see Chapter 12).

Table 15-1. I-125 alone patient characteristics (MSKCC).

	# of patients	
Gleason 4	1	(1%)
Gleason 5	7	(7%)
Gleason 6	58	(57%)
Gleason 7	36	(35%)
PSA		
0-4 ng/ml	8	(8%)
4-10	50	(49%)
10-20	32	(31%)
20+	11	(11%)

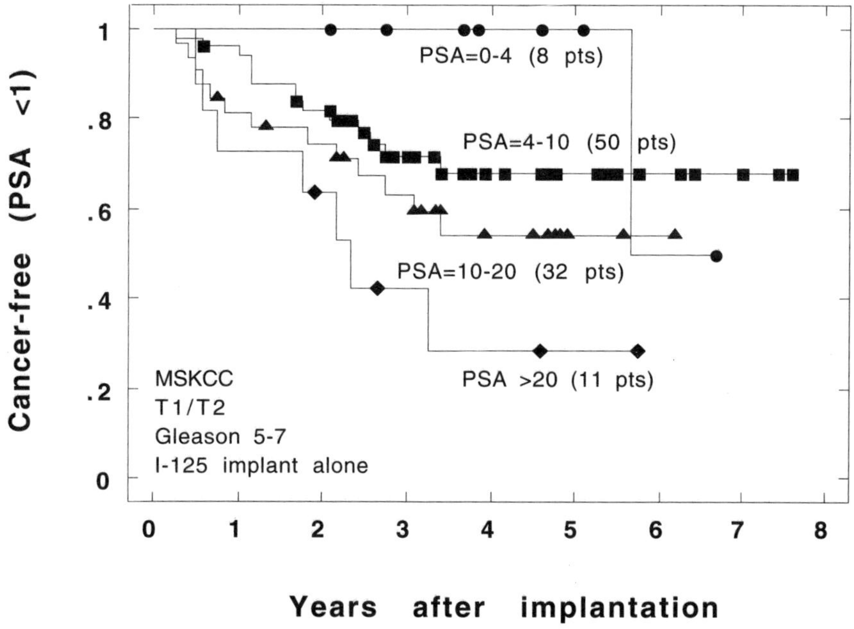

Figure 15-1. Biochemical disease-free rates after I-125 implant alone at MSKCC, stratified by pre-treatment PSA.

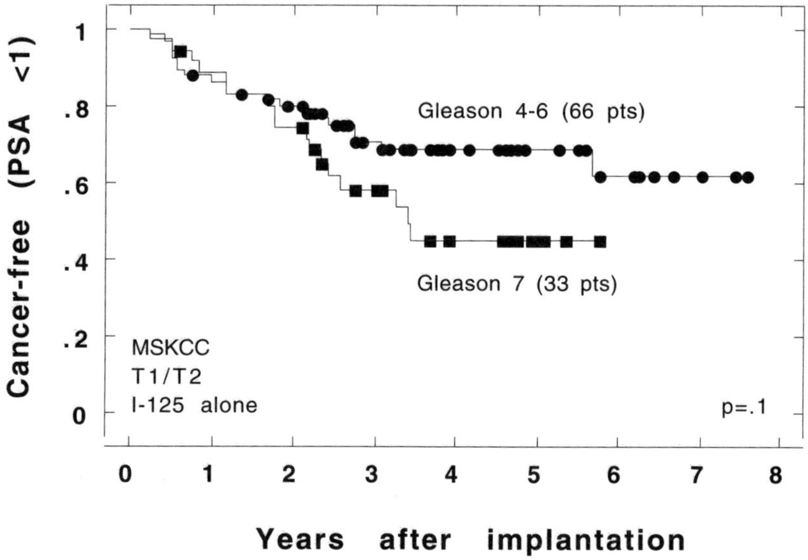

Figure 15-2. Freedom from biochemical failure after I-125 alone for patients with Gleason scores of 4 to 6 versus Gleason scores of 7. Patients with Gleason scores of 8 to 10 were not treated with implant alone.

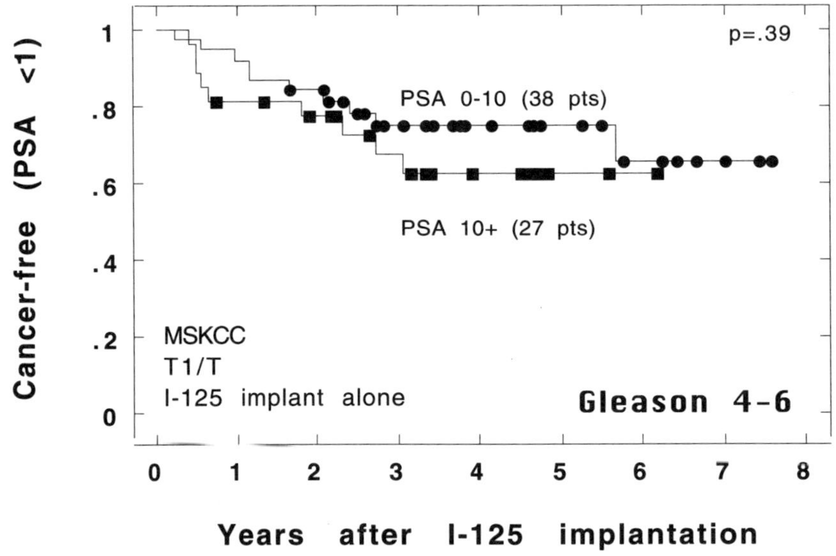

Figure 15-3a. Freedom from biochemical failure after I-125 alone for patients with Gleason scores of 4 to 6 and PSA greater or less than 10 ng/ml.

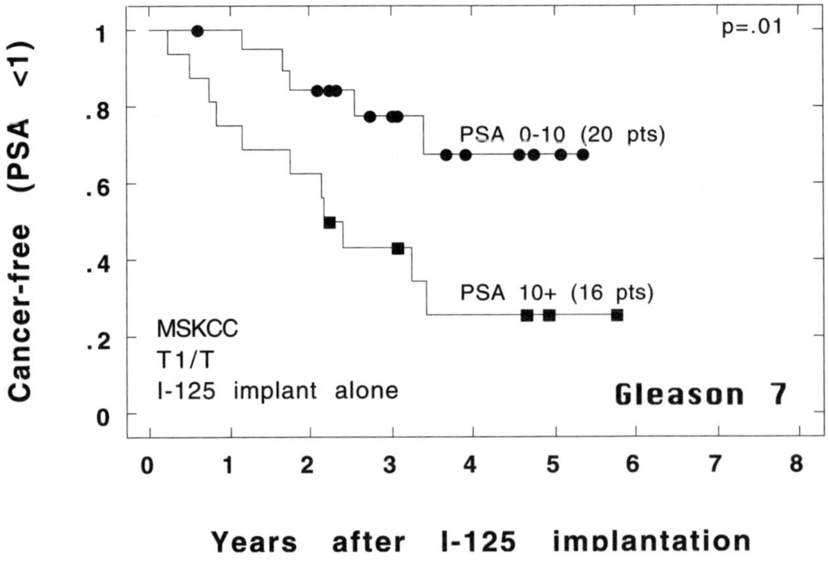

Figure 15-3b. Freedom from biochemical failure after I-125 alone for patients with Gleason scores of 7 and PSA greater or less than 10 ng/ml.

Table 15-2. Univariate and multivariate analysis of I-125 implant.

Prognostic factor	Univariate 'p' value	Multivariate 'p' value
PSA above 10	.02	.05
mm tumor in Biopsy (more than 10mm)	.028	.52
Gleason 4-6 versus 7	.1	.48

PD-103 ALONE

Published data regarding treatment with Pd-103 alone are even scarcer than that for I-125. Dattoli and colleagues have accumulated a large series of patients, primarily with Gleason scores of 6 or less, who were treated with Pd-103 alone. Patients with a pre-treatment PSA level below 10 have approximately an 80% likelihood of remaining disease-free, similar to that reported after high dose conformal external beam radiation or prostatectomy (**Figure 15-4**). The 5-year freedom from biochemical progression with Pd-103 alone is similar to that with I-125 alone. The disease-free curves plateau at each pre-treatment PSA level, suggesting that a large percentage of the patients may be cured.

PD-103 + EBRT

Dattoli and colleagues have a long experience with Pd-103 combined with supplemental EBRT.(Dattoli 1996) The series includes patients with at least one adverse risk factor, including PSA above 10, Gleason score of 7 or higher, or clinical stage T3 cancer (**Table 15-3**). With patients followed up to 5 years, the disease-free curves have leveled off above 50%, suggesting that a high percentage of such patients can be cured (**Figure 15-5**). This is particularly encouraging for patients with pre-treatment PSA above 10, for whom results with other modalities have been discouraging. Even patients with high grade tumors have done surprisingly well with Pd-103 plus EBRT so far (**Figure 15-6**).

One subgroup of patients that did poorly are those with elevated prostatic acid phosphatase (PAP). Their failure rate was over 50% at 3 years, and may be higher with longer follow-up (**Figure 15-7**). Patients with a pre-treatment PAP level above 10 have an extremely small likelihood of remaining disease-free (**Figure 15-8**). Contrary to widely held belief, some patients with moderately elevated PAP are still curable with local therapy, as an elevated PAP level may not be synonymous with distant metastases. If patients with an elevated PAP are excluded, the prognosis, even for patients with a higher PSA, are highly curable (**Figure 15-9**).

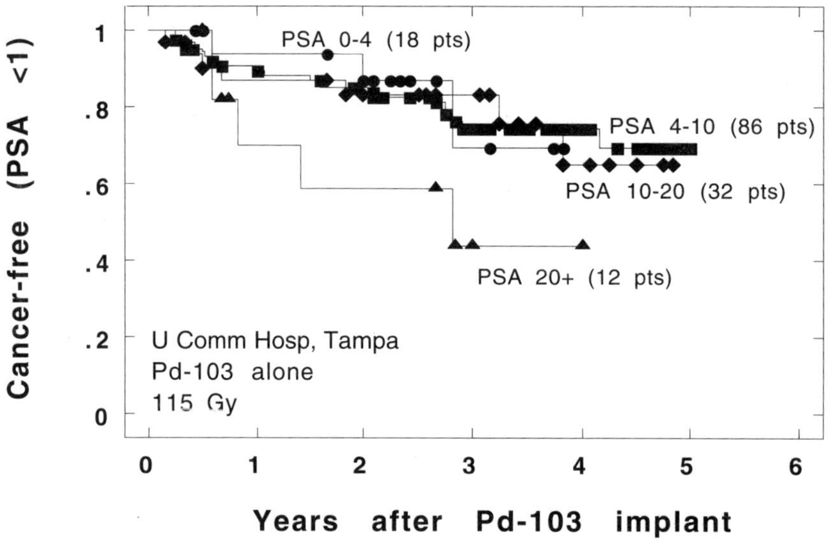

Figure 15-4. Freedom from biochemical progression for patients treated by M. Dattoli with Pd-103 alone at University Community Hospital, Tampa. The curves level off at 70 to 80%, similar to that seen with I-125 alone.

Table 15-3. Pd-103 + EBRT patient characteristics (U Community Hospital, Tampa).

	# of patients	
Gleason 4	1	(1%)
Gleason 5	7	(7%)
Gleason 6	58	(57%)
Gleason 7	36	(35%)
PSA		
0-4 ng/ml	8	(8%)
4-10	50	(49%)
10-20	32	(31%)

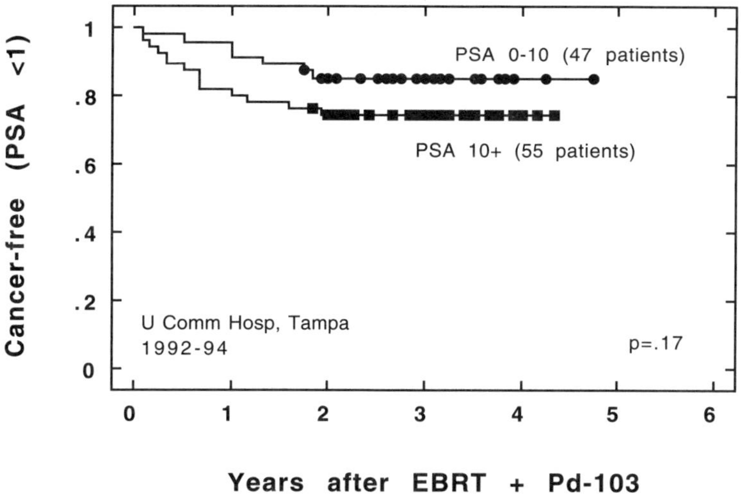

Figure 15-5. Freedom from biochemical failure for patients treated with Pd-103 plus EBRT. The curves appear to level off, even for patients with pre-treatment PSA above 10, suggesting that a large percent of patients with more advanced disease can be left disease-free, with effective local therapy.

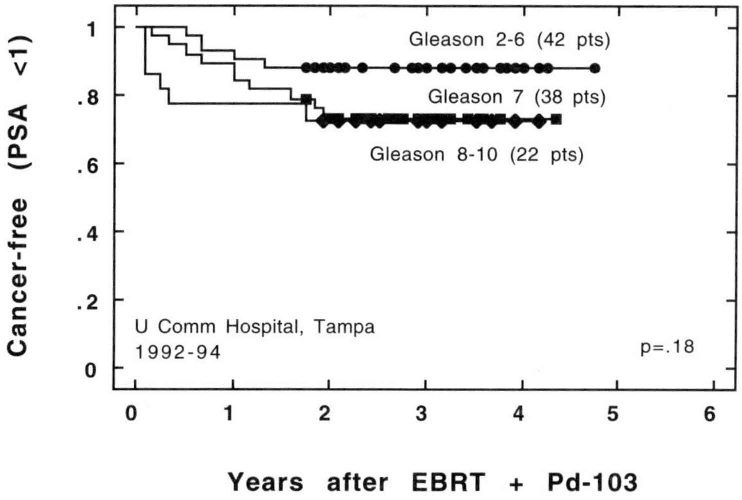

Figure 15-6. Freedom from biochemical failure for patients treated with Pd-103 plus EBRT, suggesting that a large percent of patients with high grade disease can be left disease-free, with effective local therapy.

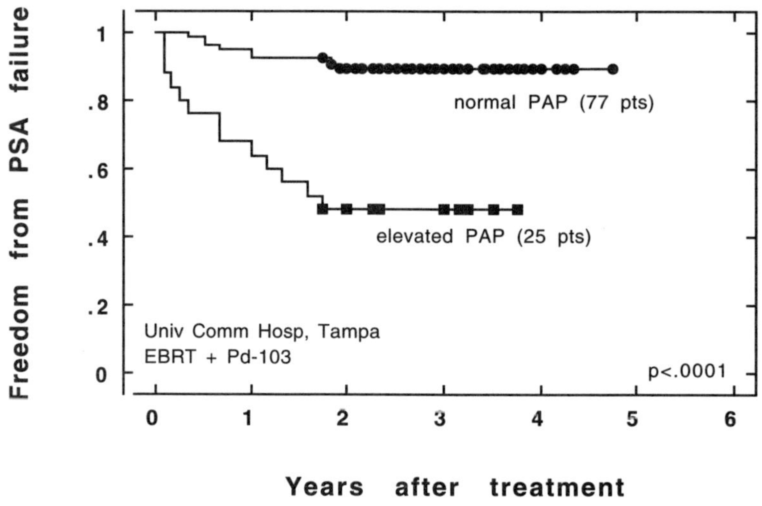

Figure 15-7. Freedom from biochemical failure for patients treated with Pd-103 plus EBRT. Patients with elevated pre-treatment PAP had a high failure rate. In multivariate analysis, elevated PAP was the strongest predictor of failure.

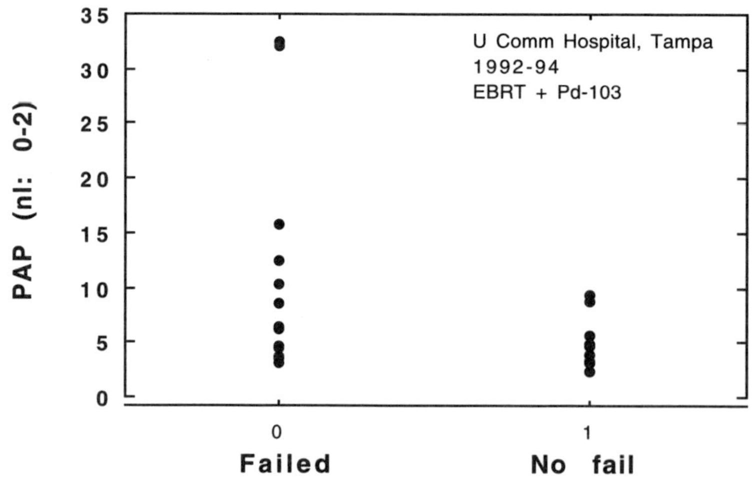

Figure 15-8. Pre-treatment PAP (including only patients with elevated pre-treatment PAP), for those patients who failed and those who did not. All patients with pre-treatment PAP greater than 10 failed.

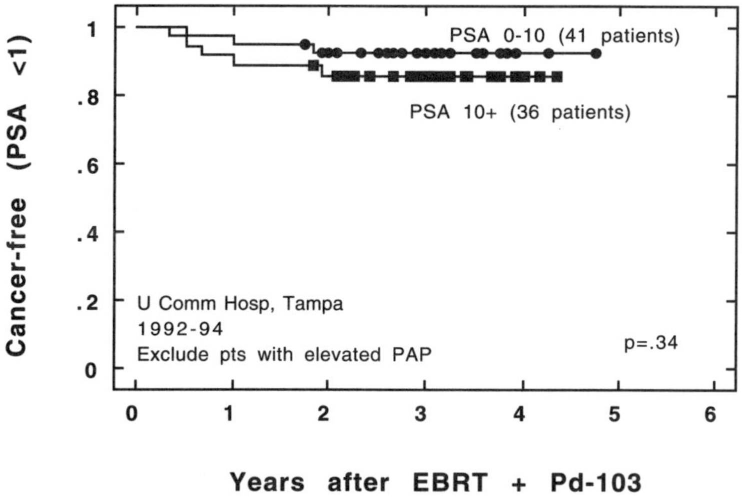

Figure15-9. Freedom from biochemical failure for patients treated with Pd-103 plus EBRT, excluding those patients with elevated PAP. When patients with elevated PAP are excluded, PSA is a much weaker predictor of biochemical failure.

Table 14-4. Univariate and multivariate analysis of EBRT + Pd-103.

Prognostic factor	Univariate 'p' value	Multivariate 'p' value
Elevated PAP	<.0001	<.0001
Gleason score	.07	.15
T2 vs T3	.08	.61
PSA above 10	.17	.71

FOLLOW-UP BIOPSIES

There is limited biopsy data following brachytherapy. The most meticulous follow-up has been reported for patients implanted at Northwest Tumor Institute (NWTI).(Prestidge 1997) Approximately half of the patients treated with I-125 or Pd-103 alone had follow-up biopsies at two years or more.

Of the patients who had a follow-up biopsy, 2% showed residual, apparently viable cancer. Another 20% showed what was believed to be indeterminate tissue, which could be interpreted as residual cancer, but with profound radiation changes that could be consistent with dying cancer. With longer follow-up, most indeterminate biopsies, when repeated, were negative (**Figure 15-10**).

Although not all patients were biopsied, those more likely to have a rising PSA or abnormal physical exam generally were. Patients with more favorable clinical status were less inclined to agree to follow-up biopsy, believing themselves cured. The selection of patients with more suspicious parameters presumably would bias results in favor of finding positive biopsies, so that the results might look even more favorable in a controlled trial.

Post-treatment biopsies have historically been commonly positive following conventional dose EBRT, but in more recent series the positive biopsy rate has been only 20 to 30%, closer to that following brachytherapy alone for early stage disease.(Crook 1995)

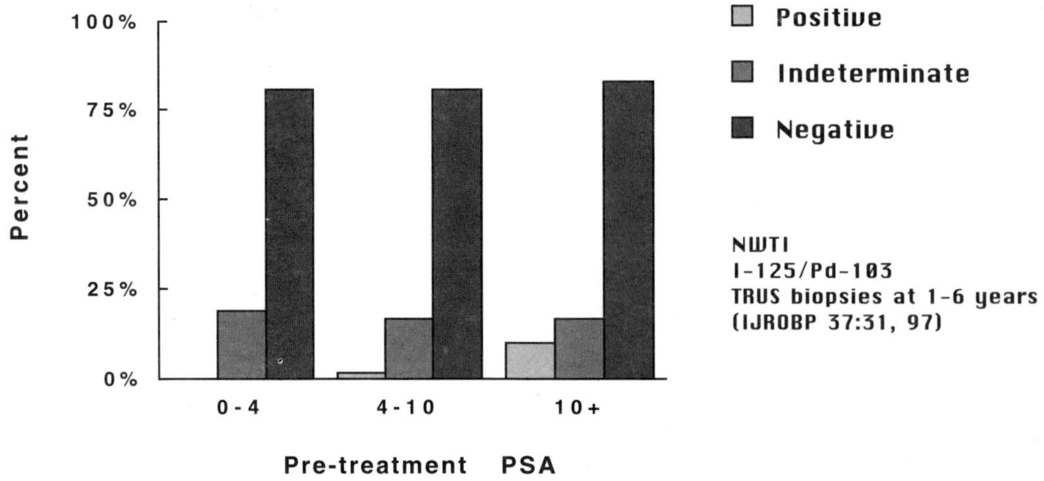

Figure 15-10. Percent of patients with negative, indeterminate or positive biopsies after I-125 or Pd-103 implant for early stage cancer.

While the lower rate of positive biopsy after brachytherapy and after more recent EBRT series is encouraging, we should pause before opening the champagne. Since the introduction of PSA, cancers are being diagnosed at much earlier stages, presumably with much lower tumor burdens than in earlier series. In fact, repeat biopsies in patients with prior positive biopsies, are frequently negative in the absence of therapy -- the tumor burden is so low in many patients that it is often difficult to find cancer even in the untreated patient![Stroumbakis 1997]

COMPARING MODALITIES

Despite regular calls for controlled trials, and for the spending of large amounts of government and private research funds, no modern controlled trials comparing surgery, EBRT or brachytherapy have been performed. In trying to compare modalities, we are left with retrospective uncontrolled comparisons. But things could be worse. Before PSA, retrospective comparisons were nearly worthless, because patients grouped by clinical stage alone are so heterogeneous. With the advent of PSA, there is remarkable prognostic agreement between institutions, within similar PSA categories, using the same modalities.[Zeitman 1994][Zagars 1995] Presumably, comparing the outcomes of different modalities for the same PSA groupings, should give some realistic indication as to the efficacy of the different modalities.

In comparing surgery with EBRT and with brachytherapy, two concepts have been remarkably consistent. First, patients with low tumor burdens (low PSA levels), have done well with modern prostatectomy, EBRT or brachytherapy. With follow-up of approximately 10 years, each modality appears to eradicate cancer in 70 to 80% of such patients (**Figure 15-11**). If there is a cure rate advantage to any of the modalities, it is not apparent within the first 10 years of follow-up. This makes sense -- if the cancer burden is small (PSA below 10), it can usually be eradicated with any moderately effective treatment.

The second consistent finding when comparing modalities in the PSA era is that patients with higher tumor burdens (PSA above 10) have a high risk of early biochemical failure, regardless of the treatment modality. It is in the higher risk patients that results with EBRT alone especially deteriorate so markedly (**Figure 15-12**). In the absence of controlled trials, the most that can be said is that low risk patients do well with any modality, at least for the first 10 years. Patients with PSA above 10 appear to do better with brachytherapy plus supplemental EBRT, but this needs to be confirmed in more centers, and preferably in controlled studies.

The possibility that brachytherapy might add to the cure of patients with more locally advanced cancer should come as no great surprise. Brachytherapy is widely believed to enhance local control of advanced solid tumors in other sites, including the cervix and endometrium.

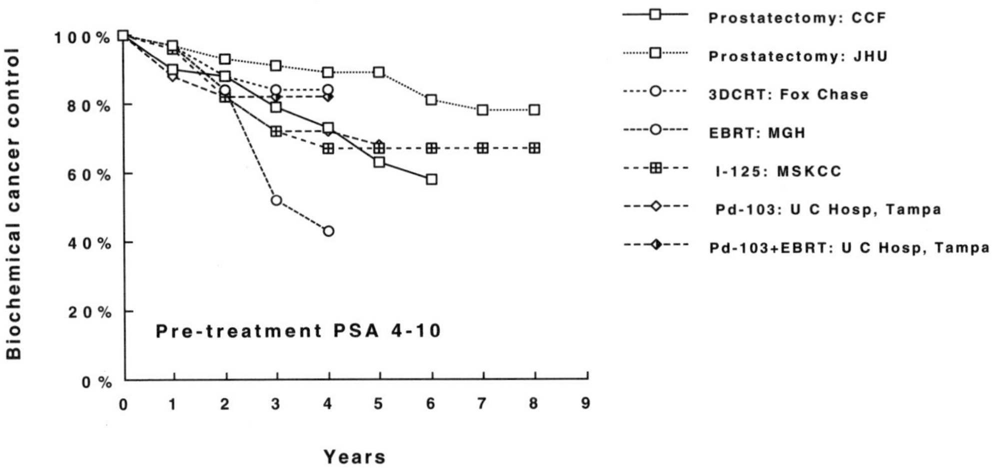

Figure 15-11. Freedom from biochemical failure in series that use stricter criteria for tumor control, in patients with pre-treatment PSA below 10.

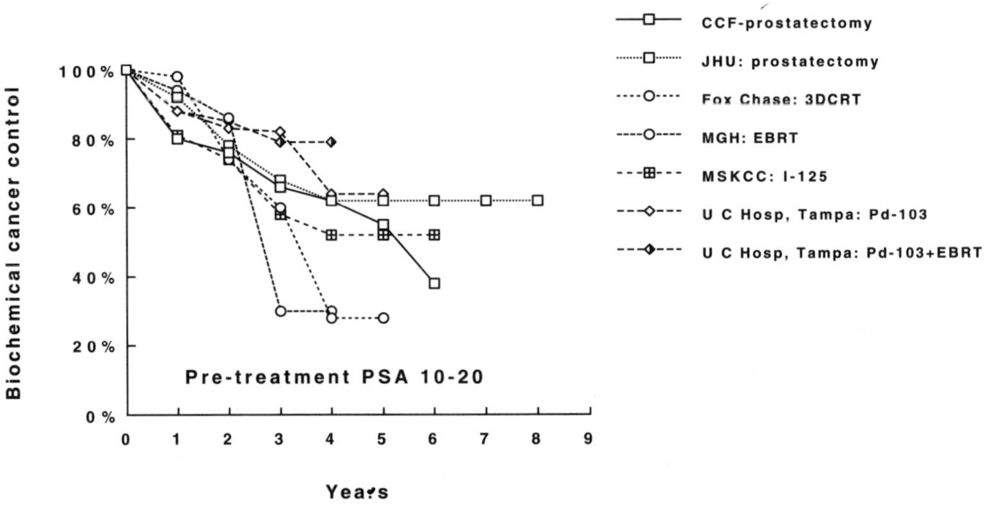

Figure 15-12. Freedom from biochemical failure in series that use stricter criteria for tumor control, in patients with pre-treatment PSA levels of 10-20.

MORE

The limited PSA-based follow-up that has been published is still dominated by a few early teams. Within the next several years multiple reports should emerge, as other brachytherapy teams accumulate more patient follow-up. What we have looks encouraging, but follow-up is still too short to know if patients are being cured, or if patients' PSA values are only being suppressed for several years.

REFERENCES

1. Crook JM, Perry GA, Robertson S, Esche BA. Routine prostate biopsies following radiotherapy for prostate cancer: Results for 226 patients. Urol 1995; 45:624-632.

2. Dattoli M, Wallner K, Sorace R. Pd-103 brachytherapy and external beam irradiation for clinically localized, high-risk prostatic carcinoma. Int J Radiat Oncol Biol Phys 1996; 35:875-879.

3. Partin AW, Pound CR, Clemens JQ, Epstein JI, Walsh PC. Serum PSA after anatomic radical prostatectomy: The Johns Hopkins experience after 10 years. Urol Clin N Am 1993; 20:713-725.

4. Prestidge BR, Hoak DC, Grimm PD, Ragde H, Cavanagh W, Blasko JC. Posttreatment biopsy results following interstitial brachytherapy in early-stage prostate cancer. Int J Radiat Oncol Biol Phys 1997; 37:31.

5. Stroumbakis N, Cookson MS, Reuter VE, Fair WR. Clinical significance of repeat sextant biopsies in prostate cancer patients. Urol 1997; 49(S 3A):113-118.

6. Zagars GK, Pollack A, Kavadi VS. Prostate-specific antigen and radiation therapy for clinically localized prostate cancer. Int J Radiat Oncol Biol Phys 1995; 32:293-306.

7. Zietman AL, Coen JJ, Shipley WU, Willett CG, Efird JT. Radical radiation therapy in the management of prostatic adenocarcinoma: The initial prostate specific antigen value as a predictor of treatment outcome. J Urol 1994; 151:640-645.

Chapter 16

Morbidity

THERE *ARE* SIDE EFFECTS

There is a false impression among many prospective patients that prostate brachytherapy has fewer side effects than external beam radiation (EBRT). The perception probably comes from the seemingly logical idea that more localized radiation of an implant should lead to fewer side effects. The perception that brachytherapy has less radiation side effects may not be correct. Brachytherapy does cause relatively prolonged radiation-related urinary symptoms. Fortunately, serious rectal or urinary *complications* are infrequent with either form of radiation.

Nearly all patients experience varying degrees of radiation-related prostatitis. Approximately half of patients use medication for several months or longer to alleviate radiation-related urinary symptoms. Proctitis, while less common than prostatitis, can occur. Patients should be amply forewarned, for their benefit and that of the physician. Fortunately the symptoms are rarely incapacitating, and do not usually interfere substantially with a patient's lifestyle.(Kleinberg 1994)

Brachytherapy-related urinary morbidity was documented in detail by Arterbery, Kleinberg, Wallner and colleagues at MSKCC in response to what was seen as overly optimistic writings regarding brachytherapy-related-morbidity.(Arterbery 1993)(Kleinberg 1994) We wanted to document the urinary morbidity in detail because we felt that patients and physicians were being given an overly optimistic impression of implant-related side effects. However, it should be noted that the morbidity and complications reported from the early MSKCC experience may partly reflect the CT-based technique employed during that time, which included generous target margins and high activity sources weighted peripherally. The degree of radiation-related symptoms is probably less with other techniques, and with more recent CT-based implants that are better executed.

ACUTE URINARY RETENTION

Urinary retention is the most common acute complication of the implant procedure. Fortunately, it usually resolves spontaneously, within one to three days. Retention is probably due to tissue swelling from needle trauma, and perhaps to the effects of anesthesia. It is not due to radiation per se, as the dose delivered within several hours of the procedure would be minimal. As might be expected, retention is most common in patients with a large prostate and in older men (**Figures 16-1 to 16-4**). Patients with greater degrees of urinary obstruction are presumably at higher risk of post-implant retention, but this has never been well documented.

Although patients with larger prostate volume are at higher risk of retention, there is a striking degree of overlap between those who do or do not develop retention (**Figure 16-2**). It is not currently possible to quantitate the risk with any certainty. Most patients, even those with a large prostate volume, do not develop post-implant retention. It is likely that yet-to-be-quantified risk factors include a combination of prostate volume, degree of functional obstruction, and perhaps anatomical configurations such as median lobe formation.

RADIATION URETHRITIS

Urinary symptoms in the first week after implantation are due to the trauma of needle insertion and catheter use. Trauma-related symptoms generally resolve rapidly. They are followed, in one to four weeks, by urinary symptoms of radiation prostatitis.

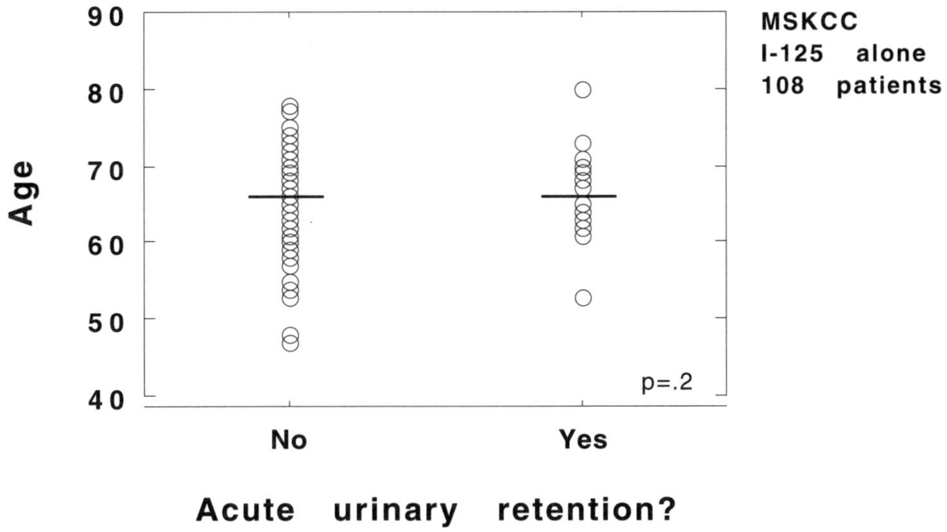

Figure 16-1. Age of patients who did or did not develop acute post-implant urinary retention. Older patients are not at increased risk.

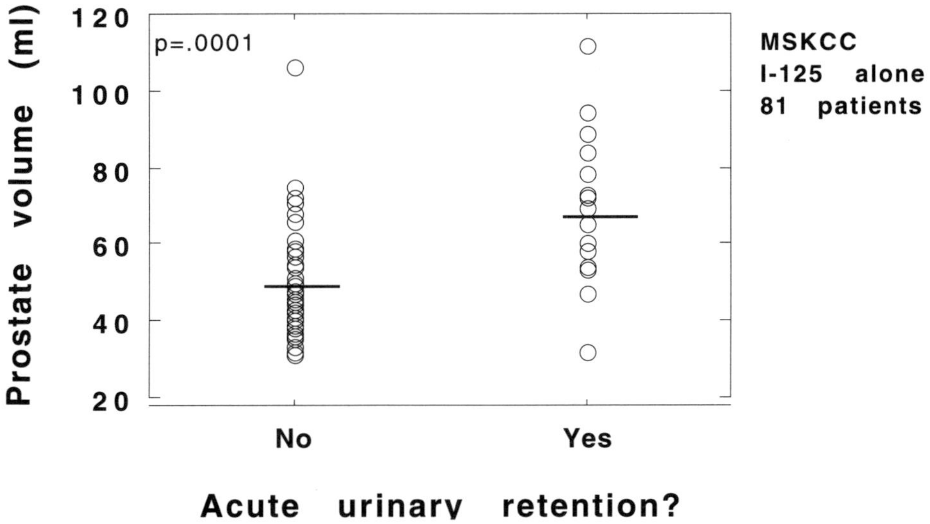

Figure 16-2. Patients with larger prostate volume are more likely to develop acute post-implant urinary retention.

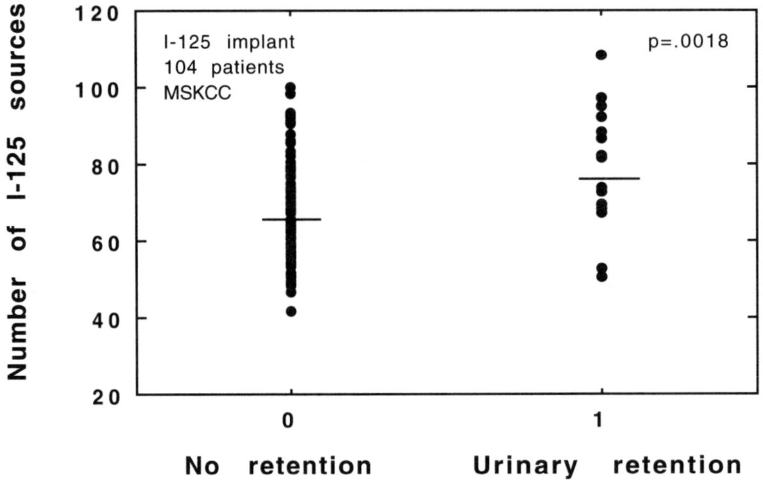

Figure 16-3. Acute urinary retention versus the number of sources implanted. Patients who required more sources were more likely to develop retention, but that is probably due to their larger prostate size, rather than the number of sources per se.

Symptoms of radiation prostatitis generally start two to three weeks after implantation. Nearly all patients develop some degree of dysuria, daytime urinary frequency, and increased nocturia. Symptoms peak at about three to six weeks for I-125 and at two to three weeks following Pd-103.(Kleinberg 1994)(Cash 1997)

Urinary symptoms arc duc to high dosc irradiation of thc prostatic urcthra and bladder neck, rather than the bladder itself. Radiation dose to bladder wall away from the prostatic base should be negligible, so that the clinical syndrome is more properly considered urethritis, rather than cystitis.

Symptoms severe enough to warrant use of alpha-blockers are more common in patients with a large prostate, but there is considerable overlap between patients who do or do not develop substantial symptoms (**Figure 16-6**). Age was not related to the likelihood of developing substantial radiation prostatitis (**Figure 16-5**). The severity of radiation prostatitis has been correlated with the urethral dose (**Figure 16-7**)(see Chapter 6).

RESOLUTION OF RADIATION PROSTATITIS

Symptoms of radiation prostatitis usually resolve within six to twelve months, but some patients have residual symptoms longer. Patients treated with I-125 alone at MSKCC have been followed closely, and assessed for their use of

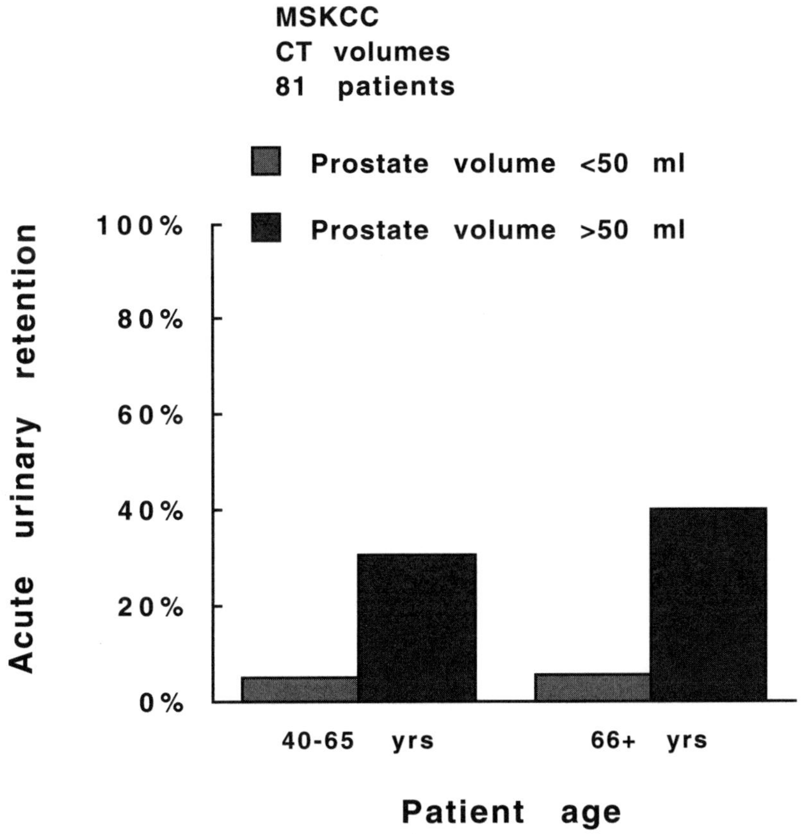

Figure 16-4. Likelihood of acute, post-implant urinary retention, versus prostate volume and age. Prostate volume is a much more important factor than age.

alpha-blockers to relieve urinary symptoms (RTOG grade 2 morbidity). Approximately half of patients used alpha-blockers for some time, and about 20% were still taking medication two years after implantation (**Figure 16-8**). It should be kept in mind that some patients in the prostate cancer age range would be on alpha-blockers for benign prostatic hypertrophy (BPH) even without having had an implant, so that the significance of 20% of patients still taking them two years afterwards may be minimal.

IT MAY NOT REALLY BE SO BAD

The substantial short-term morbidity reported from MSKCC should be extrapolated with caution. Much of the published morbidity data from MSKCC was gathered from patients treated early in the transperineal brachytherapy expe-

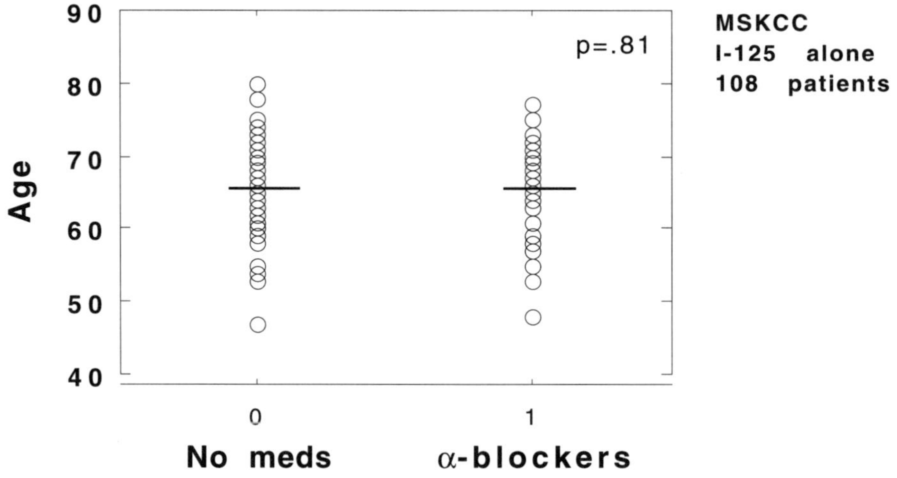

Figure 16-5. Necessity for alpha-blockers to relieve radiation prostatitis, versus patient age. Older patients were not more likely to suffer from symptoms of radiation prostatitis.

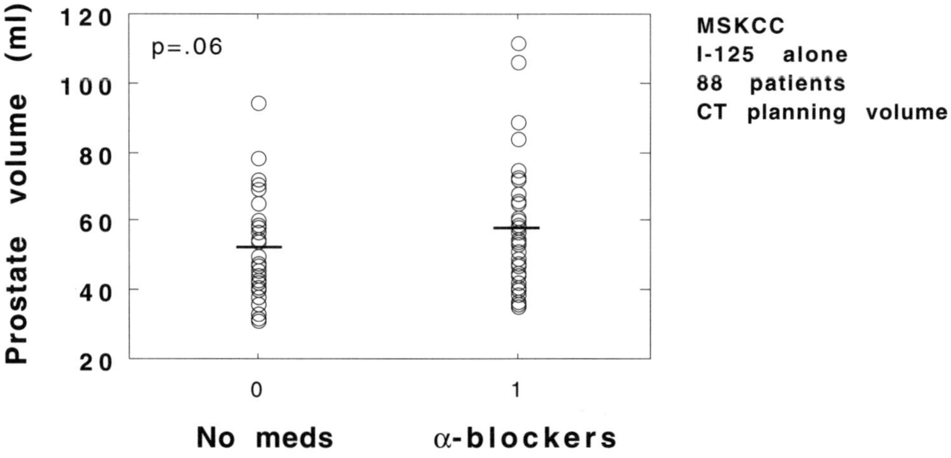

Figure 16-6. Necessity for alpha-blockers to relieve radiation prostatitis, versus prostate volume. Patients with larger prostates were more likely to suffer from symptoms of radiation prostatitis, but there is considerable overlap in the data.

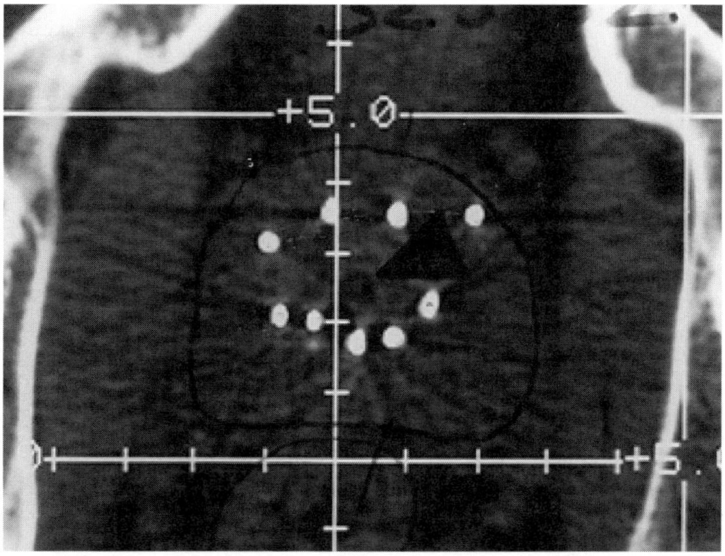

Figure 16-7. Post-implant CT scan of patient who developed prolonged, marked urinary discomfort. There are too many sources near the urethra at this level (arrowhead). This was an error in implementation, not planning. Mistakes like this increase the likelihood that a patient will experience substantial post-implant urethritis.

rience at the institution. Patients treated more recently, whose urethral dose has been kept lower, should experience less morbidity than that shown here.

BRACHYTHERAPY AS A BOOST

Acute morbidity following EBRT+brachytherapy boost has not been reported in detail. The severity of radiation prostatitis symptoms may be less than that after implant alone.

SUPERFICIAL URETHRAL NECROSIS

Investigators at NWTI noted an overall 4% incidence of superficial urethral necrosis (SUN), associated with severe dysuria and sometimes with urinary incontinence.(Blasko 1993) SUN only occurred in patients with a prior TURP. Occurrence of SUN is probably one cause of late, temporary exacerbations of urinary irritative symptoms, though this has not been documented.

Occurrence of SUN probably reflects high urethral doses that invariably occur. Homogeneous source placement practiced in the early years at NWTI probably increased the likelihood of urethral necrosis. In contrast, implants at MSKCC and University Community Hospital, Tampa, begun later, have generally been per-

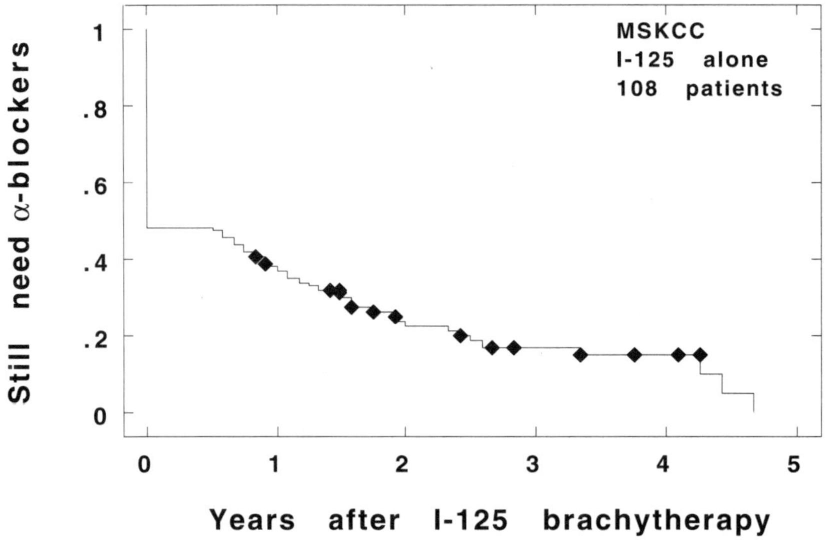

Figure 16-8. Resolution of symptoms of radiation prostatitis following I-125 implantation. Only about half of patients have substantial enough symptoms to require alpha-blockers.

formed with more peripheral source placement in an effort to keep the urethral dose lower (see Chapter 6). Accordingly, urethral necrosis has been less common.

URINARY INCONTINENCE

Significant urinary incontinence, in the absence of prior or subsequent TURP, is very uncommon. At NWTI, none of 184 patients without TURP developed incontinence despite uniform source distribution in these early patients (**Figure 16-9**). Incontinence, however, did occur in some patients who had a TURP before or after implantation. There was no obvious difference in the risk of incontinence in patients treated with implant alone versus those treated with implant and supplemental EBRT.

At MSKCC, only two of 91 patients without a prior TURP has developed urinary incontinence that required use of pads (**Figure 16-10**). Six patients described some minimal, occasional urgency or stress incontinence, not requiring use of pads in their underwear.

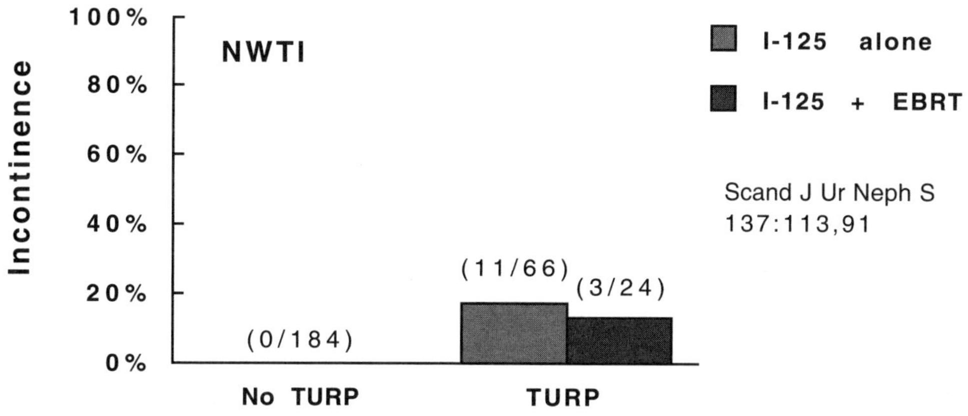

Figure 16-9. Incidence of urinary incontinence in patients treated at NWTI with I-125 alone or I-125 combined with EBRT. Patients who had a pre-implant TURP had a higher likelihood of developing post-implant incontinence.

PRIOR TURP

Reports of the risk of urinary incontinence in patients with prior TURP are conflicting. Both TURP and radiation can, in themselves, impair urinary continence. Their combination has some degree of additive, adverse effect. TURP may predispose patients to radiation-related incontinence by compromising the urinary sphincters or by denuding the urethral lining.

Blasko, Grimm and Ragde were the first to draw attention to the higher risk of incontinence in men with prior TURP.(Blasko 1993) Of 90 patients with pre- or post-implant TURP, there was a 17% likelihood of incontinence, usually associated with superficial urethral necrosis. The actuarial likelihood of incontinence has increased to 48% with longer follow-up.

The experience of NWTI with patients with prior TURP may not be representative. Of 24 patients with prior TURP implanted at MSKCC or University Community Hospital, Tampa, only two have developed urine incontinence (one mild and one severe)(**Figure 16-9 and 16-11**).

The lower incidence of incontinence in TURP patients implanted at MSKCC or University Community Hospital, Tampa is likely due to more peripheral source placement (see Chapter 6). Blasko and colleagues at the NWTI have been using a more peripheral source loading since 1994, and have noted a lower incidence of urinary incontinence (unpublished data).

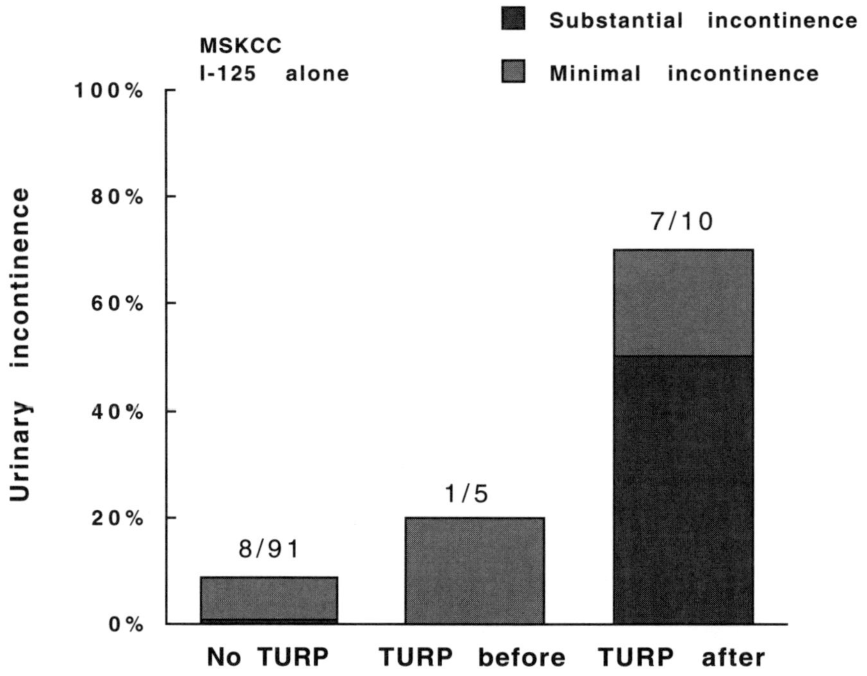

Figure 16-10. Incidence of urinary incontinence in patients treated with I-125 alone at MSKCC. The 6 patients who developed incontinence without having had a TURP before or after implant described urgency, which would occasionally lead to slight leakage if they could not get to a bathroom. This would not be considered incontinence by the LENT scoring system.(Lee 1996)

TURP AFTER BRACHYTHERAPY

Patients who undergo TURP to relieve refractory urinary retention after implantation are at increased risk of developing urinary incontinence. In the early MSKCC experience, approximately 10% of patients underwent a post-implant TURP to relieve urinary obstruction, from one to 20 months after implantation. No patient required a TURP more than two years from implantation and there does not appear to be an increased risk of urinary obstruction with long follow-up (**Figure 16-12**).

Hu and Wallner recently reviewed ten of 109 patients (9%) who underwent TURP or TUIP to relieve urinary obstruction unrelated to local tumor recurrence, from one to 22 months following I-125 implantation.(Hu 1998) Even in retrospect,

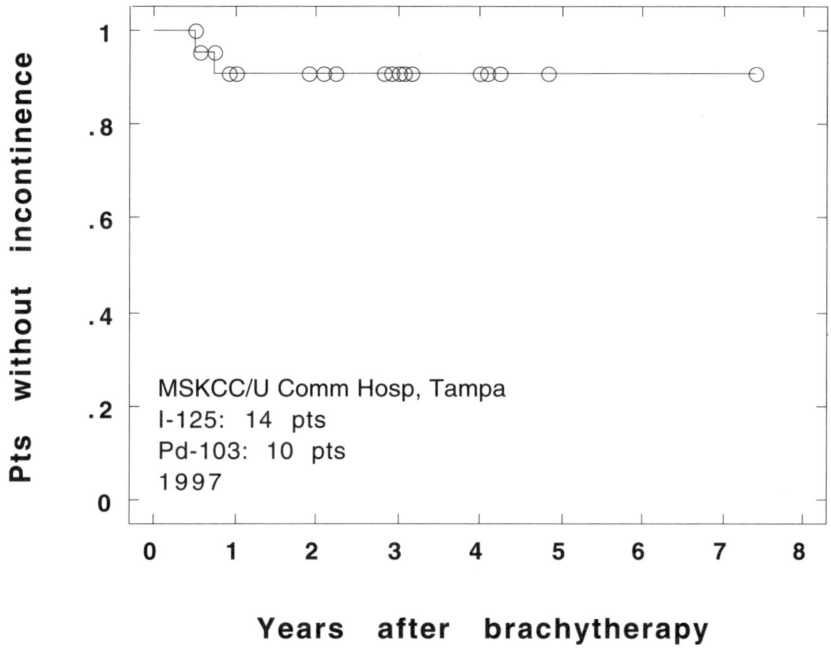

Figure 16-11. Urinary incontinence in 24 patients implanted at MSKCC or University Community Hospital, Tampa. The incidence of incontinence is much lower than that reported from NWTI, probably due to peripheral source loading. It is possible that more incontinence may develop with longer follow-up.

those patients who were destined to develop refractory urinary retention requiring TURP could not be identified by the usual pre-implant parameters. Only one of the 10 patients described substantial urinary obstructive symptoms (nocturia x 2 or more) prior to implantation. There was no clear relationship between pre-implant prostate size and subsequent need for TURP/TUIP (**Figure 16-13**).

Seven of the 10 patients developed some degree of permanent urinary incontinence following TURP/TUIP. Three patients have minimal, stress urinary incontinence and in four patients incontinence was severe. The mechanism of incontinence after post-implant TURP is unknown. Post-implant TURP may predispose patients to radiation-related incontinence by compromising the urinary sphincters or by denuding the urethral lining and radiation may exacerbate TURP-related sphincter compromise.

There was no obvious relationship between the extent of the surgical procedure (TURP vs TUIP) and the likelihood of incontinence. Equally perplexing,

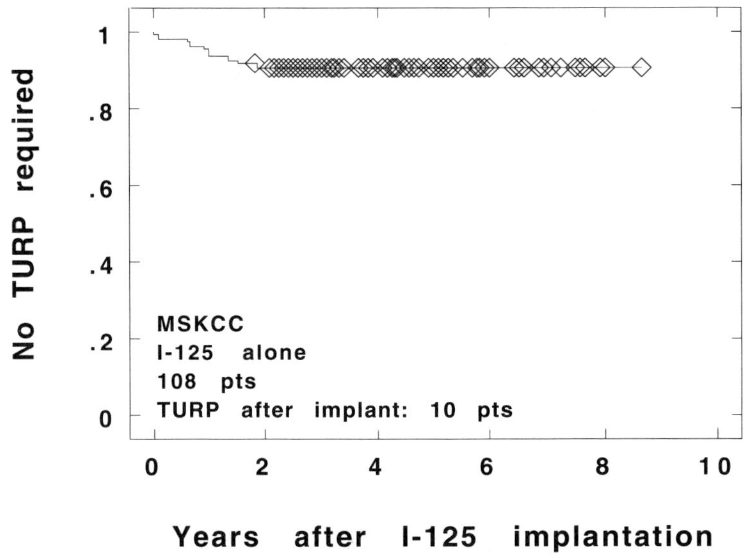

Figure 16-12. Freedom from post-implant TURP following I-125 implantation. All cases of refractory urinary retention requiring TURP occurred within the first two years following implantation.

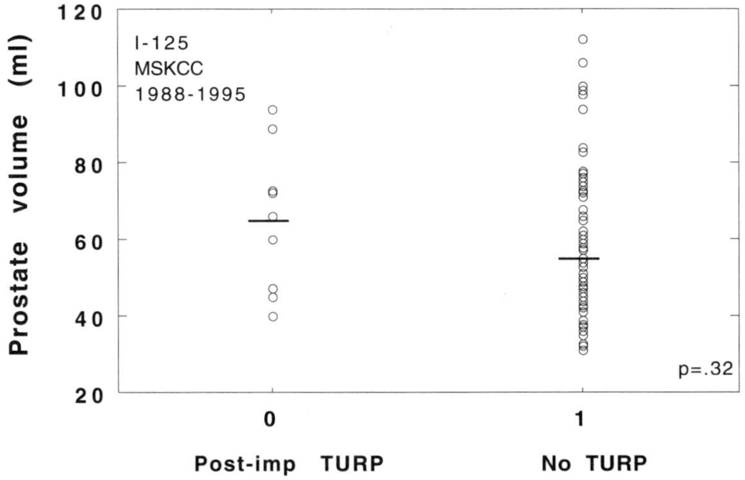

Figure 16-13. Pre-implant prostate volume of those patients who did or did not require post-implant TURP. Although the mean volume was higher for those who required an implant, there is considerable overlap between the groups, and it is not possible to predict the likelihood of post-implant retention for an individual patient.

there was no obvious relationship between the development of incontinence and the amount of tissue resected at the time of TURP or between the time from implant to TURP. There remains much to learn about the mechanism of these injuries.

In five of the patients for whom urethral dose calculations were done, the maximal dose exceeded 400 Gy, the level at which the risk of urinary morbidity rises.(Wallner 1995)

The incidence of post-implant TURP reported by Hu & Wallner is higher than would currently be expected. The current risk is probably lower because more care is being taken to keep the urethral dose within acceptable levels. Additionally, patients would now be managed more conservatively, with prolonged self-catheterization if necessary. Post-implant TURP would be postponed much longer (if not indefinitely), to allow spontaneous resolution of urinary obstruction (see Chapter 11).

URETHRAL STRICTURE

Urethral stricture has been an uncommon complication in modern brachytherapy series. One recent case appeared to be associated with excessive sources at the prostatic apex (**Figure 16-14**). There does not appear to be an

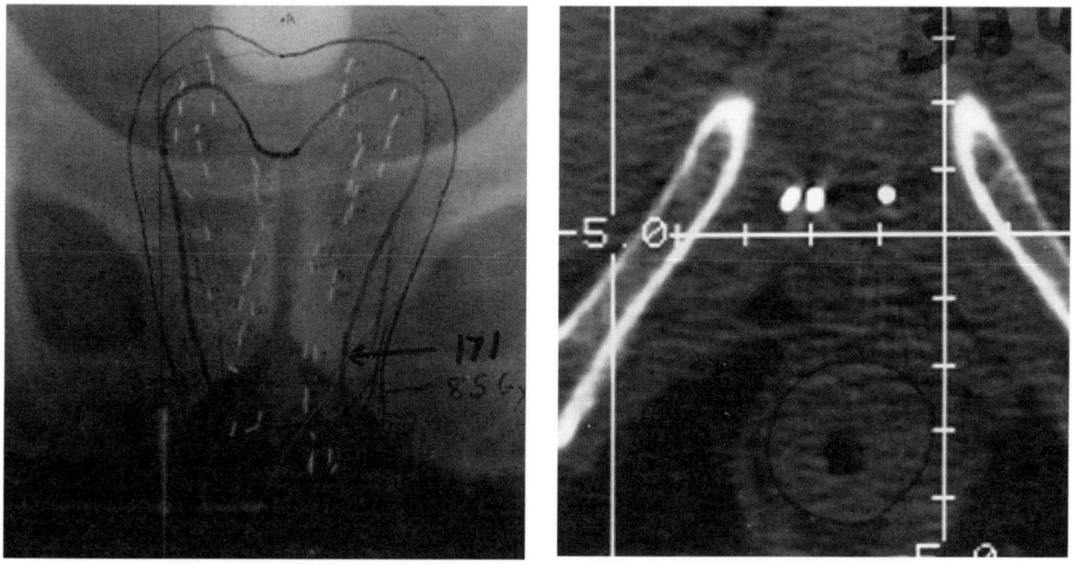

Figure 16-14. Post implant AP radiograph and CT scan of a patient who developed an apical urethral stricture 18 months after I-125 implant. An excessive number of sources were placed at prostatic apex, and probably contributed to late stricture formation.

increased late incidence of stricture formation, though this is possible with longer follow-up. However, it is our impression that the bulbous and membranous urethra are more prone to radiation induced stricture formation. For this reason, we caution against using too generous an inferior margin beyond that apex, which may increase the occurrence of urethral strictures.

PROCTITIS

Some degree of radiation proctitis is inevitable, given the proximity of the prostate and rectum. Patients commonly develop more frequent bowel movements, but not diarrhea. They rarely are bothered enough to use medication. Gastrointestinal symptoms usually resolve within a few months, somewhat earlier than urinary symptoms.

Patients commonly experience the urge to defecate when urinating, during the acute radiation reaction period. They may sit down to urinate, for fear that they may also pass stool. Although such radiation-related rectal symptoms are common, rectal incontinence and pain is rare.

RECTAL BLEEDING

Many patients will have a degree of radiation proctitis, which can be associated with mild bleeding. Minor rectal bleeding is probably more common than generally appreciated. The significance is minimal, and it has not been well documented. Rectal bleeding is probably underreported after EBRT or brachytherapy, because it is usually minor, and it may be erroneously attributed to hemorrhoids.

RECTAL ULCERATION

Fortunately, rectal ulceration is rare in experienced hands. AT MSKCC, 5% of patients treated with I-125 alone developed rectal ulcerations, all within 24 months of implantation. No case occurred more than two years after implantation (**Figure 16-15**). J. Blasko and colleagues have had only one case of documented rectal ulceration when using implant alone. No fistula has occurred, with over 10 years of implant experience.

Rectal bleeding due to proctitis is not usually painful. Rectal bleeding associated with pain may indicate a more serious condition, which should be closely followed along with an experienced colorectal surgeon. Fortunately, rectal complications are rare enough that few experienced surgeons exist. Radiation rectal ulcers nearly always healed spontaneously, within one to two years.

The likelihood of rectal ulceration or fistulas is related to the integral dose (see Chapters 5 and 9). The risk is probably a continuum with increasing dose and volume of rectal wall radiated, with no clear threshold. Patients treated at

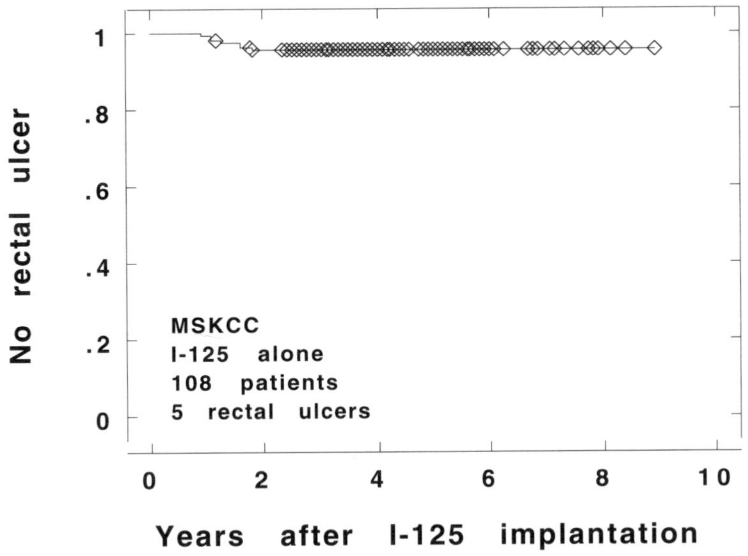

Figure 16-15. Freedom from post-implant rectal ulceration following I-125 implantation. All rectal complications occurred within two years of implantation.

MSKCC had a higher risk as more of their rectal wall was treated to doses above 100 Gy.(Wallner 1995)

The likelihood of a serious rectal reaction, in experienced hands, is extremely low. The relatively high incidence of ulcers in the early MSKCC experience was an unfortunate exception. Some of those patients had what we would now consider to be sloppy implants, which should not occur with current levels of experience.

The likelihood of rectal ulceration at MSKCC decreased as more technical experience was gained (**Figure 16-16**). We attribute this to better technique, with less likelihood of placing sources more posteriorly than intended. In the early experience at MSKCC, additional sources were commonly placed into the prostate. We believed from prior published experience with retropubic technique that the risk of fistula was miniscule. However, with the larger amount of activity placed with transperineal techniques, it is dangerous to place extra sources indiscriminantly. If extra sources are placed, they should be lateral or anterior in the prostate, away from the urethra and rectum (See Chapter 5).

There is limited information regarding rectal morbidity of I-125 or Pd-103 brachytherapy and supplemental EBRT. Iversen and colleagues treated patients with 47 Gy whole pelvic irradiation, delivering 237 cGy/day, preceded by a full

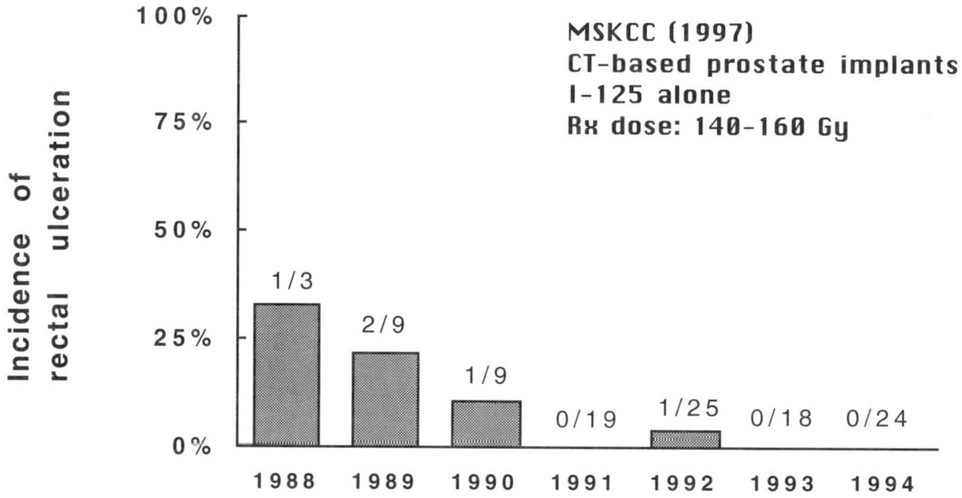

Figure 16-16. Incidence of rectal ulceration in patients implanted in early MSKCC experience. The last patient to develop a rectal complication was implanted in March, 1992.

dose (160 Gy) I-125 implant.(Iversen 1989) Severe late complications, including rectal ulceration, colostomy and severe radiation cystitis were reported in 14 of 33 patients. This toxicity would be unacceptable, but probably reflects their use of whole pelvic irradiation at high daily fractions, combined with a full dose implant. Combining full doses of brachytherapy and EBRT is not wise. Although the report by Iversen and colleagues was frightening, the incidence of rectal ulceration with implant and supplemental EBRT, as described in Chapter 6, has been negligible.

WE HAVE PROBABLY SEEN THE WORST

Modern prostate brachytherapy, using TRUS and CT guidance, has been widely practiced only for 10 years. The first few years experience, on which most of the published morbidity data is based, almost certainly indicates a higher complications rate than should currently be expected, given what we have learned about radiation tolerance and the technical experience that has been gained. In experienced hands, serious complications are surprisingly infrequent. One note of caution is that late complications may surface with longer follow-up, possibly related to very high urethral doses that can occur. But we doubt it.

REFERENCES

1. Arterbery

., Wallner KE, Roy J, Fuks Z. Patient Tolerance and Early Results with CT-planned Transperienal I-125 Prostate Implants. Int J Radiat Oncol Biol Phys 1993; 25:661-667.

2. Blasko JC, Grimm PD, Ragde H. Brachytherapy and organ preservation in the management of carcinoma of the prostate. Sem Radiat Oncol 1993; 3:240-249.

3. Cash J, Dattoli M. Management of the patient receiving transperineal Palladium-103 prostate implant. Oncol Nurs Forum 1997; 24:

4. Hu K, Wallner KE. Urinary incontinence in patients whohave a TURP/TUIP following prostate brachytherapy. (submitted) 1998;

5. Iversen P, Nielsen L, Bak M, et al. Ultrasonically Guided 125Iodine Seed Implantation with External Radiation in Management of Localized Prostatic Carcinoma. Urol 1989; 34:181-186.

6. Kleinberg L, Wallner K, Roy J, et al. Treatment-related symptoms during the first year following transperineal I-125 prostate implantation. Int J Radiat Oncol Biol Phys 1994; 28:985.

7. Lee WR, Schultheiss TE, Hanlon AL, Hanks GE. Urinary incontinence following external beam radiotherapy for clinically localized prostate cancer. Urol 1996; 48:95-99.

8. Wallner KE, Roy J, Harrison L. Dosimetry guidelines to minimize urethral and rectal morbidity following transperineal I-125 prostate brachytherapy. Int J Radiat Oncol Biol Phys 1995; 32:465-471.

Chapter 17

Potency preservation

Potency loss is the most common, permanent sequela of prostatectomy, external beam irradiation (EBRT) or brachytherapy. Brachytherapy has consistently been reported to hold some advantage over surgery or EBRT in regards to potency preservation. The true degree of its advantage is still unclear, due in part to differences in the way potency is reported from one series to the next.

DEFINITION

Quantification of the effect of treatment on potency requires a working definition of potency. The definition used in mainstream surgical literature is

the ability to maintain an erection sufficient for intercourse.

The potency statistics most widely quoted by the most respected surgeons are based on this simple practical definition.(Catalona 1993)(Quinlan 1991) Unfortunately, this simple definition leaves considerable room for interpretation on the part of the patient and the investigator. Critics of the current state of affairs have called for more detailed potency criteria and such criteria have been proposed, but their practicality is questionable.(Zinreich 1990)(Banker 1988)

SPONTANEOUS POTENCY LOSS

Analyses of the effect of treatment on potency are clouded by the fact that prostate cancer occurs in an older age group, for whom there is already a substantial incidence of impotence prior to treatment. Approximately 50% of men are already impotent by the time they are diagnosed with prostatic carcinoma.(Zinreich 1990)

The Massachusetts Male Aging Study summarized the incidence of impotence versus age.(Feldman 1994) Based on personal interviews, the study found that men between the ages of 40 and 80 will spontaneously lose potency at a rate of approximately 1.5% per year (**Figure 17-1**). In the short term, gradual "natural" potency loss should not substantially affect the potency rate changes due to therapy. However, over five years or more natural potency loss should be taken into consideration when reporting potency loss after treatment, because a substantial part of long-term potency loss may be attributed to aging, rather than to treatment itself.

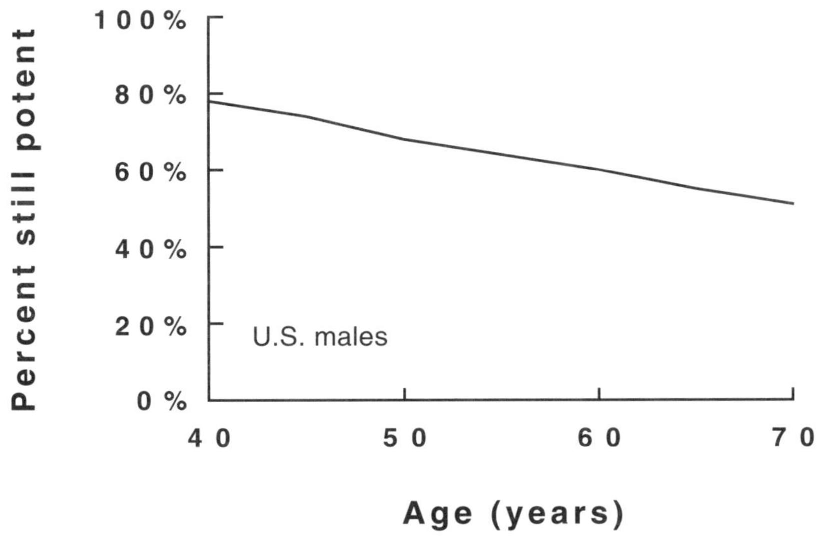

Figure 17-1. Percent of men in the general population still potent versus age. As part of the Massachusetts Male Aging Study, the data is based on personal interviews.

COLLECTING POTENCY INFORMATION

It's not easy...

Obtaining reliable potency information can be difficult . The problem may sometimes lie partly with patients' reluctance to admit potency loss. But more likely, it is due to the fact that many of the patients are older and not as sexually active to begin with. An example of how difficult collecting potency information can be is seen in the following excerpts from the hospital record of a patient followed by K. Wallner:

October, 1988 - initial consultation
"The patient explains that he has had no symptoms from this nodule."

December, 1988
I-125 implant (36 mCi)

January, 1989
"He has no erections, but this has not changed since before the procedure."

July, 1989
"....he does state that since implantation he has now maintained a full erection and complains of vague discomfort during ejaculation. These symptoms started two months after implantation and have not progressed or improved since."

December, 1989
"The patient states that he still has difficulty maintaining a full erection, but that there is no discomfort during ejaculation."

January, 1991
"The patient has had decreased sexual potency since the time of implantation and this has not changed. He is able to maintain erections occasionally, however they are soft and he is not able to obtain a sufficient erection for penetration."

January, 1992
"He also states that he is sexually potent and has frequent AM erections and is able to have intercourse and orgasm. I reminded him that he had told us one year ago he was having difficulty with sexual potency. He acknowledged that, but now insists that he feels well and is sexually active."

These excerpts show the inconsistencies that can occur from one follow-up visit to the next, and the vexing problem it can pose to a physician who is trying to determine the effect of treatment on a patient's potency. Fortunately, this example of the inconsistencies is more extreme than most.

....but it's fairly consistent

One common recommendation regarding the analysis of potency rates is that spouses should be interviewed separately because patients may not be realistic or honest in reporting their erectile capacity. However, studies have shown that patients and spouses generally report similarly about the man's erectile function.(Zinreich 1990)(Chinn 1995)

Another commonly raised concern has been that potency data should be verified with physiological testing, to make the data more objective. But from a practical standpoint it would be difficult to arrange for the physiological testing of a large number of patients. Because patients and spouses are generally consistent in their answers when interviewed separately, the necessity of such detailed physiological testing is questionable.

CAUSES

The mechanism of post-radiation impotence is not known. One report of radiation-induced arterial occlusion of the internal iliac, internal pudendal and penile arteries has been published.(Goldstein 1984) However, that was based on only two patients, and has never been confirmed by other investigators.

Impotence is probably not due to neurological compromise. Pelvic neural testing has been negative,(Goldstein 1984) and peripheral nerves should tolerate doses of 70 to 80 Gy, considering the lack of neurological damage after similar doses used for extremity sarcomas.

Another possible cause of radiation-induced impotence is venous insufficiency, due to radiation damage to the bulb of the penis (**Figure 17-2**). Venous leakage is increasingly being considered as a mechanism of post-radiation impotence, although its precise role has not been well documented.

Patients who develop radiation-induced impotence generally respond to intracavernosal papaverine or PGE1 injection.(Pierce 1991) Whether impotence is due to vascular or neural damage, vasoactive injections may work simply because

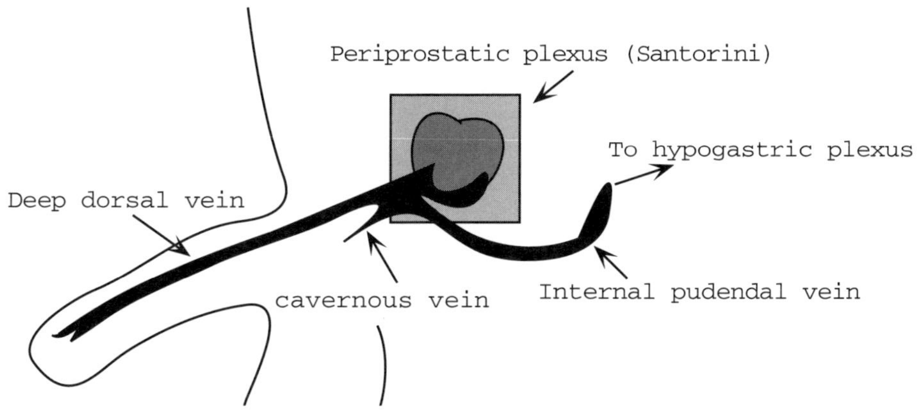

Figure 17-2. Venous drainage of the corpora. Radiation to the bulb of the penis could lead to venous leak and impotence. If venous leak is the primary mechanism, it is logical that the risk of impotence would be higher with EBRT, as a larger volume of normal tissue would be included in the high dose region.

they supplement a compromised system. The significance of this response in regard to the mechanism of impotence is unclear.

Needle trauma

A small percentage of patients are acutely impotent immediately following an implant procedure, presumably due to needle trauma to the neurovascular bundle, which is several mm from the posterior capsule (**Figure 17-3**). Varying degrees of impotence immediately following the implant procedure might be accounted for by whether one or two nerves were damaged. Some patients spontaneously recover from acute post-implant impotence at some time afterwards, presumably due to the slow healing of traumatic neurovascular damage. The incidence of and likelihood of recovery from trauma-induced impotence has not been wcll documented.

SELF-SELECTION

Potency preservation rates could be influenced by patients' perceptions of the impotence risk with each treatment option. Higher potency preservation rates have long been reported with brachytherapy, even with retropubic implants combined with a laparotomy. Accordingly, patients who are more motivated to pre-

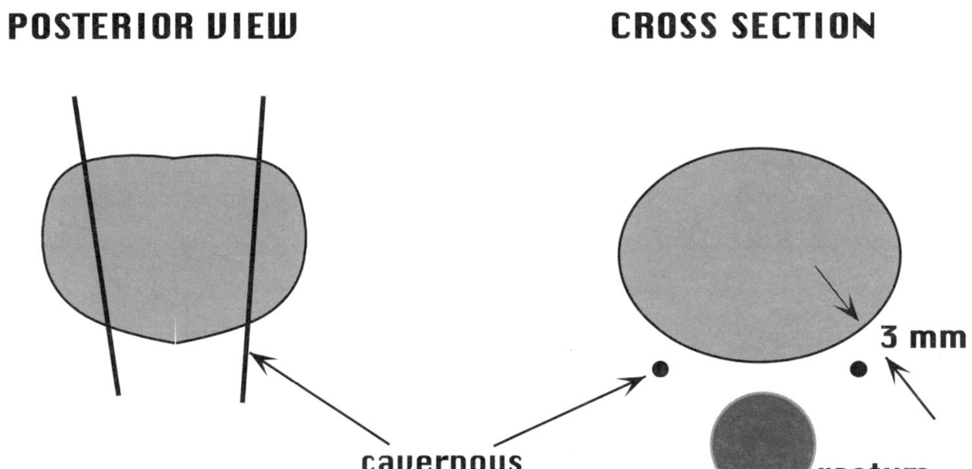

Figure 17-3. The neurovascular bundles are approximately 3 mm away from the posterior prostatic capsule. They receive a high radiation dose from an implant, potentially causing vascular or neurogenic impotence.

serve potency are probably more likely to choose brachytherapy over EBRT or surgery. Because more sexually active patients may be more likely to retain potency than potent but inactive patients,[Banker 1988] patient self-selection could become a self-fulfilling prophecy whereby potent active patients seek brachytherapy in the hope of preserving their potency, making the potency results with brachytherapy appear better by the fact that brachytherapy is being used for more sexually active patients.

POTENCY COMPROMISE BEFORE THERAPY

Men with some degree of pre-treatment potency compromise may have a higher likelihood of losing potency regardless of the treatment modality. Investigators from the University of California, San Francisco (UCSF) and the University of Chicago reported that potency-impaired patients were more likely to lose potency after EBRT. However, follow-up was limited and actuarial calculations were not used in the UCSF data.[Chinn 1995][Mantz 1997] Banker reported that patients who were sexually inactive prior to treatment were less likely to maintain potency after EBRT.[Banker 1988]

The influence of pre-treatment potency status or sexual activeness has not been consistent for surgical or brachytherapy reports. Stock and colleagues did not find a relationship between pre-treatment potency status and the likelihood of maintaining potency after brachytherapy. However, like most potency reports, follow-up was short.[Stock 1996] In addition, the effect of pre-treatment potency compromise on potency preservation following prostatectomy is unclear.[Geary 1995]

Although the importance of pre-treatment potency compromise is still unclear, patients with pre-treatment compromise should be warned that they may be more likely to develop complete impotence following brachytherapy.

ACTUARIAL CALCULATIONS VERSUS CRUDE PERCENTAGES

Statistical methods used to calculate potency preservation rates can substantially alter the results. Potency loss increases over time, so meaningful statistics require some consideration for the length of time since treatment (**Figure 17-4**). The use of crude percentages can grossly inflate the potency preservation rates. Actuarial statistics, which account for the length of time patients have been followed since treatment, give a lower, more realistic estimate of the potency rate. Surprisingly, nearly all published series have used crude rates that do not account for variable follow-up times (**Table 17-1**).

EFFECT OF ADJUNCTIVE ANTI-ANDROGEN THERAPY

Adjunctive anti-androgen therapy may increase the risk of permanent potency loss. Although this has not been well documented to date, it is a clinical

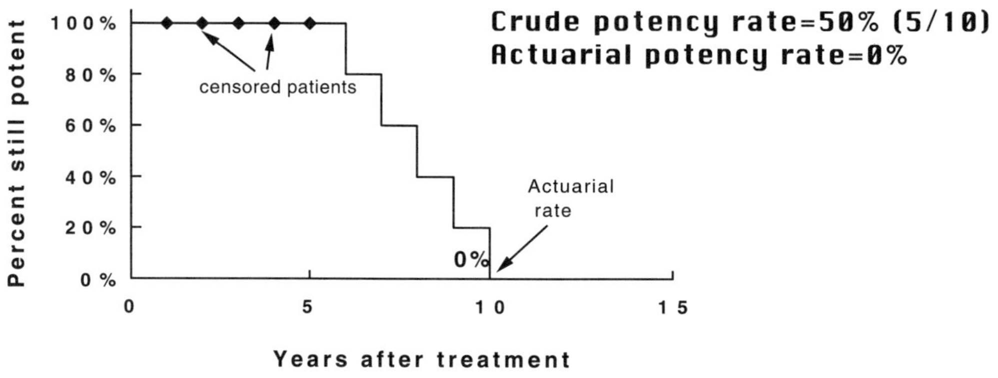

Figure 17-4. Example of crude versus actuarial potency rate. Assume that one patient is treated per year from 1985 through 1995. The first five patients become impotent in 1995, the year that the potency rate is reported. Actuarial calculation gives a potency rate of 0% at ten years, while the crude rate is five of ten, or 50%. Use of crude statistics for a time-related phenomenon like potency can be very misleading.

observation that has been repeatedly made.

EXTERNAL BEAM RADIATION (EBRT)

Despite the huge number of patients treated with EBRT over the last 30 years, there are amazingly few reports regarding potency preservation following EBRT. The lack of published reports should make one suspicious that potency preservation rates are quite low.

The largest series regarding the effect of EBRT on potency was from Stanford University Medical Center, based on a questionnaire mailed to patients.(Bagshaw 1988) Most notable in the series by Bagshaw and colleagues is the loss of potency with time. Potency was preserved in 86% of patients at 15 months after treatment, and in 50% at five years. The loss of potency decelerated at 30% approximately 10 years after treatment.

Drs. Bagshaw, Cox and Ray should be congratulated on their early interest and statistical prowess, but their results should be interpreted cautiously because they are based on an anonymous survey of a small percentage of the patients treated, and there is no mention of how potency was defined.

The relationship between potency loss and radiation volume, patient age, field size or radiation dose has not been rigorously examined. Greater potency loss

Table 17-1. Use of crude versus actuarial statistics in selected series published in mainstream medical journals. Surprisingly, most published reports use crude calculations, making the potency rates appear far higher than would be with actuarial calculations.

	NON-ACTUARIAL			***ACTUARIAL***		
	Author	*Hospital*	*Year*	*Author*	*Hospital*	*Year*
EBRT	Chinn	UCSF	1996	Bagshaw	Stanford	1988
	Banker	Sacramento	1988	Mantz`	U Chicago	1997
	Shipley	MGH	1988			
	vanHeeringen		1988			
Brachy	Fowler	MSKCC	1979	Wallner	MSKCC	1996
	Delaney	MGH	1986	Stock	Mt.Sinai,NY	1996
Surgery	Catalona	Wash U	1993			
	Quinlan	JHU	1991			
	Geary	Stanford	1995			

may occur in older patients, and as a result of larger field sizes and higher doses.

SURGERY -- THE HYPE

In the early 1980s, Walsh and colleagues reported that potency could often be preserved after radical prostatectomy if the pelvic splanchnic nerves were identified and preserved.(Walsh 1982) In the most favorable report, by Dr. Walsh at Johns Hopkins University (JHU), maintenance of potency was achieved in approximately 60% of patients, with markedly better results in younger patients. Patients younger than 60 had a 68% likelihood of maintaining potency, while patients older than 60 had a 55% likelihood.(Quinlan 1991)

The results reported by Dr. Walsh should be viewed cautiously. They have not been widely reproduced by other surgeons, and the data was not verified by an independent observer.

Like most EBRT series, no surgical series has included actuarial calculations, which would probably substantially decrease the stated rates of potency preservation.

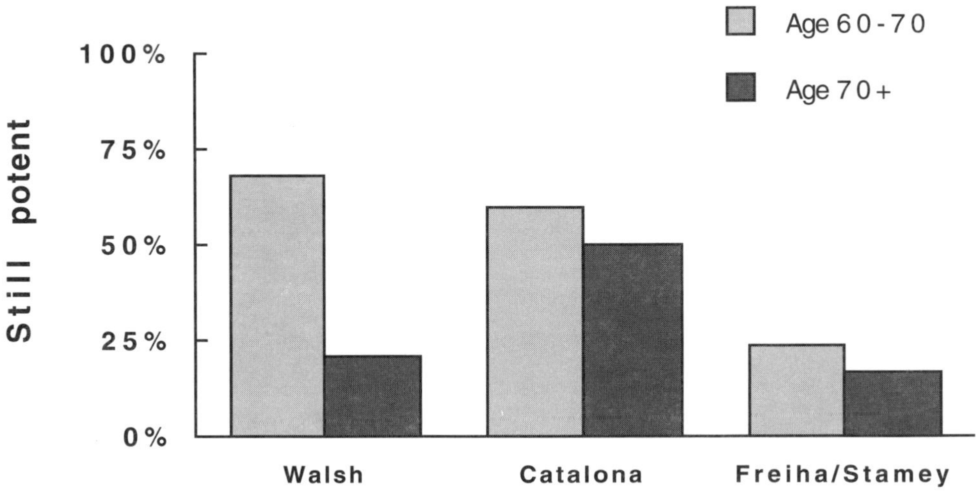

Figure 17-5. There is a large, perplexing variation in reported potency preservation rates following nerve-sparing prostatectomy by Drs. Walsh, Catalona, Stamey.

Adding to the doubt about the generalizability of the JHU potency preservation rates are reports by other respected surgeons, which show patients experiencing a much lower likelihood of preserving useful sexual function (**Figure 17-5**).(Geary 1995) Only a tiny percentage of academic urologists have ever published their own results, leaving one to wonder just how reproducible the results really are.

BRACHYTHERAPY

There is a variety of subtle and not-so-subtle changes in sexual function following brachytherapy, most of which have not been described, let alone well documented. But to avoid unpleasant surprises, patients should be told of them beforehand. (The same goes for nerve-sparing prostatectomy and EBRT patients.)

Acute reactions

Patients commonly have temporary burning with orgasm, probably related to inflammation of the terminal portion of the ejaculatory ducts or the urethra (**Figure 17-6**). This reaction may necessitate abstinence for several months. In a retrospective survey of patients implanted at Memorial Sloan-Kettering Cancer Center (MSKCC), approximately half of the patients reported some painful ejaculation afterwards. Temporary painful ejaculation is also seen occasionally with

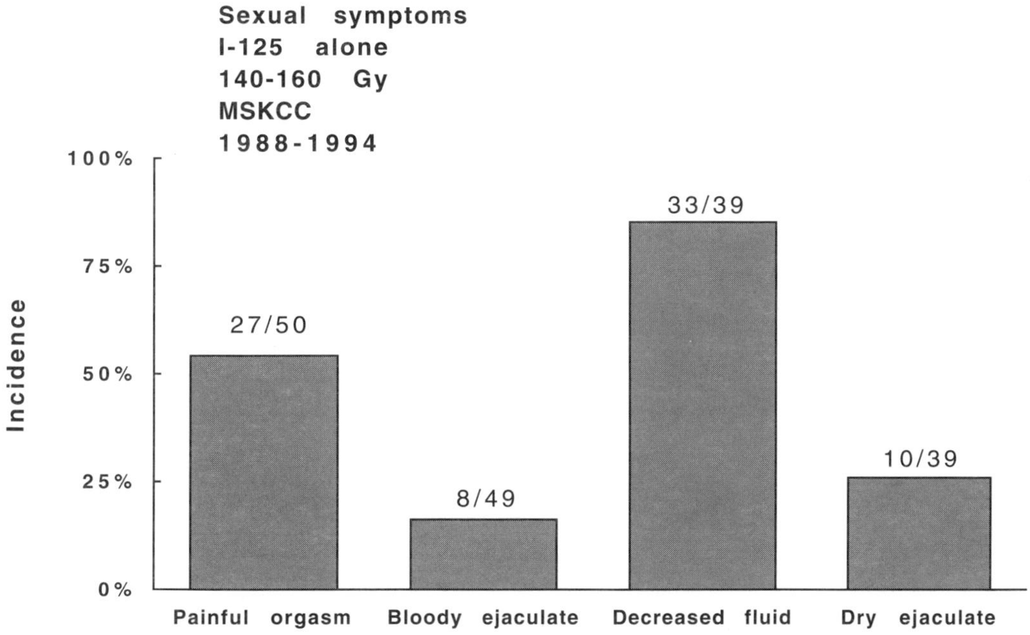

Figure 17-6. Incidence of painful ejaculation, bloody seminal fluid, or dry ejaculate in patients treated with I-125 implant at MSKCC.

EBRT, but it is probably less common and less intense than following brachytherapy.

Patients who experience painful ejaculation might take an anti-inflammatory agent prior to intercourse, though it is not clear that this helps. Fortunately, the discomfort resolves spontaneously, usually within several months.

Bloody ejaculate is very common in the first several weeks after implantation, without apparent significance.

Changes in ejaculate

Patients commonly report that the amount of ejaculate fluid diminishes in the months or years following brachytherapy (**Figure 17-6**). Dry ejaculate occurs in approximately one-fourth of brachytherapy patients.

Some patients develop intermittently bloody semen, usually several years after implantation. Hematospermia seems to be of little significance. It is probably due to radiation-induced capillary fragility. It is not routinely investigated, and no ill effects have been reported.

Erectile function

Potency following brachytherapy has not been studied through rigorous, impartial patient interviews. Most reported series have summarized the experiences of patients treated with the retropubic approach. Potency rates following

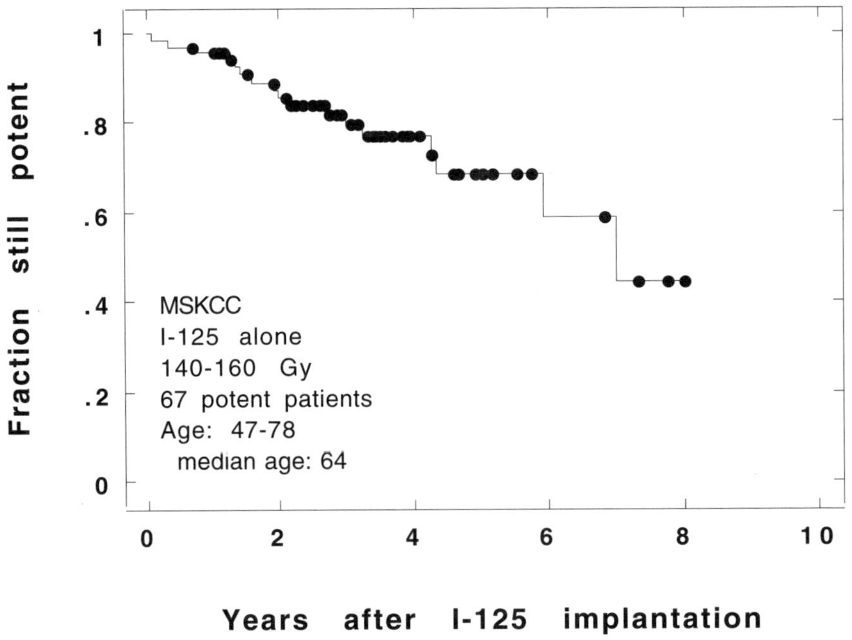

Figure 17-7. Potency preservation following I-125 implantation at MSKCC (based on the potency definition of ability to have an erection, sufficient for intercourse). Data was collected from personal interviews by K. Wallner. This graph shows the worst case scenario, in that patients who voiced concern about the quality of their erections or erectile time were considered impotent, even if they were able to achieve vaginal penetration. The data would look better with less strict interpretation of the patients' potency perception.

retropubic implantation were approximately 80%.(Delaney 1986)(Fowler 1979)(Reddy1990)

At MSKCC, the actuarial potency rate at five years following I-125 implantation in fully potent patients was 64% (**Figure 17-7**). The potency rates continued to fall over time, but only a small percentage of patients have been followed beyond five years. Younger patients may do somewhat better. Men less than 60 have had a low likelihood of permanent impotence, at least in the early post-implant years. But more developed trouble with longer follow-up (**Figure 17-8**).

POTENCY AFTER IMPLANT AND SUPPLEMENTAL EBRT

EBRT has generally been reported to lead to higher impotence rates than brachytherapy. Therefore, the potency rate following brachytherapy plus supplemental EBRT might be expected to be lower than that following brachytherapy alone. To date, there is very limited data regarding potency rates after implant and supplemental EBRT. Among 56 potent patients treated with combined Pd-103 and supplemental EBRT (41 Gy) at University Community Hospital, Tampa, the actuarial potency preservation at four years was approximately 70%. The rate was

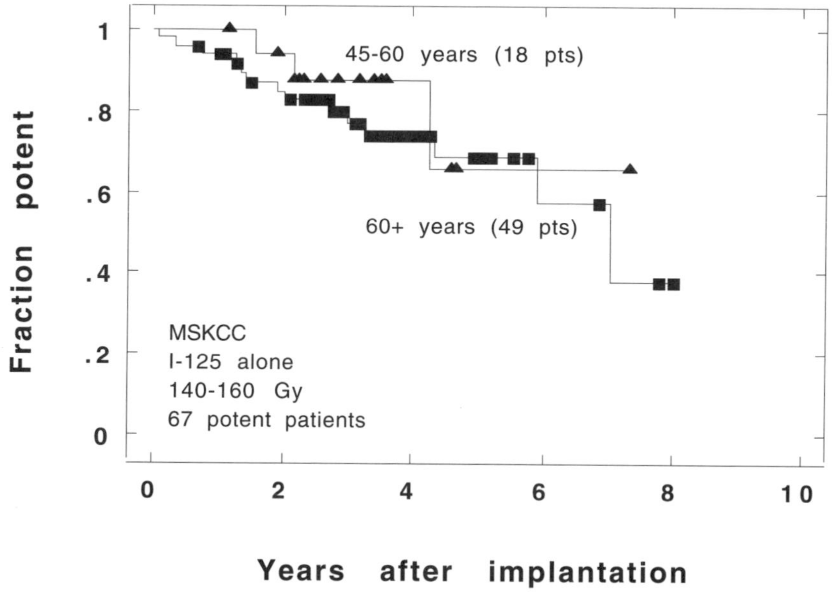

Figure 17-8. Potency preservation following I-125 implantation at MSKCC, in patients older or younger than age 60.

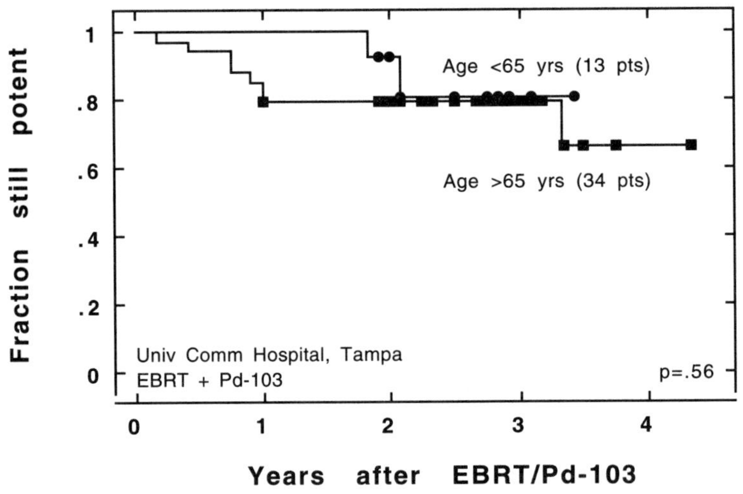

17-9. Potency preservation following Pd-103 plus supplemental EBRT at University Community Hospital, Tampa.

not clearly related to age, with those patients older or younger than age 65 achieving similar results (**Figure 17-9**).

COMPARING MODALITIES

In general, the reported potency rates following brachytherapy have been higher than those following prostatectomy or EBRT. Even in the best of surgical hands, post-surgical potency preservation is somewhat lower than that for brachytherapy (**Figure 17-10**).(Quinlan 1991)(Catalona 1993) Conclusions regarding potency preservation rates between modalities should be made with caution and qualification, considering the dearth of good quality data for any modality.

The potency rates with brachytherapy versus EBRT or prostatectomy need to be confirmed by a larger number of patients, and reviewed by independent observers. However, considering the consistency in multiple reports over many years, the potency advantage of brachytherapy is probably real.

TREATMENT OF BRACHYTHERAPY-RELATED IMPOTENCE

Although reports on the matter are limited, patients who develop radiation-related impotence generally respond to corrective measures. Treatment with vasoactive agents after EBRT is usually successful.(Pierce 1991) Five of five patients who used papaverine or prostaglandin injections after developing impotence following I-125 brachytherapy at MSKCC between 1988 and 1995 reported

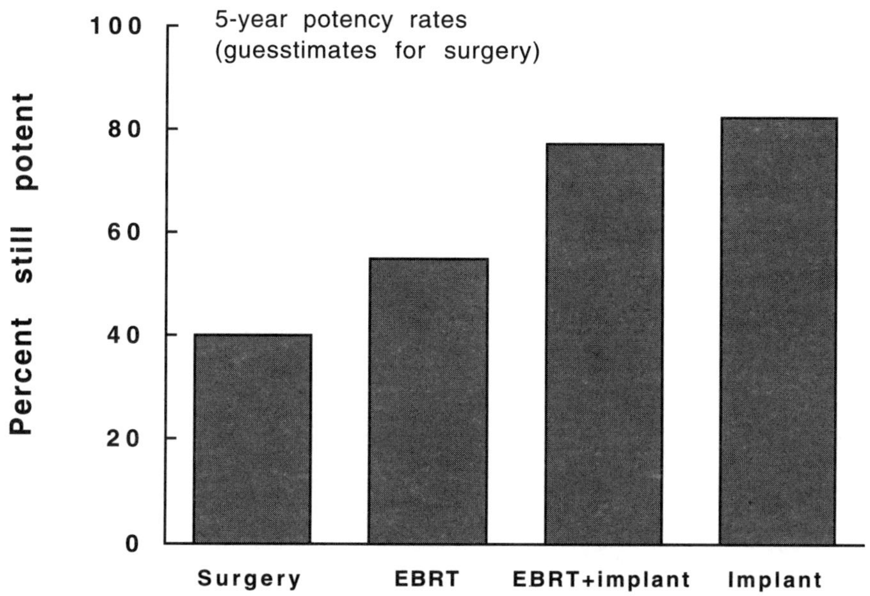

Figure 17-10. Five-year potency rates after surgery versus EBRT versus brachytherapy. The surgical rates are guesses, because longer-term follow-up has never been reported.

good results. However, enthusiasm for corrective measures should be tempered by reports of high attrition rates.(Flynn 1996)

FERTILITY

There is no published data regarding fertility after prostate brachytherapy. Probably patients are infertile afterwards, due to changes in the semen. It would be prudent to warn patients not to father children during or after treatment. Patients who desire to father children in the future should bank sperm before treatment.

WHAT CAN WE BELIEVE?

The precise effects different treatment modalities have on potency is still unclear and should be rigorously investigated by independent analysts/interviewers. In the meantime, judging from the agreement between disparate sources to date, brachytherapy probably offers some advantage in potency preservation. Just how great the advantage is is still unclear.

REFERENCES

1. Bagshaw MA, Cox RS, Ray GR. Status of Radiation of Prostate Cancer at Stanford University. NCI Monogr 1988; 7:47-60.

2. Banker RL. The preservation of potency after external beam irradiation for prostate cancer. Int J Radiat Oncol Biol Phys 1988; 15:219-220.

3. Catalona WJ, Basler JW. Return of erections and urinary continence following nerve sparing radical retropubic prostatectomy. J Urol 1993; 150:905-907.

4. Chinn DM, Holland J, Crownover RL, Roach M. Potency following high-dose three-dimensional conformal radiotherapy and the impact of prior major urologic surgical procedures in patients treated for prostate cancer. Int J Radiat Oncol Biol Phys 1995; 33:15-22.

5. DeLaney TF, Shipley WU, O'Leary MP, Biggs PJ, Prout GR. Preoperative Irradiation and 125-Iodine Implantation for Patients with Localized Carcinoma of the Prostate. Int J Radiat Oncol Biol Phys 1986; 12:1779-1785.

6. Feldman HA, Goldstein I, Hatzichristou DG, et.al. . Impotence and its medical and psychosocial correlates: Results of the Massachusetts Male Aging Study. J Urol 1994; 151:54-61.

7. Flynn RJ, Williams G. Long-term follow-up of patients with erectile dysfunction commenced on self injection with intracavernosal papaverine with or without phentolamine. Br J Urol 1996; 78:628-631.

8. Fowler FJ, Roman A, Barry MJ, Wasson J, Lu-Yao G, Wennberg JE. Patient-reported complications and follow-up treatment after radical prostatectomy. Urol 1993; 42:622-629.

9. Fowler JE, Barzell W, Hilaris BS, Whitmore WF. Complications fo 125-Iodine Implantation and Pelvic Lymphadenectomy in the Treatment of Prostatic Cancer. J Urol 1979; 121:447-451.

10. Geary ES, Dendinger TE, Freiha FS, Stamey TA. Nerve sparing radical

prostatectomy: A different view. J Urol 1995; 154:145-149.

11. Goldstein I, Feldman MI, Deckers PJ, et.al. Radiation-associated impotence: A clinical study of its mechanism. JAMA 1984; 251:903-910.

12. Mantz CA, Song P, Farhangi E, et.al. . Potency probability following conformal megavoltage radiotherapy using conventional doses for localized prostate cancer. Int J Radiat Oncol Biol Phys 1997; 37:551-557.

13. Pierce LJ, Whittington R, Hanno PM, et.al. Pharmacologic erection with intracavernosal injection for men with sexual dysfunction following irradiation: A preliminary report. Int J Radiat Oncol Biol Phys 1991; 21:1311-1314.

14. Quinlan DM, Epstein JI, Carter BS, Walsh PC. Sexual Function Following Radical Prostatectomy: Influence of Preservation of Neurovascular Bundles. J Urol 1991; 145:998-1002.

15. Reddy EK, Mebust WK, Weigel JW, Krishnan L. Iodine-125 Implantation in Localized Prostatic Cancer. Endo/Hypertherm Oncol 1990; 6:239-244.

16. Stock RG, Stone NN, Iannuzzi C. Sexual potency following interactive ultrasound-guided brachytherapy for prostate cancer. Int J Radiat Oncol Biol Phys 1996; 35:267-272.

17. van Heeringen C, De Schryver A, Verbeek E. Sexual function disorders after local radiotherapy for carcinoma of the prostate. Radiother Oncol 1988; 13:47-52.

18. Wallner KE, Roy J, Harrison L. Tumor control and morbidity following transperineal I-125 implantation for Stage T1/T2 prostatic carcinoma. J Clin Oncol 1996; 14:449-453.

19. Walsh PC, Donker PJ. Impotence following radical prostatectomy: Insight into etiology and prevention. J Urol 1982; 128:492-497.

20. Zinreich ES, Derogatis LR, Herpst J, Auvil G, Piantadosi S, Order SE. Pre and posttreatment evaluation of sexual function in patients with adenocarcinoma of the prostate. Int J Radiat Biol Phys 1990; 19:729-732.

Chapter 18

Cost

The cost of treating prostate cancer is high. Of approximately 250,000 new cases diagnosed in the United States in 1997, 70% will be clinically localized to the prostate. If all patients with localized disease are treated with potentially curative therapy, at an average cost of $12,000, the cost of primary treatment alone would be $2.1 billion per year (**Table 18-1**). The cost to treat all patients with early stage disease would be approximately 1% of the yearly budget for Medicare (**Figure 18-1**). The cost of palliative care for patients with more advanced cancers would probably be higher. Because of the staggering potential cost to society, physicians increasingly may be compelled to justify the price of treatment.

Table 18-1. Approximate annual cost of potentially curative treatment for clinically localized prostate cancer in the United States (1997).

New cases:	250,000
Clinically localized (70%):	170,000
Average cost/case:	$12,000
Total cost to treat all patients:	$2,100,000,000

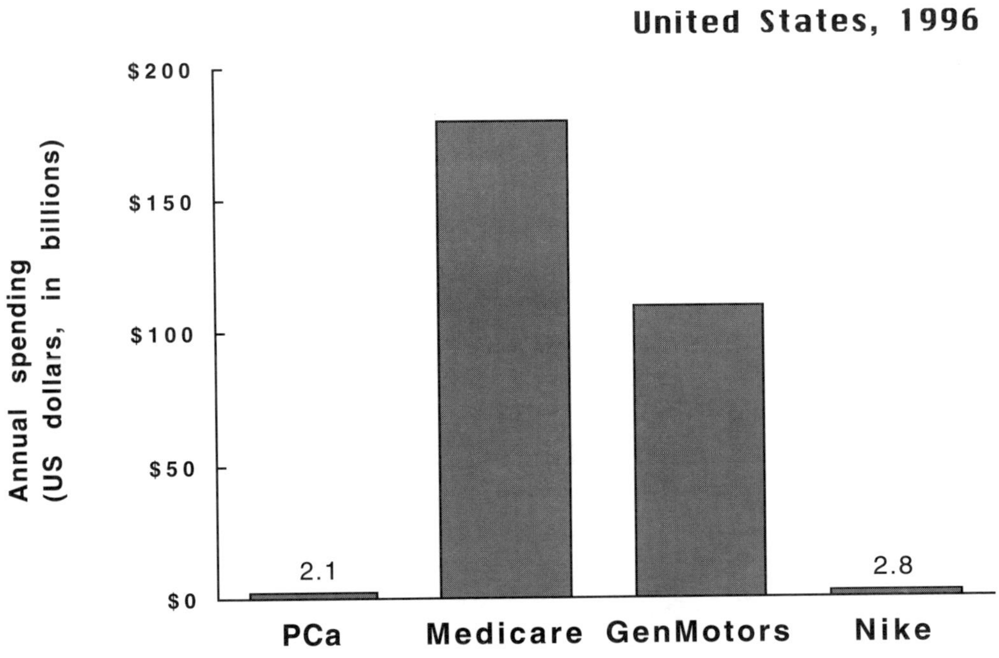

Figure 18-1. Approximate cost to provide primary, curative treatment to all patients with clinically localized prostate cancer (PCa) compared with the yearly Medicare budget, the total purchase price of General Motors cars and trucks (U.S. only, 1996), or the 1996 spending on Nike footwear (U.S. only).

PRICES -- A MOVING TARGET

The price of medical care is changing in the United States, as managed care continues to penetrate the market. Managed care probably will continue to drive down the charges for prostate cancer treatment. The figures quoted here are approximations of what is currently charged throughout the United States. Very few references for the data are quoted. Price information, especially in fee-for-service institutions, has become a sensitive issue and therefore we are not always free to reveal our sources. While the absolute numbers will continue to change, the relative prices between the various modalities will probably not change much.

TERMINOLOGY

The terminology for cost analysis is confusing. There are substantial differences between terms that are sometimes used interchangeably. *Cost* refers to the price providers pay to supply the service. Cost includes time and dollars. Unfortunately, good quality information regarding the time and dollars needed to provide therapy is sparse. *Charges* are the dollar amounts billed to the patient.

Payments are what the provider actually receives from the patient or the patient's health plan. There can be a substantial difference between charges and payments, because third party payers may be able to discount the price they pay, regardless of the amount incurred by or charged by the provider.

WHO PAYS THE BILLS?

Analysis of medical costs is complicated by the plethora of payer types within U.S. health care. There are four general categories of payers in the U.S. health market: individuals, government programs (Medicare and Medicaid), private fee-for-service (the "Blues" and other indemnity plans) and managed care (HMOs, PPOs, etc.) (**Table 18-2**). Medicare rates have a disproportionate effect on other pricing systems because they are used for guidance by non-governmental parties when setting the price of medical care. The percent of patients in various

Table 18-2. Who pays the bills?

Type of payer	Source of money	Primary price setter
Medicare	Federal tax	Health Care Financing Admin (HCFA)
Medicaid	Federal/state tax	HCFA/state agencies
Managed care	Employer/individual	Market
Fee-for-service	Employer/individual	Physician/hospital

payer categories has changed substantially, and the movement towards managed care probably will continue into the next century.

By definition, the price of a commodity is the market-based agreement between what the consumer is willing to pay and the provider is willing to accept. In a free market system, price should be arrived at efficiently. In contrast, the price of medical care is influenced by third party payers (government, insurers, employers), who stand between the physician (provider) and the patient. Because they represent large numbers of patients, third party payers have a remarkable influence on the market-derived price.

Of the four payer types, fee-for-service plans generally offer the highest reimbursements to providers, presumably covering the costs for patients to have their free choice of doctors and to be treated in the more prestigious institutions (perhaps) by the more prestigious doctors (perhaps). The cost of fee-for-service plans is inflated by cost-shifting, whereby fee-for-service patients are charged more because they are not organized to negotiate lower prices. Fee-for-service patients cannot negotiate down their costs, and are legally responsible for the amount billed by the hospital and physician. There have been sporadic attempts to control fee-for-service charges through government-mandated price controls,

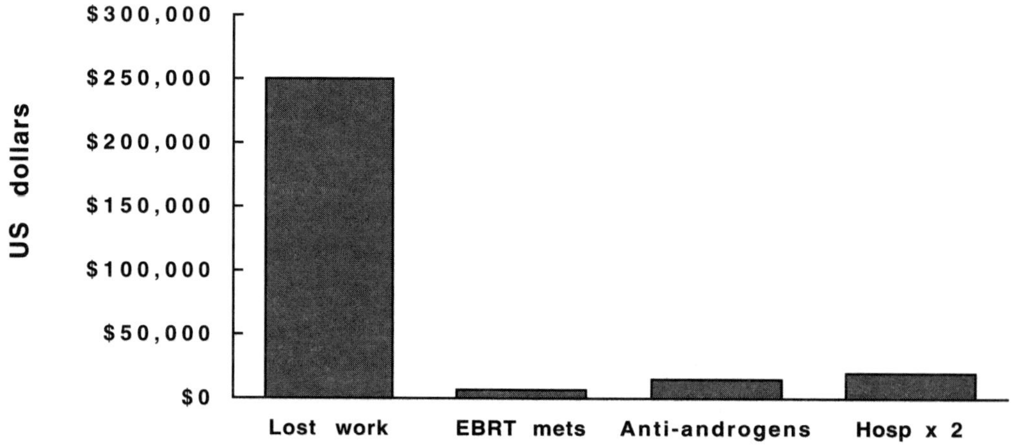

Figure 18-2. Conservative estimate of prostate cancer recurrence costs in patient who is gainfully employed, earning $50,000 per year and disabled by metastatic disease. This estimate assumes that five years of work are lost. These numbers will vary greatly, depending on an individual patient's cancer growth rate and disease progression sites.

but such efforts have consistently failed. Cost-shifting will continue to some extent, as long as there is some element of fee-for-service in the U.S. health system. As the percent of patients enrolled in managed care climbs, cost-shifting will become an increasingly impractical way for physicians and hospitals to boost their income.

THE COST OF FAILURE

Cancer recurrence is phenomenally expensive, dwarfing the cost of any initial treatment. Patients who are not cured may require palliative therapy and may have substantial loss of work time and income. A typical patient with recurrent metastatic disease might lose five years of productive work time, valued at $250,000. He would typically receive at least two years of androgen ablation at an approximate total cost of $15,000. At the more advanced stage of metastatic disease, he might be hospitalized twice for pain control ($20,000). Two courses of palliative irradiation would total $8,000. These costs do not include extra imaging studies or other palliative therapies commonly used. A conservative estimate of the additional cost for recurrence in this case would be $291,000. This dwarfs the initial treatment costs of $32,000 that might be charged for combined implant plus supplemental EBRT on a fee-for-service basis (**Figure 18-2**).

The actual cost of cancer recurrence can vary from almost nothing (if nothing is done about the recurrence) to many times the $286,000 estimated in Figure 18-8, depending on whether salvage therapy is used and how much palliative care is required. For younger patients especially, the cost of lost wages could be far higher.

COMPARING MODALITIES

There has been surprisingly little written about the cost of prostate cancer treatment. Several authors have compared EBRT and prostatectomy, showing that EBRT generally costs 60 to 70% of the cost of surgery.(Hanks 1986)(Cotter 1990) However, cost comparisons between surgery and non-surgical options have generally been muted, perhaps because of persistent doubts as to the efficacy of non-surgical treatments.

One of the few comparisons between modalities was reported by Hanks and Dunlap, from Sutter Community Hospital in Sacramento.(Hanks 1986) Based on hospital charges, the cost of retropubic I-125 implantation was comparable to that for prostatectomy. Both surgery and brachytherapy were nearly twice the cost of EBRT (**Figure 18-3**). In the Sacramento study, however, the cost of brachytherapy included the cost of an open laparotomy, which was then required for retropubic implants. Without the laparotomy, the cost of brachytherapy would have been 30% less.

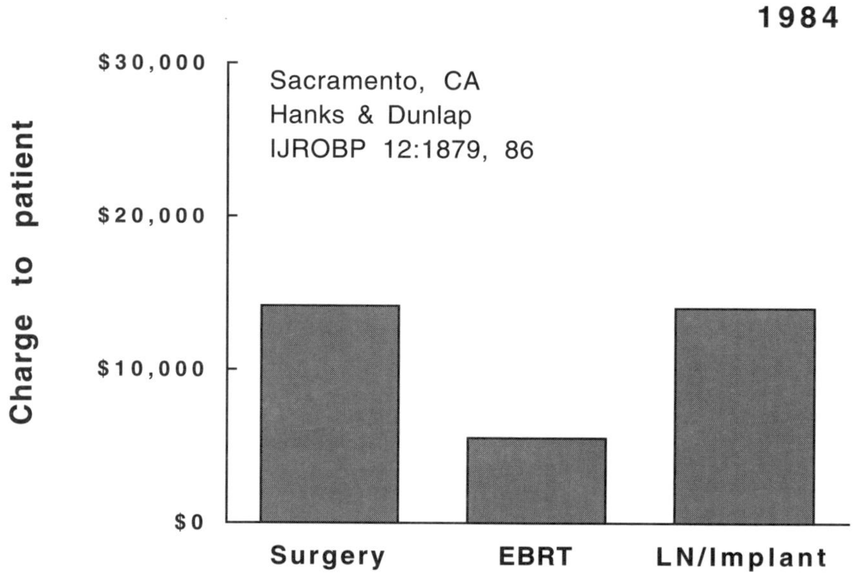

Figure 18-3. Charges for prostatectomy , EBRT or pelvic lymph node (LN) dissection/retropubic I-125 implant in Sacramento, California, 1984.

Currently, outpatient transperineal implants hold a substantial cost advantage over prostatectomy, largely because implants are performed on an outpatient basis and don't require an open surgical procedure. Implants have a cost advantage over EBRT, due to lower technical charges, including the linear accelerator use, simulation, and beam films charges that are part of EBRT (**Figure 18-4**).

PROSTATECTOMY

Surgery is an expensive therapy. Based on 1997 Medicare reimbursements, the total cost per patient is approximately \$14,000, 80% of which represents hospital charges and 20% physician fees (**Figure 18-5**).

Since most of the surgical costs represent hospital charges, substantial savings can be achieved through early abdominal drain removal, early ambulation and oral feeding, early hospital discharge, and more judicious use of laboratory tests. These goals can be achieved through aggressive pre-operative patient education and by continuous monitoring by a dedicated cost control team. With a concerted effort, substantial savings have been achieved. University of Chicago surgeons were able to decrease the average hospitalization from five days to two days, with total treatment cost cut by 34%.[Palmer 1996] Such cost savings require constant vigilance to maintain. They are being instituted widely in response to mar-

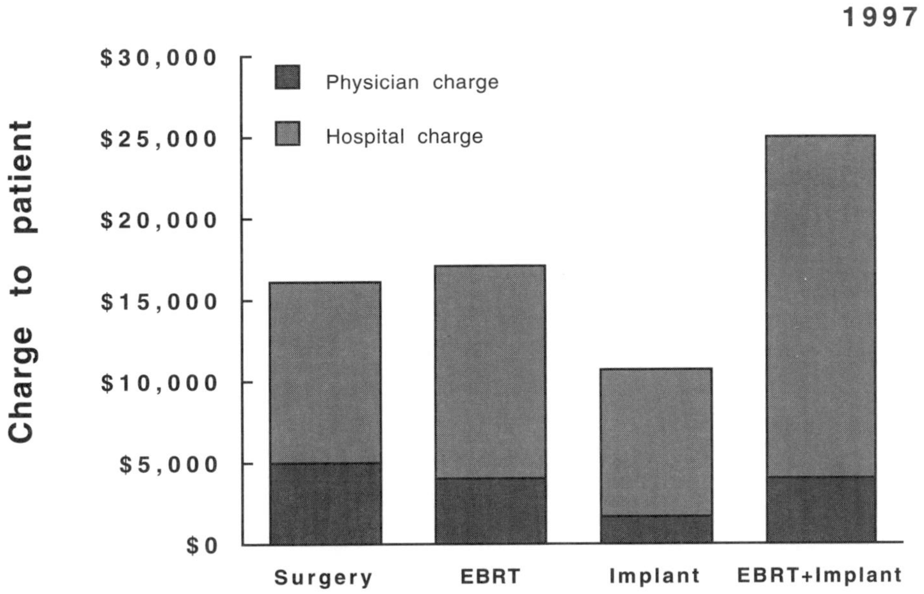

Figure 18-4. Approximate physician and hospital charges for prostatectomy, EBRT, outpatient transperineal implant and implant plus EBRT.

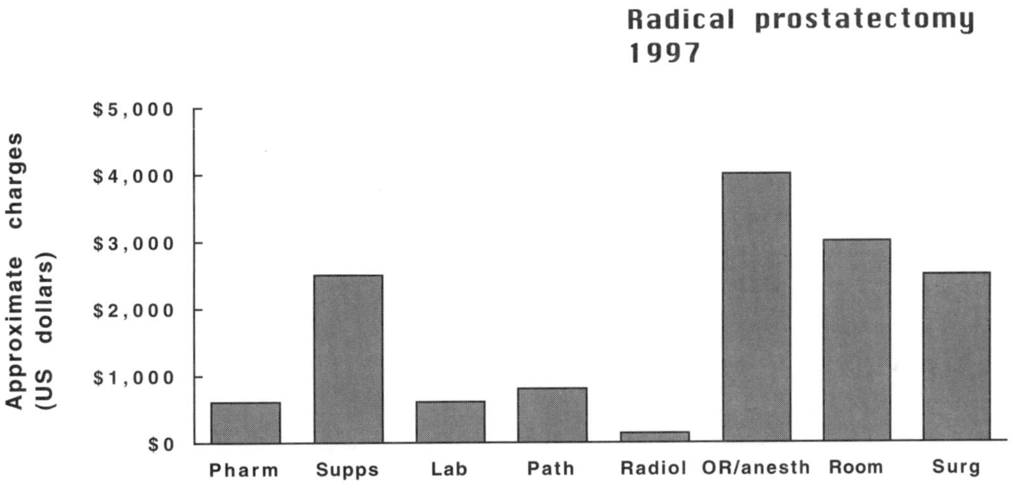

Figure 18-5. Breakdown of charges for radical prostatectomy.

ketplace pressures.

An important point to note is that if surgery offers the highest cure rate, ultimately it may be the most cost-effective treatment, because the cost of cancer recurrence can be so great (**Figure 18-2**).

EBRT

Based on current Medicare reimbursement, the per patient cost of EBRT (70 to 75 Gy) is approximately $14,000, 80% of which is comprised of hospital charges and 20% of physician fees (**Figure 18-6**).

Past analyses have determined the cost of EBRT to be lower than that of prostatectomy.(Hanks 1986)(Cotter 1990) However, the cost of providing EBRT has risen with increasingly sophisticated treatment plans and delivery systems, such as conformal EBRT, which costs between $15,000 and $32,000 per patient. Managed care plans currently may not reimburse at this charge level, but if outcome data shows that better technical delivery and higher doses increase cure rates while decreasing complications, there will be upward price pressure, because patients increasingly will insist on receiving more sophisticated therapy.

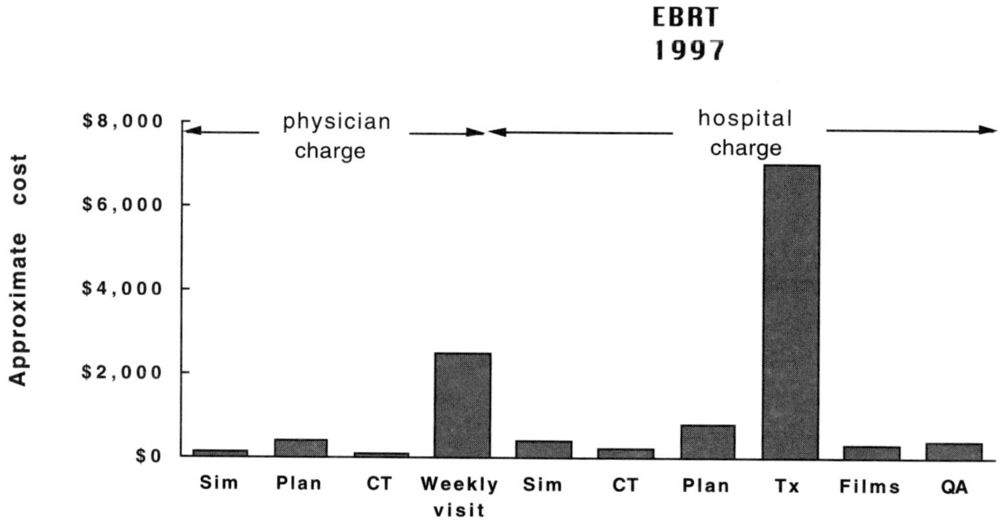

Figure 18-6. Component costs for EBRT. (Sim=simulation, Tx=daily treatment, QA=quality assurance checks)

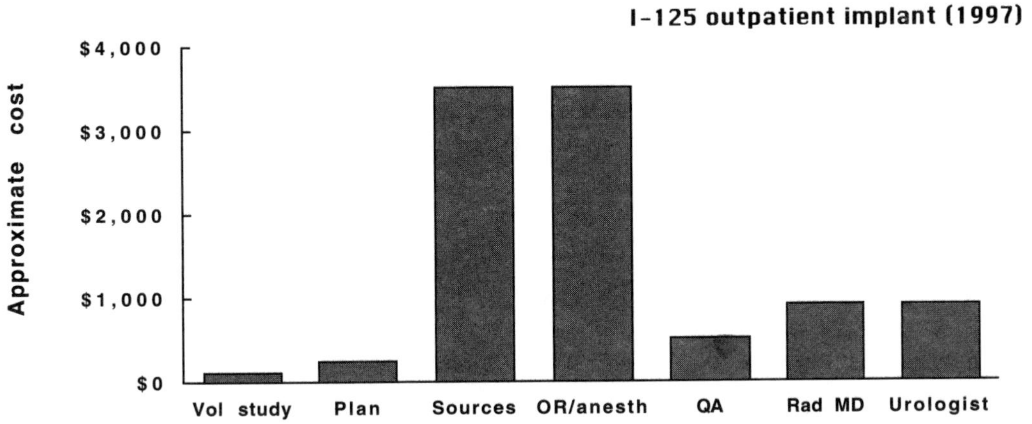

Figure 18-7. Component costs for implant alone. (Vol study=ultrasound volume study, OR/anesth=operating room and anesthesia costs, QA=post-implant CT-based dosimetric evaluation, Rad MD=physician fee for radiation oncologist)

IMPLANT ALONE

Based on 1996 Medicare reimbursement rates, the per patient cost of a permanent prostate radioactive implant is approximately $12,000, 80% of which represents hospital charges and 20% physician charges (**Figure 18-7**). This price assumes that the implant is performed jointly by a radiation oncologist and a urologist as an outpatient procedure.

The cost of the sources themselves is a substantial portion of the bill. The typical cost to the provider for I-125 is $3,000 per patient and for Pd-103 about $4,000 per patient. Hospitals may mark up the price, bringing the patient's cost to $6,000 or more. With substantial mark-up of the source price, the cost of an implant approaches that of non-conformal EBRT or prostatectomy.

IMPLANT PLUS EBRT

Implant alone is a relatively inexpensive treatment. However, when brachytherapy and supplemental EBRT are used, the cost increases substantially. The cost of the supplemental EBRT (40 to 50 Gy) is only slightly less than a full EBRT course, since a simulation is still needed and the number of treatments is decreased by only 30%. The implant cost is decreased from that of a full dose implant only by the use of 30% fewer sources than would be used for a full dose

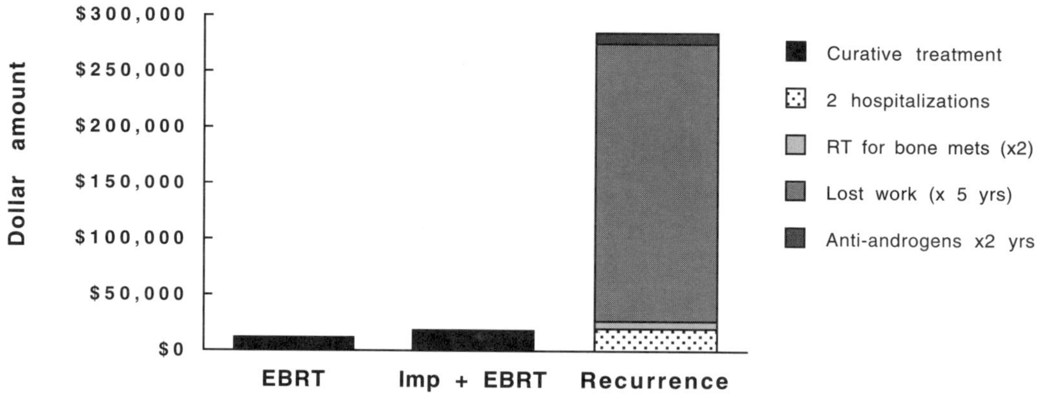

Figure 18-8. Cost of EBRT alone, implant plus EBRT and typical cost to treat a patient who develops metastatic disease. For patients who would otherwise become disabled from metastatic disease, the cost of curative therapy is a bargain.

implant. Based on current Medicare reimbursement, the per patient cost of implant plus supplemental EBRT (45 Gy) is approximately $22,000, almost twice that of an implant alone and 50% greater than EBRT.

In the long run, the only way that combined implant plus EBRT therapy will be reimbursed widely will be if early, promising results hold up with longer follow-up. If they do, the increased cost of combined treatment will be offset by savings in the steep price of cancer recurrence (**Figure 18-8**).

REDUCING THE COST OF IMPLANTATION

Several commonly used procedures of questionable benefit add to the cost of prostate brachytherapy. These procedures are not uniformly followed by all physicians, and those who do not use them do not appear to create a higher likelihood of complications or a lower cure rate. In the absence of data to support the use of such procedures, it seems prudent to discontinue them, both to save resources and to prevent complications, which can accompany any medical treatment (**Table 18-3**).

Hospitalization

Hospitalization is the single most expensive, unnecessary item that adds to the cost of implantation. A patient typically is charged $600 to $1,000 for an overnight hospitalization. Some physicians and patients would prefer overnight hospitalization because of the 10% possibility of urinary retention or the remote possibility of post-implant bleeding. However, urinary retention is not an emergency, and can be managed on an outpatient basis. And significant post-implant bleeding is rare; it has never been reported in the literature and is not a reason for hospitalization.

Occasionally, patients require hospitalization following implantation. Probably the most common are those with significant cardiac problems who need to be closely observed post-implantation. Patients with serious general health problems would generally not be advised to have curative treatment of early stage prostatic carcinoma, so that the number of people who need to be observed overnight should be quite small.

Antibiotics

Prophylactic antibiotics are nearly universally given. While this policy may seem prudent, there are little or no data to support it (see Chapter 7). The only retrospective studies that examined routine prophylactic antibiotics showed no benefit to their use. Avoiding the routine use of antibiotics could save $20 to $200 per patient, depending on the drugs used.

Post-implant cystoscopy

Post-implant cystoscopy is commonly performed to remove sources left in the bladder or protruding into the urethra, or to remove blood clots in the bladder. While post-implant cystoscopy seems reasonable, there are no data to support it as a routine procedure.

Under K. Wallner's direction at Memorial Sloan-Kettering Cancer Center (MSKCC), routine cystoscopy was never performed, without apparent detriment. If sources within the bladder are seen on post-implant films, the patient is instructed to strain his urine for one week, or until the source passes. The same policy is followed at the University of Washington. It is unusual to have sources in the bladder when the implant is performed by an experienced team.

Because the post-implant cystoscopy charge recently has been bundled into the Medicare code for urologists, reimbursement has become less of an issue. Nevertheless, ending the practice of post-implant cystoscopy would save time and money.

Post-implant complete blood count (CBC)

A routine post-implant CBC ($15) is unnecessary. Without an obvious bleeding episode at the time of implantation or in the post-operative period, the likelihood of hemodynamically significant internal bleeding is negligible.

Table 18-3. Unnecessary procedures that could be omitted to contain costs.

Item	Cost to hospital	Cost to patient
Inpatient stay (1day)	200$	800$
Antibiotics	50	100
Post-implant cysto	10	100
Suprapubic catheter	10	250
Post-implant CBC	2	15
Sterile drapes	6	12
Sterile gowns	5	10

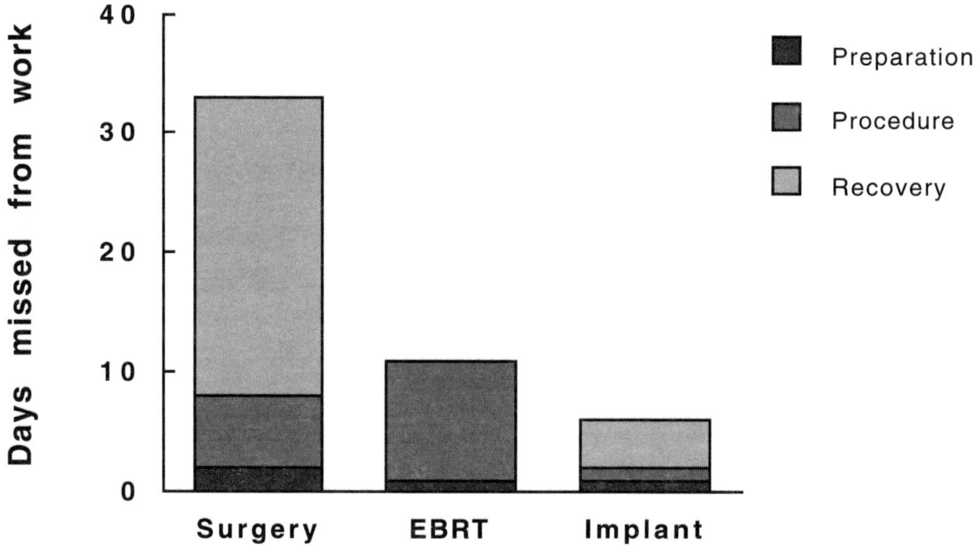

Figure 18-9. Work days missed with each modality. Numbers are estimations and could vary substantially, based on patient circumstances and physician policy regarding post-operative care.

Sterile supplies

Sterile drapes and gowns are commonly used for the implant procedure. The use of sterile drapes has never been proven to decrease the risk of infection in any type of surgery, and may actually make infection more likely in some circumstances (see Chapter 7).

Under the direction of K. Wallner at MSKCC, sterile drapes or gowns were not used routinely, with no evidence of a higher infection rate than expected.[Wallner 1996] Similarly, sterile barriers are not used at the University of Washington.

TIME OFF FROM WORK

Perhaps the largest cost of treatment is the effect on a patient's lifestyle. A full accounting of lifestyle cost has not been attempted for any treatment modality and is beyond the scope of this text. However, a relatively easily estimated factor is the time lost from work. On that basis, work time lost as a result of implantation compares favorably with EBRT or prostatectomy (**Figure 18-9**).

Work-time missed because of an implant includes the time for office visits for treatment planning volume study as well as pre-anesthesia testing. The implant itself, performed on an outpatient basis, would be one day off work. The at-home recovery time typically would be one to three days.

Work-time missed because of a prostatectomy includes time spent donating autologous blood, estimated at one day. A hospital stay ranges from two to ten days, in the absence of serious complications. The recovery time at home is generally three to six weeks, although some of that time could be spent working at home, depending on the nature of one's occupation.

Work-time missed because of EBRT is the time needed for simulation and for daily treatments. If one assumes a half day would be missed for simulation and plan verification, and two hours missed for each of the 40 treatments, approximately 11 days in total would be missed.

FOLLOW-UP COSTS

Assuming there are no complications, the cost of routine follow-up should be the same, regardless of the treatment modality used. A reasonable follow-up schedule would be PSA measurements at 6 month intervals during the first three years, and annually thereafter. In the absence of a rising PSA, routine bone scans, CT scans or biopsies are not necessary. Even less frequent follow-up PSA measurements would be adequate. Twenty-four months are needed before deciding if the biochemical response is sufficient; measuring PSA before that time is of little value (see Chapter 14). Understandably, patients are anxious to follow their PSA levels during the two years after treatment, and generally want to know their PSA response much earlier. This is understandable, but not medically indicated. In

Table 18-4. Cost of intensive versus non-intensive follow-up for first year after implant.

	Intensive schedule		Non-intensive schedule	
	Times done	Charge to patient	Times done	Charge to patient
Office visits	4	400$	2	200$
Follow-up TRUS	1	200	0	0
PSA	4	200	2	100
Total:		**$800**		**$300**

fact, the PSA often fluctuates in the first one to two years after an implant, and one could argue that patients might experience less anxiety if they simply waited a year before determining their PSA values. Avoiding unnecessary, frequent PSA determinations could save several hundred dollars per patient over the course of several years (**Table 18-4**) and probably would save patients substantial anxiety.

The PSA level is by far the most sensitive and reliable indicator of disease activity. Other routine diagnostic tests (bone scans, repeat biopsies, digital rectal exam), in the absence of biochemical evidence of disease persistence or progression, are hard to justify. Repeat biopsies should be delayed until 24 months have passed (see Chapter 14).

COST OF COMPLICATIONS

All of the cost figures discussed earlier in this chapter assume no post-operative complications. The cost of complications could be significant. The occurrence of a rectal fistula requiring temporary colostomy and reversal, for instance, could ultimately cost $50,000 or more for one patient.

No attempt will be made to compare complications between modalities. Regardless of the modality, the incidence and cost of complications varies tremendously depending on the skill of the physicians, the patient's predisposition to complications, and how complications are handled. An accounting of complication costs is beyond the scope of this book.

FINANCIAL INCENTIVES TO PHYSICIAN

There may be a marked disparity in physician compensation with different treatment options, due to differences in charges, physician time required to perform each procedure, and in the amount of uncompensated follow-up care required. To date, very little data are available from any source regarding physician compensation for specific treatment modalities.

Assuming physician reimbursement of $2000, $2500 and $1000 for prostatectomy, EBRT and implant, respectively, and total time of seven hours, four hours and four hours, respectively, the total physician income would be highest with prostatectomy, and lowest with brachytherapy. However, the disparity is less when income is compared on an hourly basis (**Figure 18-10**). These reimbursement and time estimations could vary markedly from region to region and from one physician to another. Additionally, financial incentives for the institution are far more complex to estimate and could differ markedly from those for the physician.

The physician's financial incentives are affected by the form of health insurance that the patient carries. Patients in capitated systems presumably would be discouraged from prostatectomy because they could be treated more quickly and cheaply with some form of radiation. In the absence of more definitive data that surgery is more likely to be curative, the increased power of managed care in medicine will probably encourage more use of brachytherapy, at least in patients who can be treated with an implant alone. If a combination of implant and sup-

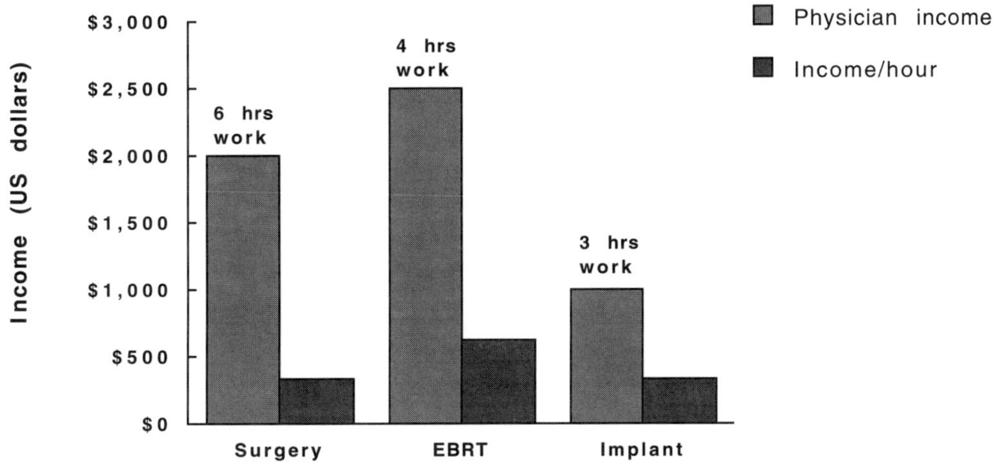

Figure 18-10. Approximate total and hourly physician income from each modality. Numbers are approximations, and will vary substantially, depending on geographic region and specific policies of the treating physician and institution.

plemental EBRT is preferable, cost comparison may favor surgery, unless definitive evidence of a superior cure rate with combined treatment emerges.

COST ISSUES ARE MURKY

Costs, incomes, and profits from complex medical procedures are difficult to define accurately. They vary by region and are constantly changing as the medical marketplace shifts increasingly toward managed care. The numbers given here are broad estimates. They are food for thought and highlight the substantial uncertainties in determining the most cost-effective treatment. Assuming that the cure rate with implant is equal to that for surgery or EBRT, implant alone (for appropriate candidates) is probably the most cost-effective therapy, but not necessarily the most lucrative for the physician or the hospital.

REFERENCES

1. Cotter GW. Surgery or radiation therapy: A comparative cost analysis for early carcinoma of the prostate and breast. App Radiol 1990; January:25-28.

2. Hanks GE, Dunlap K. A comparison of the cost of various treatment methods for early cancer of the prostate. Int J Radiat Oncol Biol Phys 1986; 12:1879-1881.

3. Palmer JS, Worwag EM, Conrad WG, et.al. Same day surgery for radical retropubic prostatectomy: Is it an attainable goal? Urol 1996; 47:23-28.

Chapter 19

The future

Prostate brachytherapy is in the midst of a phenomenal growth period. Its resurgence has met with substantial skepticism from both the surgical and radiation communities. However, as evidence confirming its comparable efficacy and relatively minor morbidity mounts, it is rapidly being embraced by both urologists and radiation oncologists. Almost unimaginable in the early 1990s, brachytherapy is rapidly replacing prostatectomy as the treatment of choice for younger, curable patients.

Early reports have been primarily by a few enthusiasts. Their early experiences, many of which are summarized in the preceding pages, have lead to widespread interest in brachytherapy within the oncology community. The primary emphases in the next five years will likely be on interpretation of longer follow-up, verification of the relatively low morbidity rates, and institution of standardized quality assurance.

LONGER FOLLOW-UP

The role of brachytherapy in prostate cancer treatment will ultimately be determined by its ability to eradicate cancer. If longer term reports show durable biochemical disease-free survival rates comparable to prostatectomy, large randomized trials comparing the modalities will not be needed. Brachytherapy will simply replace surgery as the treatment of choice because it has less adverse effects and is less costly.

The longer the follow-up, the more convincing the results are. Just how long the follow-up for brachytherapy needs to be is unclear. Ten-year follow-up, first available in 1997, will be a milestone. But for younger patients with life expectancies of 15 years or more, 10 years is not enough. Fifteen-year follow-up will be available in 2003, and will be enough to convince most patients and physicians that brachytherapy is a legitimate alternative to surgery, even in younger patients.

Although early patients will reach their 15-year follow-up mark in 2003, the median follow-up will be only 5 to 10 years. It will take at least until 2010 to have large series of patients followed beyond 15 years (**Figure 19-1**). And the wait for adequate follow-up may be even longer, because the earliest patients did not consistently get the same high-quality implants as those treated more recently (**Figure 19-2**). It could take another several years to get a 15-year follow-up on large numbers of patients who received what are now considered optimal implants.

VERIFICATION OF FAVORABLE MORBIDITY REPORTS

Early brachytherapy enthusiasts have reported both good tumor control rates and favorable morbidity rates. Morbidity reports, however, can be substantially influenced by the interpretation and bias of the reporting physician. Because virtually all early reports were compiled by the treating physicians, they should be interpreted with caution. They need to be verified by or refuted with independent quality of life studies. This is especially necessary for potency preservation and urinary incontinence rates as their evaluation is quite subjective. Such verification should be done independently of the treating physicians, and supervised by psychologists with expertise in quality of life evaluations.

BETTER QUALITY ASSURANCE

As is often the case with new techniques, early transperineal brachytherapy results have been presented primarily by enthusiasts in the field, who have ded-

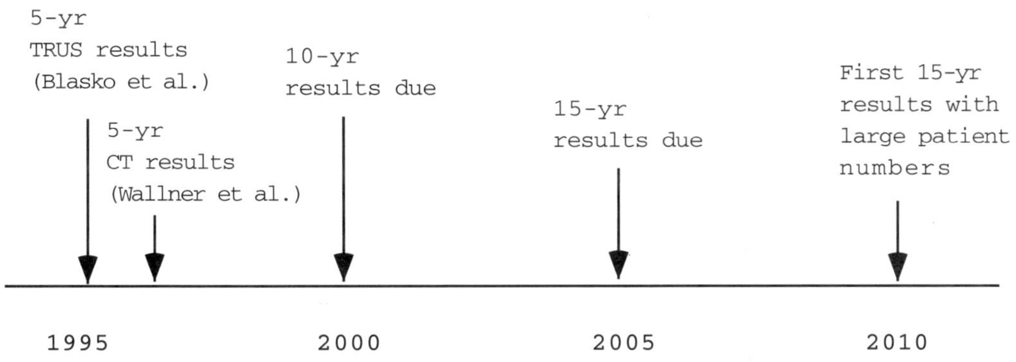

Figure 19-1. Time line for future clinical reports. Large series of patients with 15-year follow-up will not be available until 2010.

icated much of their time to perfecting the procedure. Their results may not be representative of what is achieved as the technology and skills are adopted by other, less specialized practitioners (**Figure 19-3**). Better quality assurance will be needed if brachytherapy is to meet its full potential as a widely-available, effective and relatively cost-effective treatment. Fortunately, there is the potential to use medical imaging to evaluate implant quality, to ensure the technique is carried out properly.

Ideally, a quality assurance system would be available in the operating room to verify, before the operation is terminated, that an implant has been optimally completed. Such a scenario, probably with real-time intra-operative CT scanning, is easy to visualize. Although such attempts will be complicated by prostatic volume changes during the procedure, we can do better in obtaining good, consistent implants than current practice.

TURF BATTLES

One point of controversy will probably be which specialty, urology or radiation oncology, is "in charge" of the brachytherapy procedure. Prostate brachytherapy is a radiation treatment, and so should be overseen by radiation oncologists. The physical act of placing needles could arguably be done by either specialty. Both specialties commonly have extensive experience with needle placement for biopsy (urology) or interstitial radiation (radiation oncology). But the actual placement of radioactive sources should be performed by a radiation

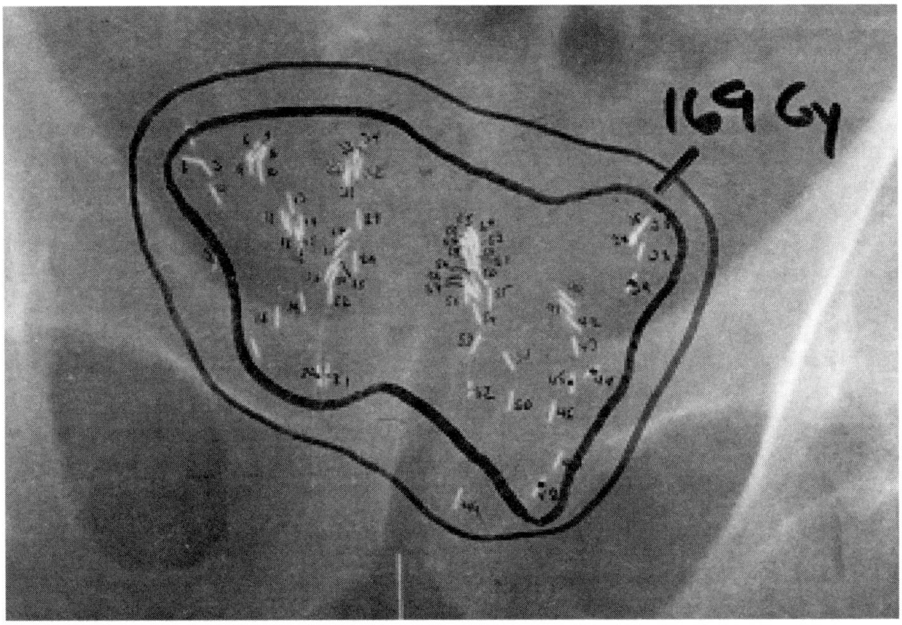

Figure 19-2. This is one of the earlier transperineal I-125 implants, performed in 1988 at MSKCC, not by K. Wallner. It is not good. Above is the anterior view, which does not look particularly bad. But to the right is the post-implant CT scan, which shows that most of the sources were superior and posterior to the prostate. Only 50% of the target is covered by the 150 Gy prescription dose. Despite this having been an obviously inferior implant compared to what is routinely achieved now, this patient was included in prior reports by Wallner and colleagues. All patients, regardless of their implant quality, were included because it would not be fair to compare brachytherapy results with other modalities if some brachytherapy patients were excluded for technical reasons. Because the earliest patients did not consistently get the same high-quality implants as those treated more recently, it could take another ten years to get 15-year follow-up on large numbers of patients who received what are now considered optimal implants.

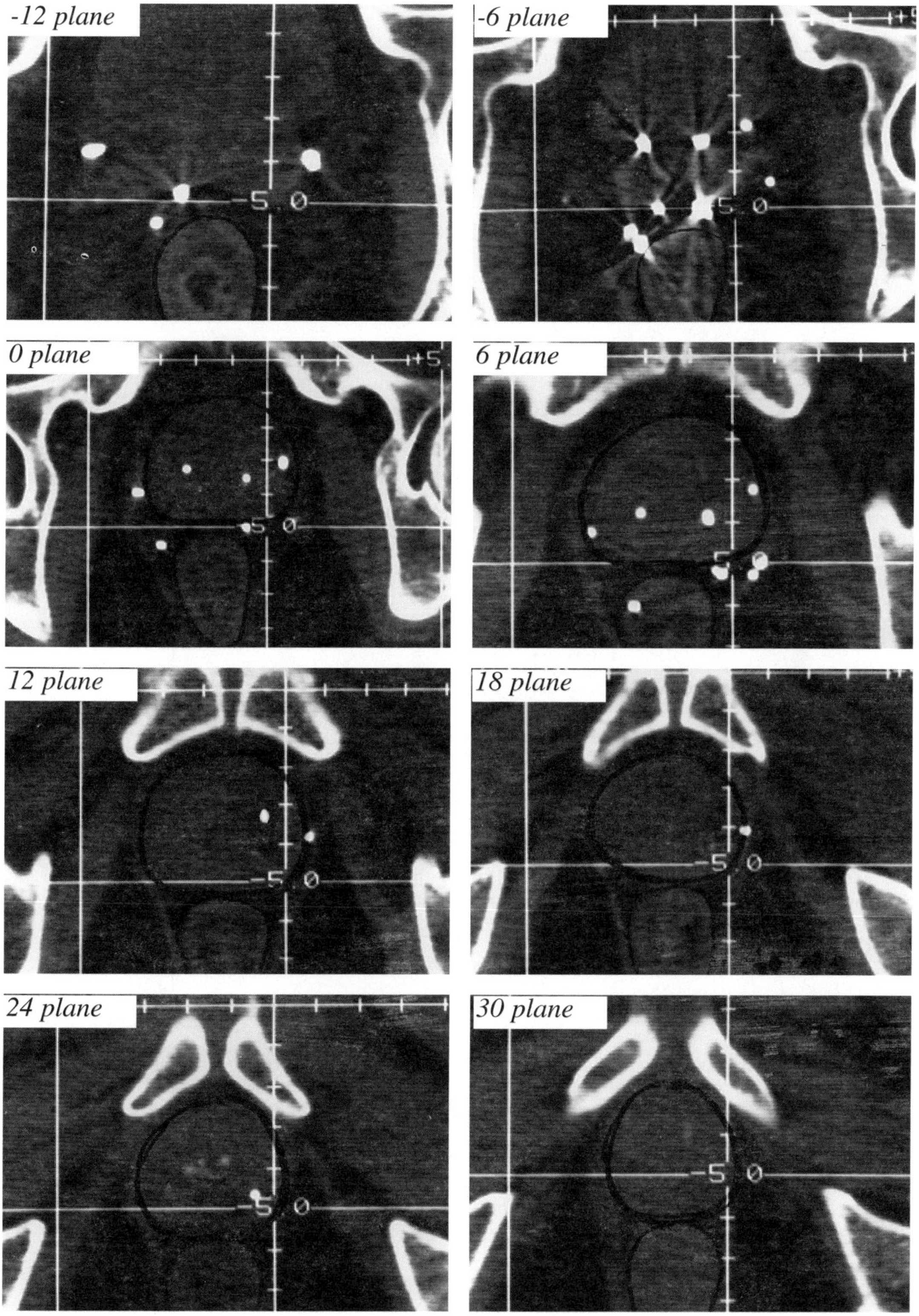
-12 plane
-6 plane
0 plane
6 plane
12 plane
18 plane
24 plane
30 plane

19.5

oncologist, who has an appreciation for the physics of radiation. Modification of the planned source placement is frequently necessary due to prostate and source motion during the procedure itself, and a radiation oncologist is the most capable of intelligently modifying the plan as needed during the course of the implant procedure.

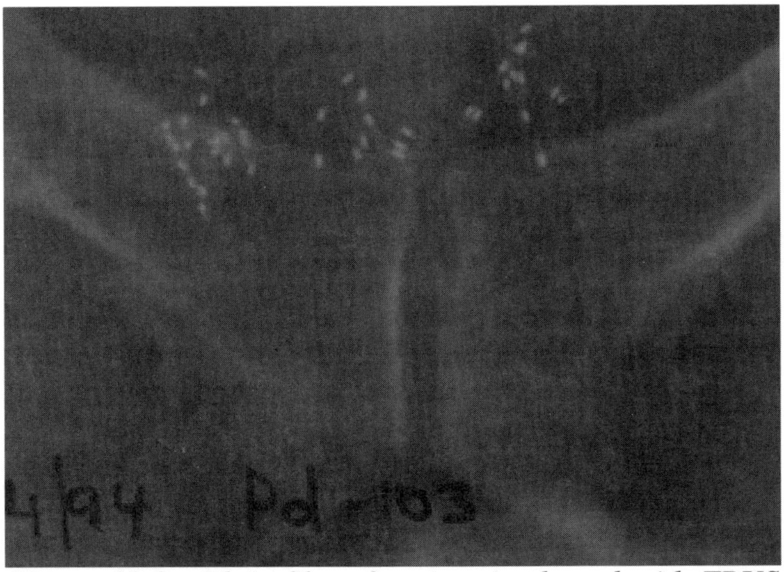

Figure 19-3. Plain film of patient implanted with TRUS guidance in the United States, 1994. The patient was diagnosed with a PSA level of 7.0 and Gleason score of 6. When this x-ray was taken in 1996, only 41 of the reported 60 sources were seen. Apparently, 19 sources were lost at some time following the procedure. Not surprisingly, the patient developed biochemical failure two years later. Also, not surprisingly, the patient is still sexually potent.

Standardized quality assurance could prevent implants like this -- either by ensuring that the physician did better work, or persuading him to send patients elsewhere. That would have been a blessing for both -- the patient might have been cured and the physician would not be facing a lawsuit.

The issue of who is in charge will probably never be settled completely. It will depend on the politics and personalities of the particular institution. Perhaps this is the way it should be, as the interest and skill of the specialists involved will vary.

ROOM TO IMPROVE

We still don't know how commonly late treatment failures will occur. For sure there will be some, as they occur after all treatment modalities. If excessive late failures do occur, it will not necessarily spell the end of prostate brachytherapy. The rectal complications, in experienced hands, are extremely low with current prescription doses. By limiting the urethral dose with peripheral loading, the prescription dose can almost certainly be taken higher, without undue risk. If needed, higher doses should increase the tumor eradication rate.

WE ARE OPTIMISTIC

We have been privileged to be a part of the the modern era of transperineal prostate brachytherapy, from its infancy to its present state of adolescence. We have seen and endured the oncologic community's gradual shift from skepticism and hostility to today's interest and support.

In our opinion, biochemical tumor control rates, morbidity, and the cost of prostate brachytherapy compare favorably with other modalities. However, only when we have a quality assurance system in place, have clearly defined the appropriate candidates for brachytherapy and have determined the optimal prescription doses, will we know the modality's full potential. Judging from what has been achieved with today's imperfect system, the results should be phenomenal.

Kent Wallner　　John Blasko　　Mike Dattoli

Index